The Definitive Guide to

Acupuncture Points

Theory and Practice

Fourth Edition

Chris Jarmey and Ilaira Bouratinos
with Lynn Pearce

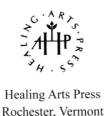

Healing Arts Press
Rochester, Vermont

Healing Arts Press
One Park Street
Rochester, Vermont 05767
www.HealingArtsPress.com

Healing Arts Press is a division of Inner Traditions International

Originally published in the United Kingdom by Lotus Publishing in 2008 and 2018 under the title *A Practical Guide to Acupoints* and in 2021 under the title *The Definitive Guide to Acupuncture Points: A Practical Approach*

Note to the reader: This book is intended as an informational guide. The remedies, approaches, and techniques described herein are meant to supplement, and not to be a substitute for, professional medical care or treatment. They should not be used to treat a serious ailment without prior consultation with a qualified health care professional.

Cataloging-in-Publication Data for this title is available from the Library of Congress

ISBN 978-1-64411-623-4 (print)
ISBN 978-1-64411-624-1 (ebook)

Printed and bound in India by Replika Press Pvt. Ltd.

10 9 8 7 6 5 4 3 2 1

Illustrations Lynn Pearce, Amanda Williams, Pascale Pollier, John Tyropolis, Michael Evdemon, and Ilaira Bouratinos
Text design and layout Medlar Publishing Solutions Pvt. Ltd., India

Contents

CHAPTER 15

Points of the Leg Shao Yin Kidney Channel 240

CHAPTER 16

Points of the Arm Jue Yin Pericardium Channel 258

CHAPTER 17

Points of the Arm Shao Yang Triple Energizer Channel 268

CHAPTER 18

Points of the Leg Shao Yang Gallbladder Channel 285

CHAPTER 19

Points of the Foot Jue Yin Liver Channel. 317

CHAPTER 20

Points of the Conception Vessel 331

CHAPTER 21

Points of the Governor Vessel 347

CHAPTER 22

Extra Non-Channel Points 366

Acknowledgements

My first thanks go to Debbie Simpson for trusting me with the work and vision of her late husband, Chris Jarmey. There is no greater honour than to be thought to hold a world and therapy view that has some similarity to that of a man who has contributed so much in his books, and brought previous clarity for students of manual therapies and acupuncture. I am humbled by this and it has given me courage to share some of my own interpretations and ideas honed over thirty years in practice within this text.

And thank you to Chris, as his words remain threaded throughout this edition. I hope they continue to inspire and bring transparency of meaning to those who may read them now, as I have read them in the past.

My deepest thanks also go to Jon Hutchings of Lotus Publishing who, as this edition took shape, has guided me through the process with patience and excitement in equal measure. The 'behind the scenes' work by him and his editing team has been professional, resourceful, accommodating to my endless changes to diagrams, and all served with a measure of good humour and enthusiasm for the project. Thank you for the opportunity Jon.

I have to thank my son, Albert, who is far too little to understand the content of this book, but one day may be proud of me. He serves to keep me grounded and yet inspired at the same time, and reminds me to continually look at the world, and that includes this work, with eyes of a child, with wonder, curiosity, questioning and non-judgement. As Albert Einstein said,

'*The important thing is not to stop questioning. Curiosity has its own reason for existing.*'

Thanks also to all my past students who have helped me learn as they learn, with whom I have shared a journey of constant fun and laughter as well as discovery, and without whom I would have been unable to contribute to this edition. It is always humbling to see a student discover their skill and touch in acupuncture, and to combine this with manual therapy has been a journey of my own discovery.

My clients, who have faithfully reported weird and wonderful effects from acupuncture treatment that have gone beyond my understanding, amazed both me and them, and shown me the power of the human condition and its capacity to heal itself if given the right kind of encouragement.

My teachers, along the way. In particular, Val Hopwood, who has been a steady ship throughout my lecturing career and from whom I have learnt so much and laughed with a lot. And to John Cross, who ignited the flame of interest in energy medicine and who has shown how much can be achieved with little but respectful input from an individual therapist.

Lastly, my two dogs, Tally and Poppy without whom I would have been melded to a chair in an office. Their faithful nature of being with me in work, and yet dragging me into the fresh air of the universe to experience it and keep learning from it cannot be ignored.

'*If you tell me, I will listen. If you show me, I will see. If you let me experience, I will learn!*'
Lao T'zu

Lynn Pearce
2021

Abbreviations

AIIS	Anterior inferior iliac spine
ASIS	Anterior superior iliac spine
CTS	Carpal tunnel syndrome
IP	Interphalangeal
ITB	Iliotibial band
MCP	Metacarpophalangeal
MND	Motor neurone disease
MS	Multiple sclerosis
MTP	Metatarsophalangeal

PIIS	Posterior inferior iliac spine
PSIS	Posterior superior iliac spine
PSNS	Parasympathetic nervous system
SCM	Sternocleidomastoid
SNS	Sympathetic nervous system
TM	Tendino-muscular
TMJ	Temporomandibular joint

Introduction and Overview

Acupuncture History

It is widely accepted that acupuncture originated in early China, within a system that we now recognise as the Chinese medical model. That model also included herbal medicine, exercise therapies such as Qi Gong, Tai Chi, diet, meditation, cupping, moxibustion and Tui Na. It is a whole-system approach, of which acupuncture generally remains part in China. Westernisation has led to a more scientific approach, but a whole-system practice remains strong and present within Chinese society.

Since finding its way into the Western medical framework, acupuncture has become more of a discrete system of its own. The application of biomedical research, on the one hand, has looked more and more minutely at a global system of treatment (which some practitioners lament). On the other hand, this research has given us more and more reasons why and how acupuncture works, which satisfies the Western model and can help determine how acupuncture can best be used.

The history of acupuncture's development is important, as this has led to the establishment of a body of knowledge that is still used today. The earliest reported text, the *Huang Di Nei Jing* (*Yellow Emperor's Classic of Internal Medicine*), presents a complex conversation between the Yellow Emperor (Huang Di, 2600 BCE) and his first minister, Qi Bo. The text is divided into two main books: the *Su Wen* (*Basic Questions*), which deals with the foundations of Chinese medicine, yin and yang, and diagnosis and treatment methods, and the *Ling Shu* (*Spiritual Pivot*), which deals with acupuncture in much more detail.

Although Huang Di lived in approximately 2600 BCE, the original book was put together in approximately 150–100 BCE. The version that has come down to us is an edited version of the original text, with substantial changes and rearrangement by a scholar, Wang Bing, in 762 CE. It remains the baseline text for all students of the Chinese medical model.

In 1973, however, tombs found at Mawangdui, in Changsha, China, were excavated and silk scrolls containing medical writings were found, pre-dating the *Huang Di Nei Jing*. These then became the oldest texts, as the tombs were sealed in 168 BCE. The meridians are mentioned as following distinct anatomical pathways, but there is little mention of acupoints.

What this highlights is the very thing we are trying to do here with the third edition of this book. Acupuncture practice is *always* evolving, and the newer concepts related to fascial tissue, embryology and current within the body have been introduced to broaden the scope of this book.

Development and Efficacy: from China to the West

While retaining the Chinese medical model explanations for points, we have expanded the underlying concepts behind these explanations in Chapter 1, although some of the more subtle theories have been removed, as they demand their own text. We have introduced sections on the Western medical approach and on point selection for both approaches. Along with the segmental reference charts in Chapter 6, the inclusion of myotomes and dermatomes in the headings for each point should help those practitioners using the segmental approach.

Chapters 8–21 have larger, more dynamic, illustrations of the meridians at the start of each chapter, enabling the student to see the relation between the course of the meridian, its connections and some of the key points, which are consistently highlighted.

In all, it is hoped that the additions to this book will provide a concise, expanded and sound anatomical base for any practitioner of acupuncture, with the rest of the text retaining the essence of the wide-reaching effect that Chinese-medicine-based acupuncture can have.

Regardless of how much knowledge we can acquire about this amazing method of treatment, as a practitioner it is worthwhile paying attention to oneself within the treatment environment.

In Chapter 25 of the *Huang Di Nei Jing Su Wen*, when asked about the principles of acupuncture, Qi Bo replies:

> '*The correct method of acupuncture is to concentrate the mind first.*'

It is sincerely hoped that this new edition will help with the background to allow you, as a practitioner, to do just that – concentrate *your* mind.

Lynn Pearce, BA, MCSP, LicAc, Cert Med Ed
Chartered Physiotherapist
Licentiate in Acupuncture
Lecturer
AACP Advanced Member
Clinical Canine Massage Therapist

About the Text Format for the Points

The following sections describe the way the text is laid out in Chapters 8 to 22. The text for each point begins with a clear title giving its name and number, followed by a calligraphic image of the Chinese ideogram. Below the title, the classification of the point is mentioned (where relevant). In an individual box, the myotome and dermatome of the point is noted.

Following the title there is a comprehensive description of the location of the point. The remaining text is presented in different sections, discussing the different treatment modalities and applications.

The following are included: location, needling, actions and indications. Further, there is a synopsis box outlining the point's major functions and the main areas affected.

Anatomical Basis

Throughout the book it is assumed that the practitioner and student of acupuncture has access to, or already has considerable anatomical knowledge. Rather than point out every potential vessel in the pathway of a point, notes are only given for particularly difficult to access points, or points with potential to do harm if needled incorrectly.

Acupoints are positioned where they are positioned for a reason. Whilst some may be in potentially delicate areas on the body, the aim in acupuncture is *not* to puncture an organ, but to affect a therapeutic outcome with sensible, educated and respectful needling. It is the therapist's responsibility to ensure that they feel safe and capable in their needling,

based on good anatomical knowledge and the motto of 'do no harm' resonates with acupuncture as much as any other medical intervention.

Title Format

Point Name-Numbers
The standard international acupuncture nomenclature is used throughout the text (see the WHO guidelines on training in acupuncture). Each point's name consists of the name of the channel and the number of the point from the beginning of the channel, e.g. ST 36.

The point name-number is also known as the *alphanumeric code*.

Chinese Point Names
The Chinese point names are written in pinyin, literally meaning 'spelled-out sounds', which is the official phonetic system for transcribing the sound of Chinese characters, e.g. *Zusanli*.

Chinese Characters
The traditional ideograms have been chosen, e.g. 足三里.

English Interpretations
The interpretation of the meanings of the Chinese names of the points is an extremely complex task requiring an equally in-depth understanding of the languages, the medical principles and the practices involved.

The interpretations in this book have been chosen to reflect their practical nature, and are common to many texts in use today. They aim to illustrate the (mostly) Chinese notion that '*the point name is there to remind the practitioner where the point is situated and what it does*', e.g. Leg Three Miles.

Main Text Format

Classification
Classification terms are given in English, followed by the Chinese term, e.g. He-Sea point. For more details, see Chapter 5.

Location Description
The locations used throughout the text are based on classical Chinese descriptions and they strive to be as clear as possible to the modern reader. Where there are alternative locations of a point, these are plainly described in the text. Variations of location according to other systems and the authors' own experiences are also mentioned where relevant.

The precision of anatomical description does not, however, relieve the practitioner of the responsibility for careful observation and palpation of the area to be treated, so that underlying structures (such as blood vessels) are protected and the most therapeutically reactive sites are located precisely. The fundamental importance of the role of palpation in point location must not be neglected. Acupuncture is an art in terms of finding the right points for an individual patient, to have the best effect.

Use this book as a guide and a map, remembering that it is not the 'territory' – that is the reality of the client in front of you.

Needling
This section details the main needling techniques, including suggestions for the *minimum and maximum depths, angles* and *directions* for insertion. Remember however that each client may require different depths of treatment due to their constitution and/or body type. Even the temperature and time of year need to be take into account, because it is easier to elicit a treatment response in the summer than in the winter, when our energies run deeper and more internal.

The text warns the acupuncturist of dangerous techniques and contraindications.

Actions and Indications
This section discusses the applications for each point, and requires that the reader have some understanding of traditional Chinese medicine (TCM) diagnosis and differentiation of syndromes. The main actions (functions) are clearly presented and accompanied by the relevant indications (including signs, symptoms and diseases). The major functions are emphasised in italic text. They are based mainly, but not exclusively, on classical Chinese medical theory.

At the end of the text for each point there is a quick reference section (a synopsis), clearly defined in a text box, highlighting the body areas, organs and functions that are deemed of most use in the clinic:

> **Main Areas**—Mentions the main body areas, tissues, organs, systems and Zang Fu affected by the point.
> **Main Functions**—Mentions the main functions of the point to complement and re-emphasise the italicised functions in the actions and indications section.

The main functions listed in the synopsis text box are often the same as the major functions that are italicised in the section on actions and indications. This means that these repeated functions are clinically of most relevance.

In some cases the synopsis of functions differs from the italicised text. This means that those functions mentioned in the text box are the most clinically relevant. The reason for this is that the italicised functions in the main text are mostly major traditional Chinese functions. For example, *regulating Qi and Blood* is a traditional function, whereas *lowering blood pressure* is not (see ST 9). Therefore, the italicised functions in the main text and the synopsis box need to be compared.

The reader must note, however, that because Eastern medicine is an 'art' rather than a precise 'science', there is considerable variation in the actions of the points, both in terms of the different traditional schools of thought, and with respect to the individual practitioner. Therefore, the synopsis of main functions and italicised text serves as a general guide only.

The functions that are emphasised have been chosen as those deemed most clinically applicable according to the authors' own experience and understanding. They are not supposed to be definitive, and they can be altered by each practitioner as he or she considers most relevant to their own practice.

Every effort has been made to include the most accurate information from principal traditional and contemporary sources. For example, the synopsis for point ST 36 is:

> **Main Areas**—Entire body. Abdomen. Chest. Mind. Stomach and Spleen. Digestive system. Lower limb. Knee.
> **Main Functions**—Tonifies and lifts Qi and yang. Nourishes Blood, fluids and yin. Boosts the immune system. Benefits the Stomach and Spleen. Regulates Qi. Calms the mind.

About the Illustrations

The illustrations aim to be as anatomically precise as possible and to show the relevant structures. The needle insertion site is illustrated with a dot. A broader area around this dot is illustrated with light-blue shading. This area displays the site where manual techniques could also be applied (where relevant). Most of the point illustrations have the shaded area, except where it has been excluded for reasons of clarity. Also, where there is more than one illustration for any given point, the shaded area is not always repeated. These shaded areas may also illustrate other possible sites for needling, acupressure and other treatment methods.

There are various possible reasons for treating outside the main point as indicated by the dot. For example, if deqi cannot be achieved at the specified point, then the practitioner must palpate this area carefully to ascertain a more reactive location to insert the needle or apply pressure. If there is distortion of the main needling site, e.g. swelling, skin eruptions, scar tissue, extreme tightness or distended blood vessels, then the practitioner must insert the needle at a different site.

The shaded area may illustrate the area in which the needle shaft may reach a deeper level, particularly when oblique or transverse needling is applied. For example, the large shaded area between the middle and anterior fibres of the deltoid muscle for the point LI 15 illustrates not only the manual techniques region, but also the area where the needle will be located when using a different needling method.

The reader may also notice that some of the dots illustrating a point appear to be slightly smaller (or larger) than others. This is because points do vary somewhat in size. For example, the jing-well points at the fingertips are smaller than large fleshy points such as SP 6 and GB 30.

Part I

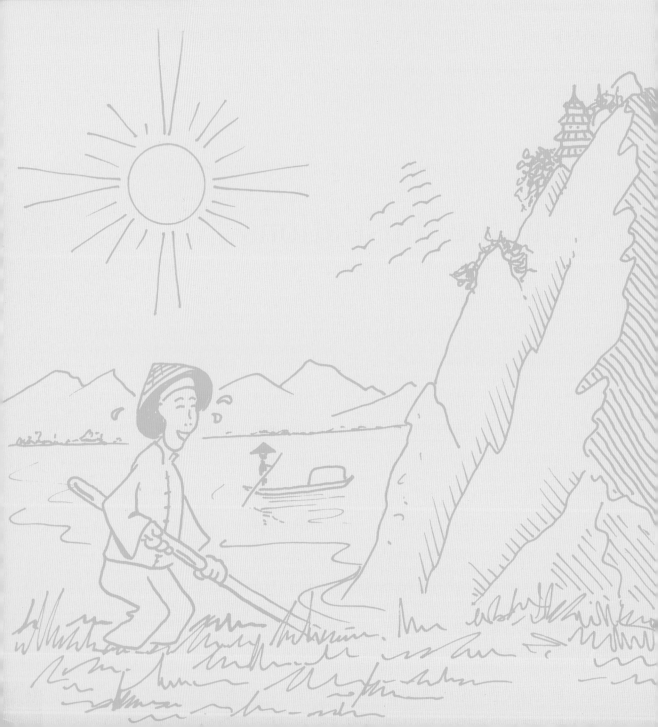

Theory

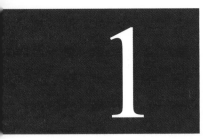

1 Baseline Chinese Medical Model Theories

While this may seem like a foreign language section for those starting out in their acupuncture practice, it is important to absorb some of the key concepts in the Chinese approach to health and illness, so as to be able to understand the functions of the points more fully, and to be able to explain the patient's responses.

To start with, the words and ideas seem very distant from a Western way of thinking, and indeed they are. The world view from Eastern traditions is based far more around the interplay of the environment and those living within it.

Illness can be caused from internal pathogens (emotions) as much as from external pathogens. Looking at health and disease from a different world view deserves respect and attention, as through meticulous observation (which is good science) has come a modality that we can use in the modern day and that has lost none of its effectiveness.

For those already versed in the complexities of the Chinese model of diagnosis and planning treatments, it is hoped that the text retains information that is clinically of use and can help guide point choice.

Qi

A Brief History of Qi (Huan and Rose) has over 180 pages dedicated to a very complex and difficult question, namely 'What is Qi?' How we answer that in the West is very different to how those with a Chinese background would answer.

Qi is not just something that 'flows around the meridians' but is the entity that 'flows and moves through all things'. Unseen, but the effects of it can be seen.

Often when asked how to describe Qi, people use the word 'energy', which is perfectly understandable, as long as we remember that energy drives all things. From the minutiae of a nuclear collision, to powering a space station, to the force that initiates our first breath. From the background to growth of plants and trees, to the clouds being pushed across the sky by the unseen wind. All of these are examples of Qi.

Medical thought hijacked the concept of Qi and put it into the body in an attempt to understand the workings of our lives, but it is much more than 'life force' as it is also often described. There is Qi in art. There is Qi in music. There is Qi in food.

Exercises to cultivate our internal Qi were developed and came to be known as *Qi Gong* and *Tai Chi*. Many other martial arts also depend on cultivating internal Qi and using the Qi of your opponent wisely. The Eastern traditions place strong emphasis on an individual's exercising in order to improve and strengthen their own Qi.

Initially, *Qi* linguistically meant the 'weather' and 'clouds'. Elisabeth Rochat de La Vallée in her book *A Study of Qi* quotes the origin as 'winds' – from four winds from the corners of the earth, to eight winds. Interestingly, these are tiles that are still seen in the game of Mah Jong today, showing a long and entwined tradition of life and environment.

From this concept of the weather comes the idea of being able to see the action of Qi but not being able to see 'it' specifically. Breathing in and out is an expression of Qi, and the vapour from cooking, which gives nourishment, expanded the notion of Qi into something that cultivates and gives rise to human action and life. One substance is transformed into another, which has additional qualities, through the action of Qi.

The radical for Qi is made up of a composite of the clouds/vapours, rising above the pot, within which is rice (of the earth) – changing from one state to another and by so doing providing the raw ingredient for energy and movement.

In medicine, then, the concept is that Qi should flow through the meridians (see meridians and channels section below). If it flows smoothly, none of the acupoints will be active, or blocked, all the organs' functions will be smooth, emotional states will be calm and there will be health. There will be 'ease' and not 'dis-ease'.

To cultivate this concept, the Eastern traditions pay much more attention to exercise, social interaction, correct behaviour, food, the earth and surrounding environment (feng shui), and much more. All of this is to have respect for the Qi that you can affect.

Artificially, and getting below the surface of the skin, we therefore have the Qi of the immune system (Wei Qi) as our defence system, the Qi in the meridians and the Qi of each organ, which can become excessive or deficient. You have the Qi you were born with – Pre-heaven/Pre-birth Qi, Ancestral Qi or Original/Yuan Qi – and you have the Qi you are responsible for obtaining throughout life – Post-heaven/Post-birth Qi.

Each organ in the Zang Fu system (see page 22) has its own Qi and, along with that, specific functions. As the Qi starts to decline, or becomes either weak or excessive from illness, then Chinese medicine

syndromes develop. For example, Kidney Qi Xu – which means 'Kidney Qi deficiency' – is a common problem of increasing age, as the Kidney Qi declines through life. Symptoms would be fatigue, feelings of timidity and fear, lack of courage, low backache and knee weakness, weakness in the bones, possible hearing difficulties (such as tinnitus), and others. These are all based on the functions of the Kidney as an organ, and the channel pathways of the Kidney and its pair, the Bladder, which cross the knees and spine.

Obviously, to live a long and healthy life the aim is to maintain and enhance the levels of your own Qi in your system, ensuring that it flows smoothly through both physical and mental exercise, good diet and avoidance of excess. For further information about this, a good source is *Live Well Live Long: Teachings from the Chinese Nourishment of Life Tradition* by Peter Deadman.

Yin and Yang

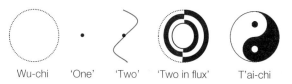

Wu-chi   'One'   'Two'   'Two in flux'   T'ai-chi

From 'nothing' (wu) comes 'something', and that something has dualistic properties (Yin and Yang). Or, simply put, from *nothing* comes *one*, which becomes *two*, and *two is the basis of all things*.

But 'nothing' is not the nothing of emptiness, of no activity – it is a space of limitlessness. This would be called the *Tao* in ancient times. This statement holds true for all creation theories, be they scientific or religious or simply the acceptance of something limitless (which is how 'wu' can be translated) and found in places of stillness and calm. Scientists invest a lot of time and money trying to find this place, both in terms of medicine and in terms of astrophysics – as much as those who meditate and spend a lifetime of inner seeking.

We may be very familiar these days with the end symbol above, without realising the importance of what it attempts to convey regarding a way of life, a way of the world and harmony within medicine and all things. As a symbol, it is elegant in encapsulating a complex philosophy.

The symbol is based on Taoist philosophy, which has a long and changeable history from Shamanic origins of 3000 BC+, and is a visual attempt to make sense of the known and experienced world of the ancient Chinese. The symbol we know today is called the *T'ai-Chi* (TaiJi) and represents the balance that is sought between the two forces of Yin (represented by the dark colour) and Yang (the light colour).

The literal translations of Yin and Yang come from the observations of nature and the sun moving through the day. Yin translates as 'the shady side of the mountain' and Yang as 'the sunny side of the mountain'. A constant flux of one flowing into the other as time progresses (Fig. 1.1).

It would be too easy to simply give a long list of opposites suggesting what Yin and Yang represent – like two sides of a coin; however, this is often the way these functions are represented. Male/female, light/dark, acute/chronic, hot/cold, strong/weak, etc. – the list goes on. The Yin-Yang symbol has

found itself translated into snappy business tools and trendy clothing/ jewelry, and has perhaps become somewhat diluted from its deeper beginnings. It is worth trying to understand that balance of the two extremes is the ideal state to aim for, no matter what field you are working in or talking about.

It may also be too simplistic to consider illness (when working within acupuncture) to be a case of opposites, but the inference of Yin and Yang is that one cannot exist without the other and there is a co-dependency. One can easily turn into the other, or be affected by an excess of one thing or a deficiency of another. Seeking harmony and ease, as opposed to dis-ease, is the goal with treatment, lifestyle changes, diet improvements, etc. – bearing in mind the whole picture.

In order for us to apply this philosophy and approach in acupuncture work, we will, however, have to restrict ourselves to certain lists and ideas that may allow us to get some idea of how to help our clients achieve that state of balanced calmness. Our aim as practitioners is to help them as *individuals* as much as with the 'condition' with which they present. Many of us who practice acupuncture therefore take a wider view of what

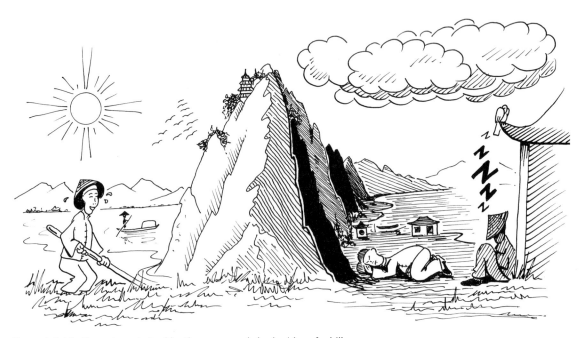

Figure 1.1: Yin-Yang characterised by the sunny and shady sides of a hill.

may be *contributing* to illness rather than just focusing on the presenting condition.

Yin is considered to be the ***foundation of action***, with ***action itself being a Yang function***. Preparing, working in the background, stabilising, running the automatic functions of health, thinking, planning – these are all Yin activities in the body.

Yang is considered to be the ***visible manifestation of the foundation work of Yin***. Muscle activity, movement (both internally of the organs and externally of the body as a whole), dynamic activity of our organs and thoughts, expression of ideas – these are all Yang actions.

As an example of how we can use this philosophy in medicine, from a Western anatomical view the parasympathetic and enteric nervous system could be considered Yin and the SNS Yang. Other examples are:

- Rest/digest/prepare = Yin; flight/fight = Yang.
- The immune system is Yin until it is fired into action, manifesting in a Yang response.
- Our thoughts are Yin, but when voiced or put into action they become Yang.
- Sitting quietly is Yin; moving around is Yang.
- Coldness, sluggish Blood flow, chronic conditions are Yin; acute, hot, sharply painful conditions are Yang.
- Flaccidity after a stroke is Yin; spasticity is Yang.
- Depression is Yin; mania is Yang. Hence, bipolar as a condition clearly demonstrates the flux that can occur between Yin and Yang behaviours, with one blending into the other as part of the same condition.

How a patient presents is crucial to making a diagnosis in a full Chinese medical model, and subsequently choosing the treatment. Seeing a quiet, withdrawn individual in your clinic, as opposed to someone huffing and puffing and fidgeting, will therefore already give you, as the practitioner, a sense of the Yin predominance in the first client (so they will need points to nourish Yin), as opposed to the Yang predominance of the second client (who may need points that calm Yang).

The difficulty comes in ascertaining *why* someone may show signs of Yin deficiency or Yang excess. That is the art of Chinese medicine diagnosis in its fullest sense, but this book is not the place to explore this very complicated system.

The individual organs are also given a classification of being predominantly Yin or predominantly Yang, as will be seen in the following section. This will form a good starting point to help with diagnosis and then treatment planning.

Shen

Shen is usually translated as *Mind* or *Spirit* but it is hard to pin down the essence of the word, much like the issues with trying to interpret Qi.

It is the 'you' which looks out at the world and wonders at it. It could be called your *soul*, the 'ingredient' that makes you human. It is everywhere within you, and thus acupuncture effects the flow of it along with the flow of Qi, Blood, Body Fluids. The word 'deqi', which is the sensation from needling, in truth means 'the arrival of your spirit'.

As such, Shen can control other aspects of your mind and other aspects of your spirit. In a way, it is like a control tower that directs other facets of your mind, such as your willpower, ability to plan and decide, and your capacity to think.

It is housed in the Heart which alone among the radicals for the organs of the body, does not have the associated symbol for flesh – thus rooting them firmly *within* the body. The Shen of the Heart (symbol below) is *not* rooted within the body.

The aspect of your mind that enables you to think with clarity and intent is called 'Yi'. Therefore, when doing a meditation that involves focusing your attention clearly upon a function such as your breathing, or a concept such as compassion, the success with which you can maintain clarity of thought and mental focus is dependent on the strength of your Yi.

In its role as a control tower, your Shen, through your Yi (Purpose), has the power to direct your Qi to fulfil your intent (Fig. 1.2).

In the Chinese tradition, spiritual aspects are housed in different organs, so Yi is housed in the Spleen, Zhi (Will) in the Kidneys, Po (the Corporeal Soul which remains within the body and through life and leaves at death) in the Lungs, Hun (the Spirits of imagination and ideas that can leave the body) in the Liver and the Shen in the Heart. But it is the Heart, which is not rooted in the body, which exerts overall control of these facets of our being.

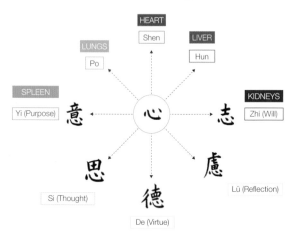

Figure 1.2: The role of the Heart in clear spiritual functioning.

It is unfortunate that the same word 'Shen' is used for both bodily expressions of spirit as well as the overriding control of spirit, and the larger concept that Shen can interact with the Shen of the environment, for example, or the Shen of your ancestors. It is both all-encompassing externally and all directing internally.

The Organ System – the Zang Fu

There is a real difficulty here, as the names for the organs in the Chinese model are, in the main, the same as those in Western medicine. But the

function of an organ in Chinese medicine goes far beyond the notion of making a body fluid or chemical. Each organ is paired with another to give a potent and dynamic function which helps drive health when everything is working smoothly and harmoniously. One organ is Yin in its action – preparing – and the other is Yang, putting that preparation into action. If there is an organ where there is movement involved, that too is usually a Yang organ.

The Chinese word for this entire system is *Zang Fu*, with the Zang organs being Yin and generally more solid and internal, and the Fu organs being more hollow and involving a more dynamic function.

There are 12 organs, each with a meridian named after it; Qi flows through these organs in a set pattern (Fig. 1.3).

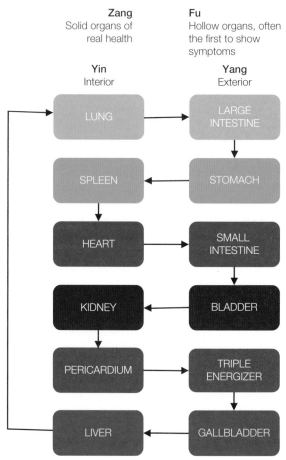

Figure 1.3: Flow of Qi through the 12 channels.

In addition to a physical function, each organ, in the Chinese medical model, is imbued with an emotion or a behaviour. Consequently, if there is an excess of an emotion seen as part of an illness, knowing the organ responsible for a balanced expression of that emotion, and which organ will be affected by an excess or a deficiency of that emotion, can help direct the practitioner to what might be needed in an acupuncture recipe. The associated emotions are:

Lung	Sadness and grief
Large Intestine	Unwillingness to let go, to move on
Stomach	'Manifests all the emotions' – stomach upsets can occur as a result of anxiety, excitement, nervousness, shock, oppression, anger
Spleen	Worry and overthinking
Heart	Joy/elation
Small Intestine	Happiness
Bladder	Caution/fright
Kidney	Fear
Pericardium	Humour and happiness
Triple Energizer	Regulation of the emotions, avoidance of sudden swings
Gallbladder	Frustration and irritation
Liver	Anger

The description of the body as a society in traditional texts, such as the *Huang Di Nei Jing*, is also a fascinating glimpse into the concept of holistic health from Chinese tradition, with no one part of the body being more important than another. The Zang Fu need to work together as one for health to be present.

There are also six Extraordinary Fu organs that get special attention in Chinese medical health. These are: marrow (the brain), bones, vessels (the circulation), Gallbladder and uterus.

The Main Meridian or Channel System

The Chinese words for the meridian (or channel) system are *Jing Luo*. These words together emphasise the concept of connectivity within the body and the provision of a theoretical pathway for Qi to flow.

Jing is variously translated as the warp (as in the warp and weave of a cloth), to pass through, threads twisted together, and a river flowing in a set path, following a set course.

Luo is translated as a net or anything that has an interwoven and interconnected structure.

Together, the two words *Jing Luo* define the meridian network as the avenue for Qi to travel within the body, through the organs, along a path, but with constant tributaries and connections. No wonder Qi is everywhere!

The *Jing Luo* covers *all* the meridian types, but for ease of definition and study, further groups of meridians have been given specific names depending on their projected depth in the body, and also on their function. The idea is to create a visual map of where Qi may prefer to flow, and in doing that, the concept of where to treat in order to deal with blockage and pathology starts to take shape.

First, each of the Zang Fu organs has a meridian associated with it and these are outlined in Chapters 8–19. These are called the *Main Meridians* and it is on these meridians that the majority of acupoints are found. There are some Extra Points (or non-meridian points) and these are given names rather than numbers and are discussed in Chapter 22.

There are also eight Extraordinary Meridians (see below), as well as Divergent, Luo-Connecting Meridians or Collaterals, Tendino-muscular (or Sinew) Meridians, and the Cutaneous Regions. Consequently, according to the Chinese medical model, Qi traverses from the skin through to the depths of the bones, around and throughout the body systems and all the Zang Fu via the meridian network. Its flow and movement maintains life and health.

The Main Meridians house all the points which the others borrow in an often more random collection, so once the main points are known, the other meridians will just take loan of them in order to make new pathways.

The Eight Extraordinary Meridians and Their Opening and Coupled Points

The *eight Extraordinary Meridians*, unlike the 12 regular channels, are not directly related to individual Zang Fu organs, although they do have a close relationship to the Kidneys, uterus and brain. They aid the flow of Qi and Blood in the regular channels by acting as reservoirs (the 12 regular channels are more like rivers).

When there is a surplus of Qi and Blood in the regular channels, this overflows into the Extraordinary Meridians. Conversely, the Qi and Blood from the Extraordinary Meridians is transferred to the regular channels as needed; this may occur in times of greater demand, such as during a chronic illness, shock or pregnancy. According to the *Huang Di Nei Jing*:

> *'The Eight Extraordinary Vessels are so named because they do not conform to the norm. Qi and Blood constantly flow through the 12 regular channels and, when abundant, overflow into the Extraordinary Vessels.'*

This is a complex Chinese medical theory and there are a number of specific texts written to help the student understand this concept further if they are interested in it, although a short description will be given here.

The filling and emptying of the Extraordinary Meridians ensure a constant and uninterrupted flow of Qi and Blood in the regular channels, so that

homeostasis is maintained. Thus, the Extraordinary Meridians do not have their own continuous pattern of circulation but rather respond to the fluctuations of the 12 regular channels. According to the *Huang Di Nei Jing*:

> *'When there are heavy rains, canals and ditches are full to the brim ... similarly, the extraordinary vessels are left out of the channel system so that they can take the overflow from the main channels.'*

The Extraordinary Meridians regulate the circulation of Essence-Jing, acting as a link between the Pre-birth Qi (Xian Tian Qi) and Post-birth Qi (Hou Tian Qi). They are mostly used for treating problems of the Essence and constitution. The Chong and Conception Vessel (Penetrating and Ren Mai) particularly influence the cycles that control growth, development, reproduction and the ageing process. Each cycle lasts seven years in women and eight years in men.

The Chong, Conception Vessel (CV) and Governor Vessel (GV) also circulate the Defensive Qi (Wei Qi) over the thorax, abdomen and back, thus aiding in the protection of the body from exterior pathogenic factors.

The *Governor Vessel*, also known as *Du Mai*, traverses the entire spine up the posterior midline, ascending to the head and face, and joining all the Yang channels at GV 14. It is considered to be the most Yang of all the channels and is also called the *Sea of Yang*.

The *Yang Qiao Mai*, known as the *Yang Heel Vessel* or *Yang Motility Vessel*, starts at the lateral aspect of the heel and travels up the lateral side of the body to join the Yin Qiao Mai at the eyes. It regulates the ascending and descending of Yang Qi and the movement of the lower limbs.

The *Yang Wei Mai*, known as the *Yang Linking Vessel*, connects and regulates the flow of Qi in all the Yang channels and dominates the exterior of the body.

The *Dai Mai*, also known as the *Girdle Vessel* or *Belt Meridian*, originates at the hypochondrium, encircles the waist and binds all the other channels.

The *Conception Vessel*, also known as the *Ren Mai* or *Directing Vessel*, ascends across the abdomen and chest, up the anterior midline to reach the face. It connects all the Yin meridians and is also called the *Sea of Yin*.

The *Yin Qiao Mai*, known as the *Yin Heel Vessel* or *Yin Motility Vessel*, starts at the medial aspect of the heel and travels up the inside of the body, following the Kidney channel, reaching the face where it joins the Yang Heel Vessel at the inner canthus of the eye. It regulates the ascending and descending of Yin Qi.

The *Chong Mai*, known as the *Penetrating Vessel*, runs parallel to the Kidney channel up the legs, through the abdomen and chest, reaching the face. It connects the 12 regular channels and acts as a reservoir for their Qi and Blood. Thus, it is also called the *Sea of Blood*.

The *Yin Wei Mai*, known as the *Yin Linking Vessel*, connects and regulates the flow of Qi in all the Yin channels and dominates the interior of the body.

With the exception of the Conception Vessel and the Governor Vessel, the Extraordinary Meridians do not have their own points, but rather share the points of the 12 regular channels. Their Qi is accessed by a special point, known as an *opening point* (also called *master point* or *confluent point*), and it is used in conjunction with a paired point or coupled point. The eight opening points are those where the Extraordinary Meridians connect to the 12 regular channels.

The Extraordinary Meridians are also grouped into pairs, much like the regular meridians, according to their Yin-Yang polarity. Each pair shares the opening and coupled point. Thus, an opening point on the upper limb is combined with the coupled point on the lower limb. These points are listed in Table 1.1.

Table 1.1: Opening and coupled points of the Extraordinary Meridians.

		Opening point	Coupled point
1.	GV	SI 3	BL 62
2.	Yang Qiao Mai	BL 62	SI 3
3.	Yang Wei Mai	TE 5	GB 41
4.	Dai Mai	GB 41	TE 5
5.	CV	LU 7	KI 6
6.	Yin Qiao Mai	KI 6	LU 7
7.	Chong Mai	SP 4	PC 6
8.	Yin Wei Mai	PC 6	SP 4

The Six Chiaos or Six Divisions

As we have seen, there are 12 regular channels, divided into six Yin and six Yang. These channels are grouped into two sets of six pairs. The first set is known as the *interiorly-exteriorly related channels*, or the *Yin-Yang paired channels*. The Yin-Yang paired channels meet at the tips of the fingers and toes, where the polarity of Yin-Yang changes.

The 12 regular channels are further subdivided into three pairs of Yin and three pairs of Yang, known as the *six chiaos* or *six divisions* (Fig. 1.4). The three pairs of Yang channels meet at the face, whereas the Yin pairs meet on the chest.

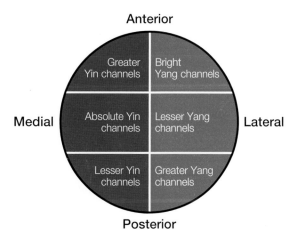

Figure 1.4: Schematic representation of the channel distribution on the four limbs.

The channels running along the anteromedial surface of the limbs are called the *greater Yin channels* or *Tai Yin*. Those traversing the anterolateral surface of the limbs are the *bright Yang channels* or *Yang Ming*. Those traversing the middle of the medial surface of the limbs are the *absolute Yin channels* or *Jue Yin*. Those traversing the middle of the lateral surface of the limbs are the *lesser Yang channels* or *Shao Yang*. The channels running along the posteromedial surface of the limbs are the *lesser Yin channels* or *Shao Yin*, and, finally, those running along the posterolateral surface of the limbs are the *greater Yang channels* or *Tai Yang*.

Thus, the six divisions reflect the similarity of the energy flowing in the upper and lower limbs. They also represent the potential pathway for external pathogenic invasion, and show the levels affected at each stage of a disease as it progresses deeper and affects the constitution more substantially (Fig. 1.5).

A pivotal level is that of Yang Ming, the Stomach and Large Intestine. If this layer is strong, if Qi is strong here, it is possible for an individual to throw off disease and prevent it from moving from Yang into Yin (i.e. from the outside to the inside), where it would cause more serious illness. Consequently, ST 36 and LI 11 are often used as a pair to improve immunity and strengthen the system as part of well-being treatments.

The Tendino-muscular Meridians (TM Meridians)

If working within musculo-skeletal medicine, these meridians have increased importance because of the close connection with known muscles and their associations throughout the body (see Fig. 1.6, pp. 27–30). It is on these meridians that Qi blockage can result in the Ashi points that indicate a place to needle. In the West this may be likened to trigger point needling. Palpable blocks/knots which are sore when pressed need to be needled in order to re-establish flow. The secret to treatment here is palpation and appropriate needling, relatively superficially, to re-establish a smooth flow of Qi.

Likewise, if anyone has studied Tom Myers' anatomy trains, then the pathways of the TM meridians are very similar to those in their depiction.

Qi is considered to flow in between the depressions and planes formed by fascia and the contours of the muscles and muscle sheaths. It can become stuck or be affected by outside phenomena, such as cold winds, and so the TM meridians can tighten up in order to prevent pathogenic factors getting into the system.

Outside				Symptoms
Tai Yang		SI	BL	Aching in the shoulders, neck, spine
Shao Yang		TE	GB	Temperature changes, increased aching down arms and into legs, fidgety
Yang Ming		LI	ST	Digestive upset, nausea, lack of appetite, feelings of heat
Tai Yin		LU	SP	Feelings of cold, further digestive upset, breathlessness, lack of movement
Jue Yin		LR	PC	Not wanting to move, feeling really ill, mental restlessness, delirium
Shao Yin		HT	Ki	Shutting down of circulation, cold, not wanting to move, lack of energy. Mania. Death

Inside

Figure 1.5: Progression of disease.

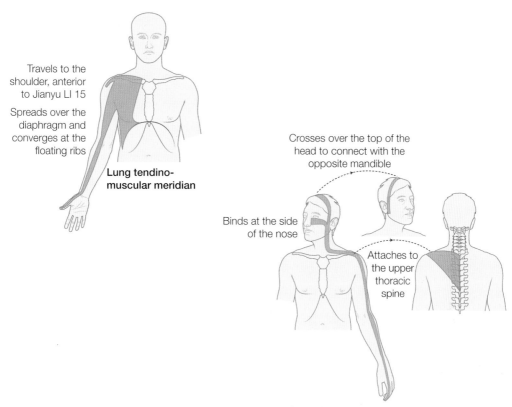

Travels to the shoulder, anterior to Jianyu LI 15

Spreads over the diaphragm and converges at the floating ribs

Lung tendino-muscular meridian

Crosses over the top of the head to connect with the opposite mandible

Binds at the side of the nose

Attaches to the upper thoracic spine

Large Intestine tendino-muscular meridian

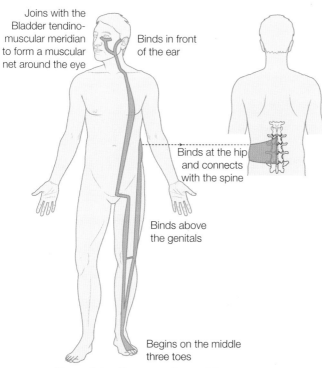

Joins with the Bladder tendino-muscular meridian to form a muscular net around the eye

Binds in front of the ear

Binds at the hip and connects with the spine

Binds above the genitals

Begins on the middle three toes

Stomach tendino-muscular meridian

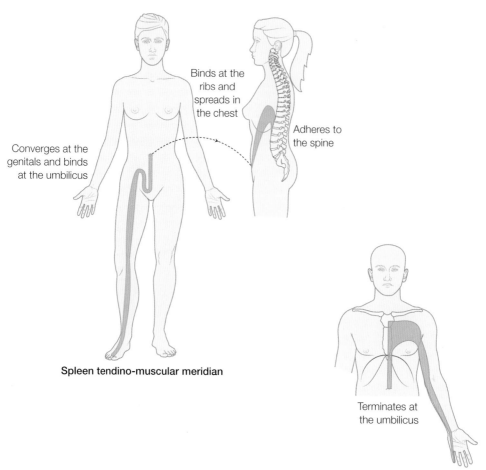

Binds at the
ribs and
spreads in
the chest

Adheres to
the spine

Converges at the
genitals and binds
at the umbilicus

Spleen tendino-muscular meridian

Terminates at
the umbilicus

Heart tendino-muscular meridian

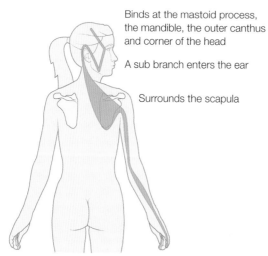

Binds at the mastoid process,
the mandible, the outer canthus
and corner of the head

A sub branch enters the ear

Surrounds the scapula

Small Intestine tendino-muscular meridian

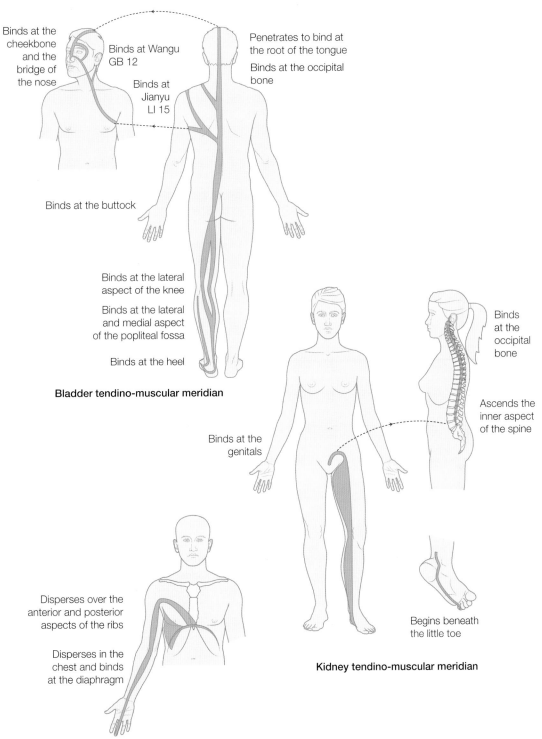

Binds at the cheekbone and the bridge of the nose

Binds at Wangu GB 12

Binds at Jianyu LI 15

Penetrates to bind at the root of the tongue

Binds at the occipital bone

Binds at the buttock

Binds at the lateral aspect of the knee

Binds at the lateral and medial aspect of the popliteal fossa

Binds at the heel

Bladder tendino-muscular meridian

Binds at the occipital bone

Ascends the inner aspect of the spine

Binds at the genitals

Begins beneath the little toe

Kidney tendino-muscular meridian

Disperses over the anterior and posterior aspects of the ribs

Disperses in the chest and binds at the diaphragm

Pericardium tendino-muscular meridian

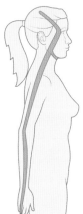

Branches to the outer
canthus and binds at the
corner of the forehead

Links with the root
of the tongue

Joins the Small Intestine
tendino-muscular meridian
on the neck

Triple Energizer tendino-muscular meridian

Meets with its bilateral
counterpart at the
vertex

Binds at the side of
the nose and the
outer canthus

A branch links with
the breast

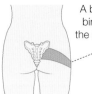

A branch
binds at
the sacrum

A branch binds in the
area above Futu ST 32

Connects
with the other
tendino-muscular
meridians at
the genitals

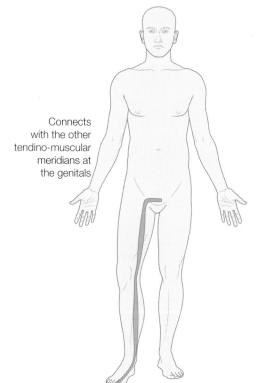

Gallbladder tendino-muscular meridian

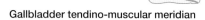

Liver tendino-muscular meridian

In Chapter 58 of the *Huang Di Nei Jing Su Wen*, Qi Bo, the first minister, explains the pathways of these meridians and what happens if there is disruption to them:

> *'The larger space between the strips of muscles is called the 'valley' and the smaller space between strips of muscle is called the 'groove'. Thus, in between the valleys and grooves, the Rong And Wei energies can pass through, and evil energies can also reside. When the evil energy invades and resides in the valleys and grooves, healthy energy can become stagnated, causing blood heat and the deterioration of the muscle. The energies will not be able to pass through and the muscle will become swollen.'*

The TM meridians have points where they move across joints or unite at points of influence, called *binding sites*. These are very useful clinically, because by 'unbinding' these areas, tightness in the muscle system can be dramatically released. This whole system of working with these meridians fits in very comfortably with the Western world of musculo-skeletal medicine.

Some key binding sites that might be of clinical use are given in Table 1.2.

Table 1.2: Some key binding sites.

Point	Binding sites
GB 12	BL, GB, ST and SI
LI 15	LI, LU, BL
GV 14	GV, SI, LI, BL
BL 10	BL, K

Blood and Body Fluids

The sole function of acupuncture when treating Blood and body fluids is to keep them moving. Without movement, there is no life. Without nourishment from the Blood to our organs, without nourishment from the fluid that surrounds our joints, without flows in the spinal canal, without removal of waste in the form of urine – we simply cannot function. All fluids are essential.

In the Chinese medical model, Qi pushes Blood around the system. Hence, Qi and Blood are completely dependent on each other: one for nourishment and one for movement of that nourishment to the rest of the body.

Blood

Blood within this medical model is not just a collection of cells that deliver oxygen and remove waste, but a more substantive substance that houses the Essence of an individual.

Clear mental activity is dependent on Blood. If, for example, there is a deficiency from Blood loss/ anaemia or a gynaecological history of heavy Blood loss over time, then some of the symptoms a client might present with may be lack of clear thought, dizziness, palpitations, insomnia and muzzy head. This is down to insufficient Blood nourishing the brain, which would be called *Blood deficiency*.

Key organs involved in the production and flow of Blood are the Spleen, Liver and Heart, and so many of their points will have reference to their effect on Blood.

Body Fluids

Body fluids are also important in the healthy functioning of all the organs. Dehydration has wide-ranging effects not just on superficial fluids, like sweat, or urine, with it becoming condensed, but on all fluids.

Key fluids, from a Chinese medical perspective, are tears, sweat, saliva, urine, mucus, joint fluid and cerebral spinal fluid.

A focus on diet and fluid intake is very important as part of a comprehensive health pattern. If there are sufficient body fluids in the superficial tissue, then Blood moves freely and does not stagnate; however, when it stagnates it causes pain. Stagnant Blood can be treated very effectively with acupuncture, but there are also excellent manual techniques, such as cupping and gua sha, which move Blood through pushing and pulling and creating space in the tissue. Massage techniques and stretching to improve Blood flow all help, and this is primarily the world of musculo-skeletal medicine.

Blood needs fluid, and fluid needs Blood – another example of co-dependency. Blood, as the more substantive part, is Yin in quality, whereas the fluids in general are Yang in quality.

The Chinese Clock

As the rhythms of nature fluctuate from day to night, winter to summer and so on, so the Qi in the channels waxes and wanes. During the daily 24-hour cycle (known as the *diurnal cycle*), the Qi surges through each of the 12 channels for two hours. It does this following the six divisions schema (see Fig. 1.4). Starting at 3 a.m. the Qi enters the Lung channel, and every two hours flows to the next, ending in the Liver channel (Fig. 1.7).

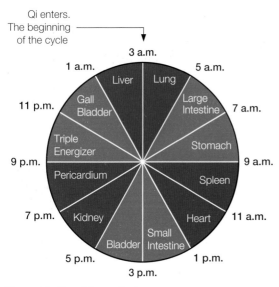

Figure 1.7: The Chinese clock.

Thus, each channel has a particular time of day during which it is fullest of Qi, and an opposite one, during which the Qi is at its lowest. A symptom occurring daily at the same time may be related to the channel that is at its peak, or the one that is at its lowest. A problem occurring around 6 a.m. may therefore be related to either the Large

Intestine channel or the Kidney channel, or to both. Treatment effects can be maximised by applying the treatment at certain times of day.

Causes of Dis-harmony – Internal and External Pathogens

What creates illness? What takes us away from a state of 'ease' to one of 'dis-ease'? Within the Western medical model, there are a myriad of pathogens that we spend thousands on research trying to combat. Pathogens in general indicate viruses, bacteria and other microorganisms or substances that cause disease. This would include environmental factors.

The Chinese medical model has two kinds of pathogens, namely *External Factors* and *Internal Factors*. While the West has increasingly accepted that physical illness can be caused by emotional and mental disruption, the Chinese have long held the view that the cultivation of our physical health, our mental health and all aspects of our environment *all together* is essential in maintaining good health. The responsibility for this falls on the individual, rather than the seeking out of a 'quick fix' in terms of medication from an outsider. Intervention from an outside agent may come after a review of the environment (feng shui), the spiritual state of the individual (which may lead them to undertake meditation or other practices), the physical state (which may lead them to undertake exercise such as Qi Gong or Tai Chi) and the diet.

Subsequent to this, or hand in hand with it, there might be acupuncture, cupping, gua sha, tui na (Chinese massage) and herbal preparations.

Underlying these factors, however, is also a person's *constitution*. This is in part dependent on the Qi inherited from the parents, and so Ancestral Qi can sometimes hold a blueprint for disease that an individual may need to manage all their life.

Table 1.3 presents a substantial, but not exhaustive, list of things to consider when diagnosing the cause of dis-ease.

Table 1.3: Things to consider when diagnosing the cause of dis-ease.

External factors	Internal factors
Climate Classically, the six climatic factors: ■ Fire: symptoms of melting/upward movement ■ Wind: symptoms of erratic movement ■ Cold: symptoms of contraction ■ Heat: symptoms of heat, rashes ■ Dryness: symptoms of stiffness, tissue deterioration ■ Dampness: symptoms of slowness, thickness All these symptoms can intermingle, and so the internal climatic picture of an individual can be complex. For example, invasion of wind and heat could cause symptoms of heat in the body that move around from place to place, as in many rheumatological conditions.	**Emotions** Classically, the seven emotions (which will each tend to affect a different organ): ■ Overjoy/mania ■ Worry/anxiety/overthinking ■ Oppression ■ Sadness/grief ■ Fright/shock ■ Fear ■ Anger
Viruses	**Constitution** If, for example, someone has weakness in the Kidneys (through no fault of their own), certain combinations of emotional states may have a more profound effect on them than on another individual. Consequently, knowing someone's underlying constitution and history is helpful in deciding where to work with acupuncture, etc.
Bacteria	
Moulds/spores	
Ingested food – poisons	
Lifestyle factors	
Lack of exercise	Poor diet/nutrition
Excessive work and lack of relaxation	Not sleeping well
Relationships	Excessive or insufficient sex – 'affairs of the bedroom'
Trauma – emotional and/or physical	

Chinese Medicine Diagnosis

When an individual presents with symptoms, in the Chinese medical model these are considered the 'branches' of the tree that represents the individual. Without attention to the 'root', a treatment is incomplete.

This can easily be understood if we take an actual example from horticulture (Fig. 1.8). How do we know a plant is unhealthy? It may bear bad fruit, or its leaves curl and darken. But we do not treat the fruit or the leaves, but instead we look at the root – more specifically, the soil in which the roots

are embedded. We feed the plant correctly, and we make sure it is in the right environment.

By directing our treatments to the root (the brain and all the biology of healing), we can enable the periphery to flourish and recover its health. (See Chapter 2 for further ideas.) Taking a careful constructed extended history, asking about *all* systems, marks Chinese medicine diagnosis out as different to the Western approach.

By including objective measures in addition, we can work out the potential root of the problem and

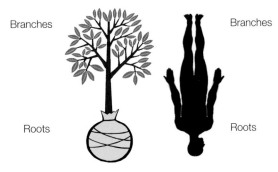

Figure 1.8: Horticultural example.

nourish/feed that aspect, as well as dealing with more immediate symptoms. So often, the condition a client presents with is not the true condition that underlies their whole health and well-being. Finding that condition is akin to being a detective and involves gleaning information about a client's past history, their underlying constitution and body type, their psyche, their parent's health, where they live, what their work and relationships are like, and so much more.

Diagnosis in Chinese medicine is structured around four key principles: look, listen, smell, and question and palpate.

Look

This starts as soon as a client enters the room. What is their demeanour? … Yin or Yang? Subdued or excitable? Skin colour/flushed? Spirit in their eyes? Dull? What is their body shape? … How might that affect their condition? What is their personality type at first glance?

As clinicians we are used to observing behaviours, which can give away a lot about a client's condition. Are they moving away from pain? … Or holding an area, giving it pressure? (This suggests Blood stagnation.)

The five sense organs can be useful, and there is a whole school of facial diagnosis that is not within the realm of this book (but a good starting point for further study is *Face Reading in Chinese Medicine* by Lilian Bridges).

Tongue diagnosis also fits in the 'look' principle, with observation of the tongue body and colour as well as the coating and cracks. What shape is it?

Does it have indents at the side? The latter a very useful indicator of poor fluid movement around the body, as the dents are formed from a tongue which is swollen. This is very common in premenstrual women, who may suffer with bloating and fluid retention, but the tongue will return to its normal shape after the onset of the menses.

Tongue diagnosis is a surprisingly accurate reflection of internal health, with each organ being represented in a different area of the tongue (Fig. 1.9).

Key features to look for in tongue diagnosis are:

Colour of tongue body. Too red suggests heat in the system. Too purple suggests Blood stagnation. Too pale suggests Blood deficiency. Salmon pink is the ideal colour for the tongue body.

Position of tongue. A tongue which is sideways when stuck out suggests Internal Wind as an internal factor of disease. This kind of tongue is seen in those with migraine that predominates on one side, as well as in those who have had (or are about to have) a stroke (wind stroke).

Colour of certain areas of the tongue. A red tip, for example, might suggest that the individual has too much heat in the Heart. Rather than this being a cardiac condition, it often represents too many thoughts rising to the top and causing heat and mental restlessness. Thus, insomnia results from too much internal stress.

Cracks. These are indicative of the state of Qi in the relevant organ. A central crack in the tongue, commonly seen if the immune system is under stress, is suggestive of Spleen Qi deficiency. The deeper the crack, the more severe the deficiency. A small crack in the Lung area would indicate asthma or another Lung condition. With correct treatment, the idea is to see these cracks reverse and become less pronounced.

Coating. The tongue should have a thin white coating – a result of normal digestion. A *thick* coating suggests that the individual is responding to the invasion of a pathogen, and the ensuing battle between Wei Qi (Defensive Qi) or the immune system is ongoing and a good thing. Scraping of the tongue is not recommended. A *yellow* coating

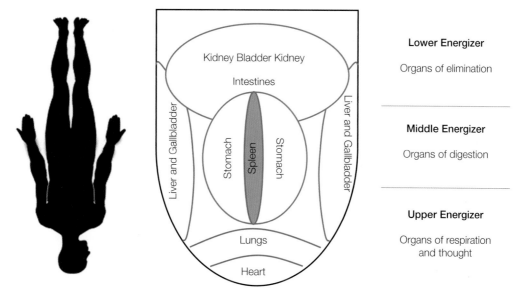

Figure 1.9: Organs represented by different areas of the tongue.

suggests heat in the system, whereas a *white* coating suggests cold. For example, a thick yellow coating at the root of the tongue might suggest an infection in the bladder or intestines, which could manifest as cystitis, or diarrhoea and an upset stomach.

Strange as it may seem to Western diagnostic tradition, a good tongue diagnosis can often help identify where the root of a problem may lie and in which organ, how deeply the system has been invaded, and how well the individual's own immune system is dealing with it. Such a diagnosis helps the practitioner deal with the organ-based dysfunction more accurately and gives him/her an objective sign that should improve as the client improves.

Listen

Listening to a client's speech can tell you a lot about their fundamental energy levels. The language they use can also give an indication of their state of mind. A low, feeble voice, for example, is suggestive of a deficiency of some kind, while a loud, blustery voice shows an excess.

Breathing rate and intensity are also good indicators for conditions of the Lung. There is a strong relation with the Heart and Kidney here in terms of clinical presentation (e.g. fluid build-up may present in the Lung but be down to poor Kidney function and sufficient fluids not being offloaded).

Smell

This may be something that has been lost over time in Western practice, but there once was a time when the smell of urine was used to identify diabetes and would have been a regular clinical test. Asking a client about the smell may be helpful – urinary tract infections and Kidney conditions result in urine that can smell like ammonia. Obviously, urine smelling of pus/sweat can indicate an infection somewhere.

Question and palpate

Systematic questioning about the origin of the current problem, past history/previous episodes, and past medical history as far back as can be remembered is something the Western medic will be more familiar with.

Chinese diagnostic questioning, however, tends to cover a larger range, as it seeks the *root* of a problem. Often a practitioner will go through each system, regardless of whether or not it has anything immediate to do with the presenting problem, and, by doing so, build a picture of the individual in front of him/her.

Therefore, working through all the respiratory, cardiac, digestive, intestinal, urogenital, gynaecological, neural and musculo-skeletal systems has a place in creating a complete picture of a client's health and constitution.

How a client describes pain can be helpful in directing the practitioner to the correct treatment. Obviously, there is locality, which may indicate certain organs, but there are also particular qualities that help establish the cause:

- Distending pain (Qi stagnation)
- Sharp, local pain, often muscular (Blood stagnation)
- 'Heavy', deep pain (damp within the system)
- Colic (obstruction of Qi)
- Pain like a tight rope in the tissues (cold invading the channels)
- Hollow pain (Blood deficiency).

Palpation covers a variety of techniques. The simplest of these is palpating along the lines of the channels and finding areas of pain, or tissue fullness or emptiness. This is an art – not only in terms of palpating but also in terms of interpreting the findings.

Many successful manual therapists have developed this skill to the point that as soon as they engage with the client's skin, they know whether or not that tissue is moving freely. By following the channel, any acupoints that are blocked or empty can be found and needled. This method was in fact the way classical Chinese medicine practitioners were taught and remains an extremely successful therapy approach to this day.

Pulse diagnosis falls into the palpation category and is a whole clinical area on its own. There are many excellent texts if the reader wishes to take this further, and it is appreciated that what follows only touches the surface of this as an effective technique.

It might be difficult for a Western-trained medic to go with the concept that there are 12 pulses to be found at the wrist – six superficial, which represent the health of the Yang organs, and six deeper ones at the same sites, which represent the Yin organs. Within those 12 are 28 different qualities of pulse. The author has endeavoured to continue to try taking the pulse of every client over the years, and while some differences in quality have been felt, even after 28 years of practice only a few distinct different pulses have so far been ascertained with confidence. Pulse diagnosis is truly an art.

Figure 1.10 shows the positions for taking the pulses and the names of the regions and organs each pulse represents.

The pulse rate is important, but it is more about the *quality* of the pulse and the relationship each area has with the ones above and below it as well as deep to it.

One of the common pulse types that can be felt, even with limited training, is the *wiry pulse*, which usually occurs in pain conditions (often on the

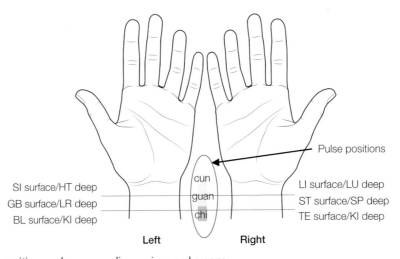

Figure 1.10: Pulse positions and corresponding regions and organs.

GB pulse position if the pain is within the muscle system). It feels like a steel guitar string – often completely different to surrounding pulses.

Other words that go with describing pulse types are:

- Surging (excess of heat)
- Rolling (damp and poor fluid movement)
- Hesitant (stagnation of Qi and Blood, Blood deficiency)
- Soft (pathogenic dampness)
- Weak (Qi deficiency)
- Abrupt (excess of Yang, stagnation of Qi and Blood).

It is said that those who have mastered the art of pulse taking will be able to tell if a woman is pregnant or not through there being an 'echoed' second pulse on the Spleen section – in other words, two pulses. This skill takes years and years to master, as can be imagined.

What should now be apparent after reading this chapter is that Chinese medicine diagnosis is a treasure hunt. The treasure is the root of a client's presenting problem, but also, perhaps, the root of the issues that have plagued them throughout their life. This approach pays attention to *who* they are and not just *what* they have got.

Treatments based on information that comes from such a wide range of objective and subjective reports may have a better chance of success than the isolated approaches of simple trigger point needling, or the recipes that do not involve all this digging and do not treat the person but rather a condition.

2 The Western Medical Approach

What is Western Medicine and Western Acupuncture?

Allopathic medicine, biomedicine, conventional medicine, mainstream medicine, orthodox medicine – these are all names given to the Western approach of treating disease and providing care for patients.

As a system, Western medicine is characterised by the use of the scientific method, and in the modern day, the use of evidence-based practice. Drugs, surgery, radiotherapy, and manual therapy also play a role. Interestingly, much like Chinese medicine, the Western approach has a long tradition of development, starting with the use of plants and herbs in pre-history. This remains a common thread throughout its development, as many of the drugs we use today are plant based.

One comparison which may be made between Western and Chinese approaches is that the Western approach *focuses on the pathology of the disease* that is giving the symptoms in the patient, whereas the Chinese model *focuses on the health, healing and long-term management of the patient as an individual*.

Western medicine has been forced to look outside of the body, to the environment, and to the mind/body more so in recent years. Instead of focusing purely on internal disease and causative factors, examining ever smaller and smaller pathogenic factors, such as bacteria and viruses, it has had to take a leaf out of the Eastern tradition; it has had to look around at the effect the environment has on the health of both the mind and the body and take a more holistic approach that considers the patient rather than the disease.

Acupuncture in the West is called *medical acupuncture* or *clinical acupuncture*, but it is only the reasoning behind needling that is different rather than the needling itself. After all, acupuncture (*acu* = 'needle', *puncture* = 'to go through') as a technique remains the same for practitioners of any school. (I do pay homage here, however, to the clinical masters of acupuncture who show great skill and ability in interpreting the sensations and feedback from a patient, and in no way am I suggesting that acupuncture is merely a technical exercise.)

Clinical reasoning in the West focuses on the signs and symptoms that a patient presents with. Along with the results of tests and scans, the understanding of anatomy and the understanding of pathology and microbiology, in the main the Western practitioner may actually end up using acupuncture in a similar way to the Chinese practitioner. In the process of looking at the evidence for acupuncture, the start point has often been the Chinese medical explanation.

Questions then arise as to *why* should a particular point do this? And, *how* does a particular point do this? What happens in the body that is measurable when someone has acupuncture? What happens in the brain when someone has acupuncture? Using functional MRI imaging, CT scans, PET scans, blood tests, etc. has enabled the Western medical practitioners to build a portfolio of medical evidence in the same way that repeated observations over thousands of years in the Chinese medical development has.

Deqi may not be considered to be the sign of the arrival of Qi at a point for a Western-trained practitioner, but more a stimulation of a certain type of nerve fibre. The intended result, however, is the same: the relief of symptoms and the restoration of health.

What is key is that the nervous system, together with the control it exerts throughout the body, is considered the fundamental mechanism by which acupuncture works.

Deanne Juhan, in the introduction to *Job's Body* (1987), tells us:

'Neural activity is the most pervasive organizing principle in the body. There is no cell whose environment is not directly sustained or adjusted by the activities of the nervous system. It ultimately determines the plasticity of all the other tissues and systems, and it is itself the most radically plastic of all the systems in the organism.'

Suggested Mechanisms of Action

Neurobiology
The discovery of endogenous opioids – such as β-endorphin, dynorphin and enkephalin – and the evidence that they have an effect on pain relief and well-being, and are released into the bloodstream in response to acupuncture, has opened a real window into understanding the biology of acupuncture.

As these substances are produced and circulate, there is a reduction in the chemistry of stress biology (adrenaline, cortisol), a reduction in pain perception and a switching-on of descending inhibitory neural impulses that travel down the spinal cord and affect aberrant incoming neural messages as well.

In addition, there are documented favourable effects of acupuncture on gut motility, on natural killer (NK) cell activity within the immune system and on mast cell activation, which can account for the anti-inflammatory effect of acupuncture. The immune system is challenged into action with acupuncture,

and so there is the switching-on of the self-healing mechanisms.

Neurohumoral effects are also seen in response to the neural messaging of acupuncture to various parts of the brain after the primary sensory cortex, causing a release of hormones. The hypothalamus in particular has a key role to play in switching on many hormones via the pituitary gland. The crossover in terms of definition between neurotransmitters and hormones may be contrived, but what is clear is that the stimulus that acupuncture creates causes a chemical release of various substances, from within the brain and in local tissue, and this can affect very specific target organs and bring about a change in an individual's health.

Neural Connections

Intimately linked with neurobiology, the increased knowledge about the spinal and central nervous systems' anatomy and where neural connections are made within the brain, from the use of fMRI and other investigations, has helped us understand how an individual's behaviour may change as a result of acupuncture. Stimulation of these inhibitory systems of the brain has a role in pain relief. Areas such as the hypothalamus, the raphe nucleus magnus in the medulla, the insular cortex, the pre-frontal cortex and the cingulate gyrus all have connections with the primary sensory cortex, where the sensation of acupuncture is first received into the brain.

With activation of the descending cortical pathways, the effect of acupuncture in managing the incoming sensations from pain or damaged tissue has been demonstrated through alteration at the spinal level. This is the cornerstone of the gate control theory of pain as introduced by Melzack and Wall (1965) and subsequently improved upon by many researchers. Katz (2015) and Mendell (2015) give good overviews of how this original concept has changed as a result of new discoveries of how the human pain system works.

If we look wider afield from just a specific spinal segment, the health of a human being is always a delicate balance of neural connections and

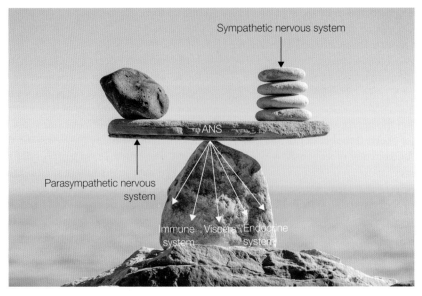

Figure 2.1: The delicate balance of the autonomic nervous system.

messaging between key systems of the autonomic nervous system (ANS). The sympathetic system (flight–fight) and the parasympathetic system (rest–digest) are the two main systems, but these are affected by the enteric system of the gut as well (Fig. 2.1).

The neural connections and the resultant neurobiological mechanisms they activate within the human body control the immune response in part. The aim is for balance of the immune system, doing enough to ward off pathogens but not too much to cause internal damage.

Maintaining a delicate balance is what we all strive to achieve, as practitioners for our clients and as individuals ourselves living in an increasingly stressful world. Increased stress levels, we know, can weaken the immune system and allow illness in or to manifest from within.

The *back-shu points* are very useful in terms of targeting the sympathetic system, and many treatments that work on the whole system will involve these points. Likewise, the *abdominal points* affect the parasympathetic system, along with points in the region of the cranial or sacral output of the sympathetic chain.

Segmental Acupuncture (a Continuation of Neural Connections)

In terms of Western assessment, most pain pictures and some other circulatory and neurological conditions will have a component of *spinal pathology* or at least *sensitisation of a spinal pathway*. The problem may have originated in the spine, or it may have originated in peripheral tissue, with an altered feedback loop potentially developing over time and sensitising the segmental nerve supply. This means that all tissue supplied by that segment is overly reactive and could involve myotome, dermatome, sclerotome or viscerotome (see Chapter 6).

Any of the above-mentioned tissues could be the start point for an injury that feeds back into the spinal cord. An altered message from the aberrant structure will be sent, via the peripheral nerves (Aδ fibres primarily), into the spinal cord level that supplies it, with an altered message then being sent back out to *any* of these tissue types. Consequently, long-term adaptation within the system starts to develop.

One segmental disruption in an organ could thus give rise to segmental disruption throughout all the muscles supplied by that segment. This was the basis of the development of trigger point

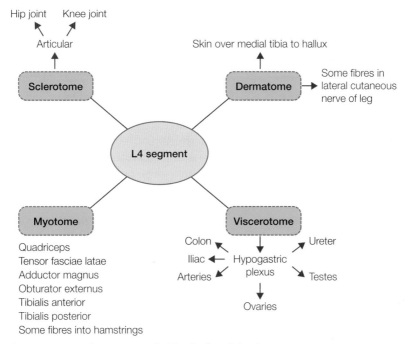

Figure 2.2: Range of tissue types and organs supplied by the fourth lumbar segment.

acupuncture in James Kellgren's inspired article in 1938, when establishing that organ dysfunction could give rise to muscle pain at a distance from the affected organ (Kellgren, 1938). For example, acupuncture within the muscles supplied by L4 may have an effect with regard to pain reduction when other tissues supplied by L4 are the source of pathology (Fig. 2.2).

Often, *central sensitisation of the entire neural network* also starts to occur, which makes it harder to get to grips with resolving these symptoms. The practitioner then has to reconsider the points and the effects on global biology in an attempt to dampen down the pain system and improve well-being.

A Word on Trigger Points

Since Kellgren's original work, and the combined thoughts and approaches of a number of key proponents of this way of working, trigger point acupuncture has become an easily trainable way of bringing acupuncture into the world of musculo-skeletal pain and providing often very quick and dramatic results (see also page 85).

Janet Travell, Michael Kelly and Michael Gutstein were all working independently in the 1940s and 50s and their resultant work gave rise to the trigger point theory, which is still being reviewed and revamped (Shah, 2016).

Patients presenting with myofascial pain can benefit from this kind of acupuncture, but the main problem is that this approach *does not treat the root of the problem*. It may well be all that is needed if the muscles system appears to be the only source of the problem. More often than not, however, the trigger point areas will recur in the same places, and so a thorough musculo-skeletal assessment should accompany a full whole-patient assessment.

There are numerous articles, as a quick search of PubMed will reveal, discussing 'What is a trigger point?', 'Do they exist?' and 'Are they transient developments within muscle?', along with many investigations into the pathology surrounding them, including biopsies and ultrasound scanning. Whatever the take on them, those working with myofascial pain syndromes will often use trigger point needling to great effect.

There are also a number of different techniques described for trigger point needling, ranging from extremely superficial (which must work on a neural feed to the area) to much deeper needling in order to disrupt the trigger point and deactivate it. Many books and articles covering this topic exist, and it is not within the remit of this book to give anything but an introduction to the concept.

Dry Needling

Acupuncture is *acu puncture*. A needle will go through the skin in varying depths dependent on the style of acupuncture being used. While developing her work, Janet Travell coined the term *dry needling*, which involves the use of hollow wide-gauge injection needles. Initially, she injected saline into areas of muscle overactivity, but it soon became apparent that the needle itself was the source of the change and not the chemistry.

Nowadays, practitioners treating with this kind of approach use the single, solid, filiform needle employed by most acupuncture practitioners. They do not use a 'hollow' needle, with a bore down the centre but no chemical within it: this would be more correctly called a *dry needle*. Consequently, Travell's term is misleading, and if a practitioner says they are using 'dry needling' they are in fact using acupuncture (unless they truly are using a wide-gauge hollow needle!).

Fascial Mechanisms

The study of fascia and its role in allowing free movement, transmission and nourishment of all cells embedded within it is a growing field of medicine. Among those practicing manual therapy – but also exercise and movement therapies, such as yoga, tai chi and Pilates – this field of work is becoming increasingly researched and valuable.

Collagen, elastin and the ground substance of fascia can distribute and organise itself into multiple systems. This has provided a physical structuring within the body that has up until now been somewhat ignored in our understanding of anatomy. In addition, the concept of the *interstitium* (Benias et al., 2018) reinforces the fact that the spaces in between tissues are as important as the physical structures themselves. For example, the air within a balloon makes it into a functional balloon; and, more importantly, the space to fill that balloon up with air is always there.

For the acupuncture practitioner it has given new potential understanding as to how Qi may travel around the system, what meridians may be, how fluids move to nourish the internal system and how acupuncture can affect all of this.

The meridian system is one that binds together the body. The word *fascia* comes from the Latin, meaning 'to bind or hold together', and the *Jing Luo* – the name for the meridian system – does exactly that. It binds but allows movement within it.

Within the Western model, the spaces in between fascial planes, and the way fluids move around the body, encased within fascial structures, explains why a line of acupuncture points, for example, may give a better result than random local needles if following an anatomy pathway. Helen Langevin and her team (Langevin 2002, Langevin 2007) have carried out vast amounts of work on the connections between acupuncture and fascial tissue, with suggestions that many acupoints are located in grooves between two structures, and that tissue distortion with acupuncture can travel considerable distances, via a fascial network, throughout the tissue being needled.

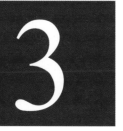

Needling – Considerations for Treatment and Responses

Tools of the Trade

Acupuncture needles (Fig. 3.1) come in many gauges and lengths, as well as different handles and coatings. They are filform, meaning solid.

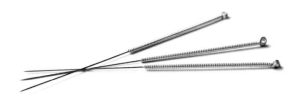

Figure 3.1: The most commonly used needle has a shaft of stainless steel (a supposedly inert metal from the point of body/metal interactions). The handle can be made from stainless steel, copper or plastic.

It is also possible to get gold, silver, zinc, and copper needles and with experience the acupuncture practitioner can match the patient type, treatment type and needle to ensure the best outcome. Gold needles in particular may be used if the client has metal allergies to cheaper metals, so that in itself is not a contraindication to acupuncture.

There isn't a 'one size fits all' needle, so it is important to consider what you as a practitioner are trying to do for the client, and choose the most appropriate tool. Dealing with a client with a weak constitution may lean you toward thinner and possibly coated needles, which will insert much more gently. But, a drawback here means there is less of the needle shaft to engage with the tissues, so it may not have such a therapeutic effect if treating a musculo-skeletal problem where you may want some tissue distortion.

Packaging also varies from single use needles with their own guide tube, to multiples of needles and one guide tube, to needles on their own and no guide tube. Again, preference will emerge for the practitioner in terms of the numbers of needles they may be using, and the body area/skill of the practitioner regarding insertion.

Good-quality needles are flexible, have a very sharp tip and pierce the skin painlessly. It is recommended that only CE-certified needles be used. This ensures codes of practice with regard to sterility and needle strength.

Needle Sizes
The size of needles varies by manufacturer. Common needle sizes are listed by length and diameter in Fig. 3.2.

LENGTH OF NEEDLE	Common (but not exclusive) areas for use	THICKNESS OF NEEDLE →								
		Chinese gauge	#44	#42	#40	#38	#36	#34	#32	#30	#28
		Needle diameter (mm)	0.12	0.14	0.16	0.18	0.20	0.22	0.25	0.30	0.35
		Japanese gauge	02	01	1	2	3		5	8	
		Plastic handle colour									

Length (mm)	Inches		Increasing length means increasing diameter or the needle becomes too flexible to insert and handle.
5		Ear	
7	0.25	Ear and face	
13	0.5	Face and wrists/ankles	
15	0.6	Face and wrists/ankles	
20	0.8	Wrists and ankles	
25	1	HTJ/inner BL points in thin clients. Otherwise, a general needle.	
30	1.2	General	
40	1.5	General – bulkier muscle areas	
50	2	General – especially the lumbar spine	
75	3	Buttock/deep trigger points	
100	4	Buttock/deep trigger points	
125	5	Buttock/deep trigger points	
150	6	Buttock/deep trigger points	

Figure 3.2: Needle sizes.

Note: The actual needle length and cun relationship is an approximate one because sizes vary from one manufacturer to another. Throughout the text, guidelines for needling depth are based on the above chart.

Considerations Before Treatment

After carefully assessing the patient's history and current condition, and ruling out any specific or general contraindications, the acupuncture practitioner must take into account the following factors:

■ The needling sites, skin condition/infection/ thickness of skin
■ Proximity to vital organs, vessels and other sensitive areas
■ Characteristics of the needles that will be used, including size and gauge
■ Angle of needle insertion
■ Depth of needle insertion
■ Manipulation technique(s) used
■ Intensity of stimulation given.

Other precautions to take account of include:

■ Seeing that the patient is in a comfortable position, adequately supported by cushions before needling. It is *always* preferable to treat a patient lying down, regardless of the body part being treated. If BP drops then the client is already in a safe place, and recovery measures should be easily able to take place (e.g. raising legs above the level of the heart)
■ Ensuring that the patient remains still and does not change position during needle retention.
■ Applying aseptic needling techniques conscientiously.

The therapist must be sure that he/she has gained full consent from the client before applying acupuncture and written that in his/her notes and signed and dated it.

How to Needle

What is important in needle insertion is finger force. This is the impetus given at the moment of insertion and students should practice this over and over. It is key to a pain-free insertion of a needle through the skin. Slow unsteady insertion will cause discomfort, whereas a speedy, either tap or push (dependent on whether or not guide tubes are being used), makes the whole process more comfortable and effective. Most of the free nerve endings that register sensory pain are in the surface of the skin and the aim is to go beyond these as soon as possible, so as to recruit deeper fibres and elicit the sensation of deqi.

In traditional practice, firm pressure of the guide tube on the skin (if using one), or firm pressure from the non-needling hand (called the 'listening hand') makes the process of insertion more comfortable for the patient.

Do not touch the shaft of the needle as this will end up in the patient and sterile technique is essential. The practitioner will have washed his/her hands as the last thing before needle insertion (alcohol gel is accepted).

In unwrapping the needle from the packet, again, do not touch the shaft and have the work area designed so that patient and equipment are close. This would include having cotton wool (in case of a bleed), and the sharps bins close to hand.

Techniques

Needling Angles
The relevant angle and depth of needling (Fig. 3.3) must be carefully determined after an analysis of the following:

■ The normal anatomy of the area to be treated and any observable distortions or pathological changes at the needling site.
■ The desired result; i.e. *where* is the target? Where is the most likely place to elicit deqi?
■ The underlying condition of the patient.

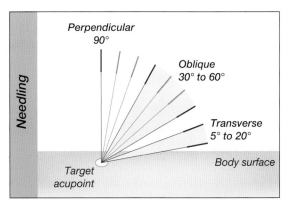

Figure 3.3: There are three main angles of needle insertion that may be modified according to the treatment requirements.

1. ***Perpendicular insertion (90 degrees).*** The most common insertion angle. Especially suitable for thick fleshy areas. More tonifying.
2. ***Oblique, diagonal or slanted insertion (30 to 60 degrees).*** Suitable where the flesh is thin or where an internal organ or vessel lies deep to the location. Oblique insertion is also used to penetrate muscle fibres. Effective to move Qi in a particular direction. More dispersing.
3. ***Transverse insertion (5 to 20 degrees).*** Suitable for thin areas with little flesh and for subcutaneous or transcutaneous needling. Most of the head, face and neck points are needled transversely. Transverse needling is also used to join points and in aesthetic acupuncture.

The angle chosen will determine how far the needle can be inserted so as not to exceed the maximum correct needling depth. For example, points on the scalp can be needled to a depth of up to 0.2 cun, but at a *transverse angle* the needle may be inserted up to 1.5 cun.

Needling Depth
Dependent on style of acupuncture, this will vary (see section on manipulation below).

The needle depths recommended throughout the text are considered for adults of varying body type within the norm and they are based on a classical Chinese needling style. They do not take into account the following cases, for which the practitioner will have to modify the needling depth accordingly:

- Obesity (deeper needling required)
- Emaciation (more superficial needling required, or only subcutaneous or transcutaneous needling applicable)
- Extreme deformity (acquired or inherited).

	Shallow insertion	Deep insertion
Body type	Thin, weak	Robust, obese
Age	Elderly, children	Middle years

The **minimum depths** are recommended to obtain deqi. Nevertheless, in a substantial proportion of cases, deqi is, or can be, obtained more superficially, subcutaneously or even transcutaneously. In general, however, the minimum depths are too superficial for large body types.

The **maximum depths** are recommended to obtain deqi in large-build body types. This means that in a small body type, these depths should not be reached (use the minimum depths).

The importance of **not** exceeding the maximum depths cannot be emphasised enough. Surpassing these depths poses **considerable risk of injury**.

It is important to gauge depth by feeling the Qi reaction at the needle (Fig. 3.4). If there is no reaction superficially after manipulating, then progressively increase the depth in order to achieve deqi. Sometimes deqi can be achieved more superficially and sometimes more deeply.

The maximum depths have been chosen to be on the cautious side of some traditional Chinese needling recommendations that prescribe deeper needling. For example, certain Chinese doctors needle thoracic and upper back points (much) more deeply and at more dangerous angles than is recommended throughout this text. In practice, this means that one can, albeit extremely cautiously, and only after adequate experience, needle more deeply in specific cases.

Manipulation

Dependent on the style of acupuncture being used, manipulation may range from strong to none at all.

Japanese style needling is extremely superficial, and as a result, very thin gauge needles can be used. The skin is barely breached and so the needling is called cutaneous or subcutaneous. There is no seeking of the kind of deqi that is commonly thought of for Chinese-type treatments. In fact, if the client feels anything at all it is often much more tingly and electrical in its nature, and also often travels away from the point. There is also warmth and this is also apparent to the practitioner should they hover their hand above the needled area. Superficial needling can have surprisingly powerful effects and is excellent in terms of improving blood flow away from acute conditions/injuries.

Chinese style needling has a range of manipulation styles and in classical practice these are given names like 'nourishing', 'tonifying', 'dispersing', 'reducing' and more. This is a very difficult skill to explain as it comes with years of practice and understanding what the effect in the tissue/organ is aiming to be. There are many extended texts to help with getting to grips with these variations for application.

In general however, *nourishing and tonifying techniques* are *gentle, involve clockwise rotation of the needle and long needle retention time. Reducing or dispersing techniques* are *fast, involve quicker*

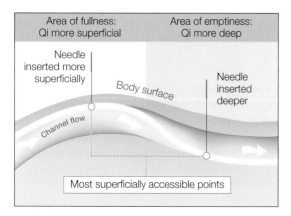

Figure 3.4: Needle depth variation in area of fullness and emptiness along the course of the channel.

anti-clockwise rotation and have short needle retention time.

The *'even'* technique is a mixture between the two and involves the needles being inserted to obtain deqi and then left alone. After 5 minutes, they are stimulated and then left alone again. This is repeated throughout the session of maybe 20–30 minutes – like a see-saw. This is commonly used in practice.

The commonest actual manipulation of the needle is called 'lift and thrust' which involves the practitioner essentially seeking out the deqi reaction and building it up much like a pump within the tissues. In practice there is a lifting and slight rotation of the needle as this is performed, in and out (although not outside the skin of course – the needle stays within the tissue at all times). Once deqi has been obtained the angle of the needle can be altered, and directed in the line of the channel so as to direct the Qi to where it needs to go.

All of these techniques would be applied after a period of 'watch and wait', as deqi can slowly build without stimulation and it is essential to respect the innate nature of the body with healing and not interfere too much.

Periosteal Pecking

As a method of manipulation, periosteal pecking is probably one of the most uncomfortable in all acupuncture types for the patient, but the results on tendinopathies and ligament attachment site problems can be profound.

As the name suggests, the needle is inserted with respect until the unmistakable feel of bone, as opposed to the usual soft tissue sensations that the clinician is feeling for. Once at this junction, the needle is moved up and down through a *very small amplitude*, 'pecking' on the bone. Exploring the small point of insertion in a circular motion can be useful. Time duration for this is very short – about 30 seconds is enough to have a therapeutic effect. Patient tolerance is also only about this length of time at the most.

Some of the common sites where this technique can be valuable are the lateral epicondyle in

tennis elbow, pes anserinus attachment on the medial tibial condyle, Achilles tendinitis on the calcaneum, the greater trochanter in hip problems and the external occipital protuberance in headache from muscle pull.

Care needs to be taken with this technique, as the intensity of the stimulus can be quite a 'shock' to the system, so always treat the patient in lying. Classically, the lateral epicondyle can cause the biggest response, as it is supplied by C6 and can make the patient feel quite faint.

Electro-acupuncture

By adding electrical current to the needles, manipulation can effectively be maintained throughout a session, reducing the need for constant manual stimulation.

The human being uses current continually. Every cell has a resting potential on its membrane. Every message is transmitted neurally through an alteration in polarity. Electricity is everywhere. Some sources feel that Qi is essentially the current of our internal biology. What is interesting is that we need current in order to function healthily, and so the addition of current to an acupuncture treatment adds a whole new dimension and allows us to be more selective in the type of neurotransmitters we encourage to be released in the central nervous system.

Dr Tim Watson reiterates the need for the body to have current with this comment from *Electrotherapy: Evidence-Based Practice,*

> " ..there is a concept that biological tissues demonstrate electrical characteristics and that this bio-electrical activity is ... integral to their form and function. It would appear that without this activity, characteristics, behaviour and response to adverse events, the body would not be able to deal with the environment as efficiently as it does."

Watson, T. (ed.) 2008, *Electrotherapy: Evidence Based Practice.* Churchill Livingstone.

The key frequencies which have an effect on pain, blood flow, tissue relaxation and tissue healing range between 2–15 Hz, whereas higher frequencies up to 150Hz have an effect on pain. Initial work by Jisheng Han in the 1980s and 90s (Han 1990) identified specific pathways for the release of endorphin, enkephalin and dynorphin with different frequencies, and his work has been expanded considerably. Electro-acupuncture is often used in research studies as it is repeatable, and ensures uniform stimulation to a needle. The principles of electro-acupuncture are the same as the principles for the use of TENS (Transcutaneous Electrical Stimulation). For further reading on this subject, David Mayor's book, *Electro-acupuncture: A Practical Manual and Resource*, is recommended.

Dose

This is a difficult subject because there are so many variables to consider within an acupuncture treatment. The question of what makes an effective dose can only be answered truly per patient. Just as with drug therapy, some patients need high levels of a drug to have an effect, whereas another patient may need a third of that dose.

Sadly, the resources available within the clinical situation, such as time allowed per treatment/room

sharing etc. often have to be taken into account in terms of the time each patient is allotted for their session.

The STRICTA guidelines (MacPherson H et al. 2010) written to aid those in acupuncture research, list the components of a treatment that can effect outcomes as:

- Patient sensitivity
- Style of acupuncture. Japanese, Chinese – this will affect the depth of needling
- Type of needles (coated/thick or thin gauge?)
- Sought after response. Local twitch response with trigger point, deqi with others
- Number of needles
- Needle stimulation (manual or electro-acupuncture)
- Length of time for retention
- Frequency of treatment planned
- Total number of sessions.

Consequently, finding the right dose for a patient involves taking all these factors into consideration. In an ideal world, where there are no limits on time or approach, and considering what the patient needs, see Fig. 3.5.

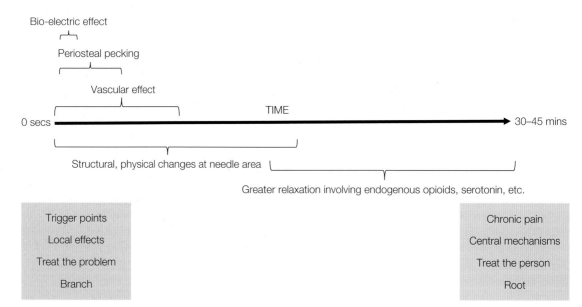

Figure 3.5: Suggested time required for specific effects.

Where Not to Needle

Facial Points

These are very sensitive and bruising can easily occur. Nerves, blood vessels and glands are very superficial, especially in thin people.

Circulatory System

Puncturing blood vessels carries the risk of internal bleeding or clot formation (especially in predisposed patients). Care should be taken when needling areas of poor circulation and vascular disease, because there is an increased risk of infection or accidental puncturing of an artery (sometimes aberrant). This may lead to bleeding and haematoma formation, as well as to arterial spasm or more serious complications, particularly when pathological change is present, e.g. aneurysm or atherosclerosis. Bleeding caused by the puncturing of a superficial blood vessel may be stopped by direct pressure.

Thorax, Abdomen and Back

Deep needling of abdominal, thoracic and back points has the potential danger of puncturing the pleura or peritoneum and injuring vital organs. Cautious needling, preferably obliquely or horizontally, is of utmost importance. Maximum attention should be paid to the direction and depth of needle insertion.

Lung and Pleura

Injury to the lung and pleura caused by excessively deep insertion into points on the chest, back or supraclavicular fossa may result in traumatic pneumothorax. Coughing, chest pain and dyspnoea are the usual symptoms and occur abruptly during the manipulation, especially if there is severe laceration of the lung by the needle. However, symptoms may develop gradually over several hours after the acupuncture treatment.

Intestines

Puncturing the intestines carries substantial risk of severe infection.

Liver, Spleen and Kidneys

Puncture of the liver or spleen may cause a tear and internal bleeding. Symptoms include local pain and tenderness, and rigidity of the abdominal muscles. Puncturing a kidney may result in lumbar pain and haematuria. If the damage is minor, the bleeding will stop spontaneously, but if the bleeding is serious, a decrease in blood pressure and shock may ensue.

Central Nervous System

Inappropriate manipulation at points between the upper cervical vertebrae, such as GV 15 (Yamen) and GV 16 (Fengfu), may puncture the medulla oblongata, causing headache, nausea, vomiting, sudden slowing of respiration and disorientation, followed by convulsions, paralysis or coma. Between other vertebrae in the midline, above the first lumbar, excessively deep needling may puncture the spinal cord, causing lightning electric pain perceived in the limbs or the trunk below the level of puncture.

Dangerous Points for Needling

The following list contains the seven most dangerous points for needling mentioned in the 'Guidelines on Safety in Acupuncture' (WHO traditional Chinese medicine guidelines, 2001). These points are mentioned as 'being potentially dangerous and requiring special skill and experience in their use'. These points are listed as:

BL 1, ST 1, CV 22, SP 11, LU 9, GV 15 and **GV 16**.

Many other points discussed in this text could be dangerous if needled at the wrong angle/depth and without due regard to the underlying anatomy. These include:

LU 1, LI 17, LI 18, ST 9, ST 10, ST 12, ST 13 to ST 18, SP 12, SP 17 to SP 21, SI 14, SI 15, SI 17, BL 11 to BL 23, BL 41 to BL 51, KI 25, KI 26, TE 17, TE 21 GB 2, GB 3, GB 20, GB 24, GB 25, LR 13, LR 14, CV 2, CV 3, CV 12, CV 14, CV 15 and **CV 23**.

Specific Contraindications

Certain areas should not be punctured, e.g. the fontanelle in babies, the external genitalia, nipples, tongue, gums, umbilicus or eyeball. Clearly, nerves, blood vessels and internal organs should not be punctured.

Needling should not be applied to: scar tissue, wounds, swellings (such as cysts), lipomas, skin growths, moles, eruptions, boils, lesions, infections or lymphoedema. Instead, other points should be chosen, either along the same channel pathway or adjacent to the problem area.

Needling should be performed with extreme caution, or not at all, on patients with bleeding and clotting disorders, or on those who are taking drugs with an anticoagulant effect, depending on each individual case. Patients with a Factor 2 level of 25% and above are safe to needle in the case of prothrombin deficiency.

If on anti-coagulants then an INR of between 2–3 is considered normal. Higher levels indicate poor clotting and the client should not be needled.

Absolute contraindications to needling are:

■ Tissue viability – infected, fragile, thin skin. Areas affected by diabetes or other neuropathy which may compromise the body's capacity to heal following an 'insult' such as a needle.
■ Unstable Epilepsy/Diabetes/Heart conditions.
■ Spontaneous bleeding or bruising.
■ Acute haemorrhagic stroke (until the client is stable and no further risk of bleed and notably GB 20).
■ Overly anxious, or mentally incapacitated patients such as Alzheimer's/Dementia/mental health issues. Much of this may revolve around consent issues from the patient.
■ Unwilling patients may be needle phobic or religious reasons may prevent them to consenting to acupuncture.
■ Pacemaker (contraindicated for electro-acupuncture).

Points Contraindicated for Needling ST 17, CV 8. HT 1.

Untoward Reactions and Accidents

Accidents and untoward reactions are generally avoidable if all aspects of the treatment are properly considered and adequate precautions are taken (see also previous sections). However, the practitioner ought to be able to effectively manage such a situation should it occur. It is impossible to know where every capillary and approximately 3% of interventions will bleed. This is nothing to be alarmed about dependent on where the needle is.

Accidental injury to important organs requires urgent medical or surgical help.

Stuck Needle

In certain, albeit rare, cases it is possible for the needle to get stuck in the tissues, making it difficult to remove. It may be difficult or impossible to rotate, lift and thrust, or even to withdraw the needle. This can occur as a result of: muscle spasm; rotation of the needle with too wide an amplitude; rotation of the needle in only one direction causing muscle fibres to tangle around the shaft; or movement by the patient.

The patient should be asked to relax. If the stuck needle is due to excessive rotation in one direction, the condition will be relieved when the needle is rotated in the opposite direction. If the cause is muscle spasm, the needle should be left in place for a while, then withdrawn by rotating it or massaging around the point, or another needle inserted nearby to divert the patient's attention. If the stuck needle results from the patient having changed position, the original posture should be resumed and the needle withdrawn.

Broken Needle

Breaks may arise from poor-quality manufacturing, erosion between the shaft and the handle, strong muscle spasm or sudden movement of the patient, incorrect withdrawal of a stuck or bent needle, or prolonged use of galvanic current.

If a needle becomes bent during insertion, it should be withdrawn and replaced by another. Excessive force should be avoided when manipulating needles, particularly during lifting and thrusting. The junction between the handle and the shaft is the part that is prone to breakage. Therefore, when inserting the needle, *a quarter to a third of the shaft should always be kept above the skin*.

If a needle breaks, the patient should be told to remain calm and still, so as to prevent the broken part of the needle from going deeper into the tissues. If part of the broken needle is still above the skin, remove it with forceps. If the needle is at the same level as the skin, press around the site gently until the broken end is exposed, and then remove it with forceps. If the needle is completely under the skin, ask the patient to resume their previous position and the end of the needle shaft will often become exposed. If this is unsuccessful, surgical intervention may be necessary.

Local Infection
Negligence in using strict aseptic techniques may cause local infection. If infection is observed, appropriate measures must be taken immediately or the patient referred for medical treatment. Needling should be avoided in areas of lymphoedema.

Fainting (Syncope)
During acupuncture treatment, the patient may feel faint. This is because acupuncture will draw blood away from the centre of the body, thus causing a drop in BP. The needling procedure and the sensations it may cause should therefore be carefully explained before the treatment. For those about to receive acupuncture for the first time, a lying position with gentle manipulation is preferable. The complexion should be closely monitored and the pulse frequently checked in order to detect any untoward reactions as early as possible. A very good indicator of physical response that can be paid attention to, is to watch the patient's ears. A global response of the body to acupuncture will be indicated as the top two-thirds will go red. This is because of an autonomic response, and the ear is supplied by the trigeminal nerve, which is usually active in pain and stress states. Also check the palms and soles for sweating.

Particular care should be taken when needling points that may cause hypotension (e.g. LR 3 and LI 4), and points around the neck that may cause excessive parasympathetic activity (e.g. GB 20 and BL 10).

Symptoms of impending faintness include: feeling unwell; a sensation of dizziness; movement or swaying of surrounding objects; and weakness. An oppressive feeling in the chest, palpitations, nausea and vomiting may ensue. The complexion usually turns pale and the pulse is weak. In severe cases, there may be coldness of the extremities, cold sweats, a fall in blood pressure and a loss of consciousness. Such reactions are often due to nervousness, hunger, fatigue, extreme weakness of the patient, an unsuitable position or overly forceful manipulation and fortunately they are rare.

If warning symptoms appear, stop inserting needles and stay rested in the first instance. If the patient still feels unwell, remove the needles and readjust the patient so they can lie flat with the head down and the legs raised. Let them settle and the BP will invariably reset itself. Offer warm, sweet drinks. The symptoms usually disappear after a short rest. In severe cases, first aid should be given and, when the patient is medically stable, the most appropriate of the following treatments may be applied: Press GV 26 with the fingernail or strongly massage GV 20.

What is interesting is that the responses of red ears and sweating are also indicators of a good treatment. It shows that the effect the needle has had, has affected the autonomic nervous system and you need to reach this level to have a global response for the patient.

Convulsions
All patients about to receive acupuncture should be asked if they have a history of convulsions. Remember that unstable epilepsy is an absolute contraindication. Patients who do have such a history should be carefully observed during treatment if you decide to go ahead. If convulsions occur, the practitioner should remove all needles and administer first aid. If the condition does not stabilise rapidly, or if the convulsions continue, the patient should be transferred to a medical emergency centre.

The Concept of Deqi

In Chinese, 'De Qi' literally means 'the arrival of Qi'. The term is used to describe the situation where the Qi of the point and channel is being mobilised for therapeutic purposes.

In order to explain deqi, we must first describe an acupoint, called *Xue* in Chinese and *Tsubo* in Japanese, as a specific place where the energy from the channels and body tissues gathers and converges. Acupoints are likened to vessels whose function is to hold and contain the Qi, but also to offer an opening or doorway that allows the Qi to flow harmoniously from the inside of the body to the outside and vice versa. The point is the entrance connecting the outside with the inside, thus allowing the practitioner to achieve therapeutic results by activating the Qi and Blood of the channels via the body's surface. (See Chapter 2 for an alternative explanation.)

Because the Qi fills up the acupoint, it inevitably flows outwards to the body's surface through the 'opening' of the 'vase' (Fig. 3.6). In this sense, acupoints are the 'gates' or 'windows' of the person's physical and energy body. It is for this reason that there is an inherent connection between the external and internal environment and a continuous ebb and flow of Qi.

When an acupoint is stimulated for therapeutic purposes, its 'door' must first be 'opened' to access the channel passing through it. When correct stimulation is applied, the Qi is activated in the desired channels and areas of the body, offering appropriate therapeutic results. It is thus inevitable that when the channels and areas are being properly activated, a 'Qi sensation' is felt, indicating that the Qi is being mobilised. This can be likened to opening the door or window into the passageway of a building: when it has been opened, the 'breeze' can be clearly felt.

According to the *Huang Di Nei Jing*: 'The sensation of hitting the point of Qi is like walking on an open street, but striking the juncture between the muscle and the bone causes nothing but pain in the skin.' 'When walking on an open street, one is unrestricted and moves freely with no obstruction. When deqi is achieved in this manner, there is no obstruction and thus there is no pain.'

Deqi sensation has been described in many ways by millions of people throughout the millennia. Some of the most widely used descriptions include: 'a relieving ache or pain', 'a spreading sensation', 'numbness', 'tingling', 'distension', 'pulling', 'dullness', 'heaviness', 'warmth', 'dull ache' and 'soreness'. Strong deqi can also produce a sensation of electricity or intense pain extending around the point and along the channel pathway.

An interesting paper in the *Journal of Alternative and Complementary Medicine* by Peter White et al. '*Southampton Needle Sensation Questionnaire: Development and Validation of a Measure to Gauge Acupuncture Needle Sensation*' 2008, presented 16 commonly used words, by patients when trying to describe deqi.

These were:

- Deep ache
- Dull ache
- Uncomfortable
- Heavy
- Pressure
- Bruised
- Stinging
- Tingling
- Warm
- Spreading
- Fading
- Numb
- Twinge
- Throbbing
- Pricking
- Electric shock.

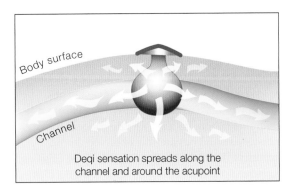

Deqi sensation spreads along the channel and around the acupoint

Figure 3.6: Modified acupoint character depicting the point like a vase.

This paper references two others who have also tried to quantify the deqi sensation. Vincent et al 1989 and Park et al 2002 and the descriptions are remarkably similar. Hui et al. has also tried to characterize the response (Hui et al. 2007), as has Philips 2018.

Other indications of deqi include: changes in the depth and rate of breathing, in pulse rate and rhythm and in body temperature; abdominal rumbling, sighing, coughing, sweating, itching or lacrimation; emotional changes such as sadness, crying or laughing; and visible flushing or other colour changes of the skin surrounding the point. So it is both a sensation and a reaction.

Deqi sensation varies from person to person and is different from one channel or point to another. Moreover, it depends on the state of the person's underlying condition and constitution, and the nature and location of the disease, as well as other physical, environmental or psychological factors (such as medications used now and in the past, the environmental temperature and weather, time of day, food intake, stress levels, etc.).

Each point is connected to different energetic and neural pathways and consequently produces different sensations. Some produce strong sensations, whereas others do not. Moreover, apart from the intensity of the sensation achievable at a point, there are many variations in the '*quality*' *of the sensation*. The latter is attributable to the different intrinsic *energetic characteristics* ascribed to the channels and points by the numerous classical Eastern medical practitioners of the past four millennia or more.

Additionally, current research suggests that deqi is apparent on many levels, which we are normally unaware of, thus boosting our understanding of more subtle biological functions. This helps to confirm many traditional theories regarding the movement of Qi in the body, thus aiding the modern practitioner achieve a deeper understanding of the nature of the channels and of Qi.

Specific Therapeutic Deqi

It becomes apparent that because an acupoint may have *a number of different functions, it must*

also have a similar number of distinguishable deqi manifestations. This means that the specific deqi sensation achieved must be for the *specific therapeutic purpose for which the acupoint was chosen.* Thus the sensation varies, depending on the desired result. Three different aspects of deqi are briefly analysed:

1. The specific area(s) it reaches.
2. The direction the sensation travels in.
3. The particular quality of the sensation.

1. Areas affected by deqi

When treating disorders of specific body areas, *it is important that the deqi sensation reaches the affected sites* because treatment will not be as effective if this does not occur. This becomes even more apparent when treating painful conditions. One could even go so far as to say, that if the sensation does not reach and extend over the entire area of pain, the treatment has little or no effect at all.

However, with reference to the above, it important to consider that stimulation of distal points may not necessarily elicit deqi at the affected area, and is still an effective treatment choice.

2. Direction of sensation

The direction the Qi sensation travels in varies greatly from one case to another. However, in general, the sensation travels in the following directions, often simultaneously (see Fig. 3.6):

■ Extending (radiating) out around the point. *Considered more tonifying.*
■ Travelling distally towards the fingers and toes along the course of the channel (applicable mainly to points on the limbs, but may also be induced from treatment applied to spinal and paraspinal points). *Considered more dispersing.*
■ Travelling proximally up the limb towards the chest, abdomen or back (applicable only to points on the limbs). *For specific internal disorders. Can tonify and harmonise.*
■ Extending inwards into the thoracic cavity or abdomen (applicable only to points on the chest, abdomen, back and neck). *For specific internal disorders. Can tonify and harmonise.*

■ Extending outwards across the back, chest or abdomen (applicable only to points on the back, chest and abdomen). *For specific disorders.*

■ Extending from the back to the chest and abdomen (applicable only to spinal and paraspinal points). *For spinal nerve disorders and internal complaints.*

It is common that a sensation is perceived in a completely unrelated area of the body that does not seem to have any relationship with the channels, areas or conditions being treated, or with the patient's history. Although there is no general explanation for this phenomenon, it may be simply interpreted as a re-adjustment in the flow of Qi within the energy system brought about by the organism's innate tendency to preserve homeostasis.

When treating systemic disorders with points on the limbs, it is most effective to achieve the sensation travelling proximally towards the target organs and areas. Proximally achieved deqi seems to have better therapeutic results, particularly when treating disorders with manifestations of deficiency. When treating local channel disorders and pain using proximal and distal points, the sensation should traverse through the diseased area and beyond, distally towards the fingers and toes.

3. Quality of sensation

The quality of the deqi sensation varies from person to person and from location to location. Deqi may be difficult to achieve and varies greatly in patients who are on analgesic, anti-spasmodic, anti-inflammatory, anti-depressant or other forms of medication. Also, persons who are under (a lot of) stress or who have psychological disturbances may react unexpectedly to deqi. They may be hypersensitive to any method of acupoint therapy, reacting in an extreme manner. However, the opposite may also occur, making it impossible to obtain deqi.

Also, there seems to be a certain (small) percentage of the population who do not seem to be able to feel deqi. Another (small) percentage of the population seems to achieve an extremely strong sensation with the slightest stimulation, thus requiring that treatment be applied extremely lightly

and superficially (no deep pressure or needling required).

If there is no sensation at all, one of the following may have occurred:

■ The needle was not applied at the right location (the point was mislocated).

■ The needle was not applied correctly (the needle was applied either too superficially or at the wrong angle, or in some cases the needle tip went too deep through the acupoint).

■ The needle manipulation was applied without Qi projection (the practitioner's Qi is weaker than that of the recipient).

■ The patient was extremely deficient in Qi and Blood.

■ The patient had neurological damage or cerebral transient ischaemic attack, or had taken drugs that alter sensation, such as sedatives, analgesics or anti-depressants.

■ The needle was too thin or too short.

If none of the above were applicable, the wrong point was chosen for treatment. Choose a point from an area or channel that is more reactive or full of Qi and Blood.

If there is 'pain'

Two questions should be asked when your client uses the term 'pain':

(1) Does the pain feel sharp, like something is being bruised or injured by pressure, or pricked by a needle, like an injection? *This type of pain may be considered 'unwanted pain' and indicates wrongly applied treatment.* Having said that, the author finds that the two unwanted sensations that a patient may report can be 'sharp' or 'stinging'. Usually this means the needle is in close proximity with a capillary on the surface, and if the needle is pushed through a little deeper this sensation usually stops. If it doesn't, the needle needs to be removed and it would not be uncommon for this site to bleed slightly. Another needle should be placed just a little way away from this first site as soon as possible, or the psychology of that point may take over and your patient will be anxious and not want you to needle there. In which case, that point will be

lost to you in therapy, because the client has a bad experience, and that will stay with them.

It is often unavoidable to feel a small prick when a needle is being inserted. Although this indicates minor tissue damage, it is not dangerous, except when major blood vessels are punctured.

(2) Is there also a sensation of 'relief', 'release', 'warmth', 'pulling', 'stretching' or 'something opening up' at the same time? *This type of pain, as long as it is not excessive, may be considered a 'good pain' and indicates that the Qi is being mobilised.*

Terms such as 'dull spreading pain or aching', 'tingling' and 'heaviness' indicate deqi and should be distinguished from the other presentations of pain (such as those caused by incorrect pressure or clumsy needling). So the two words of 'sharp' or 'stinging' are ones we want to avoid, but any other description is fair game, and patients will say the weirdest things in their descriptions.

Some people are more sensitive to pain than others. In general, the following applies:

- Men are more sensitive to pain than women.
- Children and the elderly are more sensitive than middle-aged people.
- Those suffering from stress are usually more sensitive.
- Women during the menstrual and premenstrual phase tend to be more sensitive.
- Athletes tend to be more sensitive.
- People with a sedentary lifestyle tend to be more sensitive to pain.
- Diabetics and those on long-term corticosteroid use have more sensitive skin and blood vessels.
- In the morning the skin may be more sensitive than towards the end of the day.
- In cold temperatures the skin and muscles tend to tighten up, causing both acupuncture and acupressure to be more painful.
- Pain sensitivity can also vary significantly between different races.

Additionally, a small percentage of the population is extremely sensitive to pain for reasons that are not clear, and are thus put down to constitutional or psycho-emotional factors.

In any case where there may be heightened sensitivity to pain, the practitioner should apply all forms of treatment lightly and gently. Use the thinnest suitable needles and apply all other techniques softly and gently.

Electric pain during pressure (or sudden shooting pain)

The pressure was (wrongly) applied directly to a nerve that is either inflamed or located at a very superficial level (usually in thin bony areas). Excessive and wrongly applied pressure may cause inflammation of the nerve. Pressure is *contraindicated* on areas of neuralgia.

Sharp pain or pricking during needle insertion

Unskillful needling, particularly inserting the needle tip too slowly, (remember finger force) or at the wrong angle to the skin, causes a strong pricking sensation. Use of a blunt, bent or excessively thick needle can also do the same. In addition, using too thin a needle can cause a strong prick because the shaft is too flexible and thus more difficult to insert, particularly if the skin is thick or tight.

Inserting the needle too quickly below the subcutaneous layer into the deeper tissues is dangerous and can result in damage to nerves, blood vessels and even internal organs. The needle should always be inserted slowly to the correct depth, so that if pain or a strong sensation occurs, deeper insertion is avoided.

It is generally normal for a small prick to be felt when a needle is inserted, although a competent acupuncturist should usually be able to needle without causing any pain. Using a guide tube helps to minimise the risk of causing a prick, because the needle tip can be inserted more quickly and easily. It is recommended to use a guide tube on very sensitive patients and for very thin needles (0.14mm to 0.22mm).

Pain when the needle is inserted deeply

This can be due to hitting pain receptor nerve fibres, in which case the needle should be lifted until the tip is in the subcutaneous layer and carefully re-inserted in a different direction. This could also indicate injury to a blood vessel, particularly if accompanied by a burning sensation.

Pain during needle manipulation

This usually occurs when the needle is rotated with too wide an amplitude, or during lifting and thrusting manipulation, and is normally due to it becoming entwined with fibrous tissue or muscle fibres. To relieve the pain, gently rotate the needle back and forth until the fibre is released. Work by Helene Langevin suggests tissue damage can start to occur after two full rotations, and manipulation may not need to be as strong as previously thought. (*Connective Tissue Fibroblast Response to Acupuncture: Dose-Dependent Effect of Bidirectional Needle Rotation*, 2007.)

Burning pain during needle retention

This means a vessel has been punctured. The burning pain sensation is from the bleeding in the tissues. Remove the needle and apply pressure to the point. Additionally, a cold compress can be applied.

Sharp or electric pain during needle retention

Sharp pain occurring while the needle is in place is commonly caused by it changing position or bending due to the patient moving, and is relieved by resuming the original position. If this is not the case, it means needling was done too suddenly, too deeply, at the wrong angle or in the wrong location.

Consequently, the needle could have pricked a blood vessel or be close to a nerve.

In an extreme situation, this could mean the needle has damaged the nerve. In such a case, the patient may feel the pain for several weeks after the needling. As far as thoracic points are concerned, remove the needles immediately if there is pain associated with breathing.

Excessively strong sensation, electric or spreading pain during needle retention

This could be indicative of either a strong deqi sensation, or of the needle tip being close to, or touching a nerve sheath. Compare the anatomy of local channel and nerve pathways to ensure that deqi manifests along the channel, not the nerve pathway.

Pain after withdrawal of the needle

This is usually due to unskilled or excessive manipulation and is caused either by bruising or by nerve damage. In the former, the pain will subside after a few days. However, if a nerve has been damaged, the pain may continue for several weeks. There are also many cases where pain is perceived after the withdrawal of the needle but subsides very quickly in minutes or a few hours. This generally indicates a continuation of the Qi sensation.

To relieve pain, apply stationary pressure to the affected area. Also, suggest to the patient that they might like to apply arnica lotion if bruising is suspected.

How to Locate Acupoints

Cun Measurements

The traditional method of locating the points includes a comprehensive measurement system that uses **Body Inches**, or **Proportional Anatomical Measurement Units**. These units are relative to the size of the area being measured and are called *cun* in Chinese. For example, 1 cun on the abdomen may be a slightly different size to 1 cun on the forearm or face; and 1 cun on an adult differs greatly from 1 cun on a child.

- 1 cun is approximately the length of the middle phalanx of the middle finger.

- 1 cun is approximately the width of the IP joint of the thumb.
- 3 cun is approximately the width of the four fingers at the level of the first IP joint of the index finger.
- 2 cun is approximately the length of the middle and distal phalanges of the index finger.
- 1.5 cun is approximately the width of the index and middle finger at the level of the first IP joint.

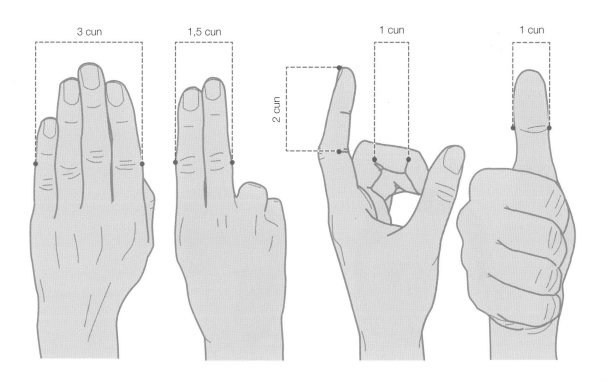

Cun Measurements According to Body Area

Head and face	
Anterior to posterior hairline	12 cun
Glabella (between the eyebrows) to anterior hairline	3 cun
Glabella to posterior hairline	15 cun
Left to right ST 8 (at the corner of the forehead)	9 cun
Left to right mastoid processes	9 cun
Eye, inner to outer canthus	1 cun
Chest	
Anterior midline to tip of acromion process	8 cun
Anterior midline to nipple	4 cun
Distance between the nipples	8 cun
Distance between the midpoint of the clavicles	8 cun
Centre of axilla to inferior border of eleventh rib	12 cun
Back and neck	
Lower border of C7 (GV 14) to posterior hairline	3 cun
Posterior midline to medial border of scapula	3 cun

Medial border of PSIS to posterior midline	1.5 cun
Abdomen	
Umbilicus to xiphisternal junction (sternocostal angle)	8 cun
Umbilicus to upper border of pubic symphysis	5 cun
Anterior midline medial aspect of ASIS	4 cun
Upper limb	
Upper arm, anterior axillary fold to cubital crease	9 cun
Forearm, cubital wrist crease (or LI 5 to LI 11)	12 cun
Lower limb	
Upper border of greater trochanter to knee crease	19 cun
Protuberance of greater trochanter to knee crease	18 cun
Gluteal crease to popliteal crease	14 cun
Patella, superior to inferior borders	2 cun
Medial malleolus to knee crease (or inner eye of the knee)	15 cun
Lateral malleolus to knee crease (or outer eye of the knee, or ST 35)	16 cun

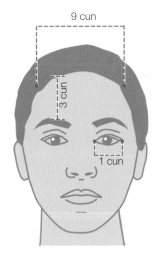
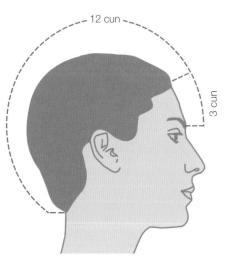

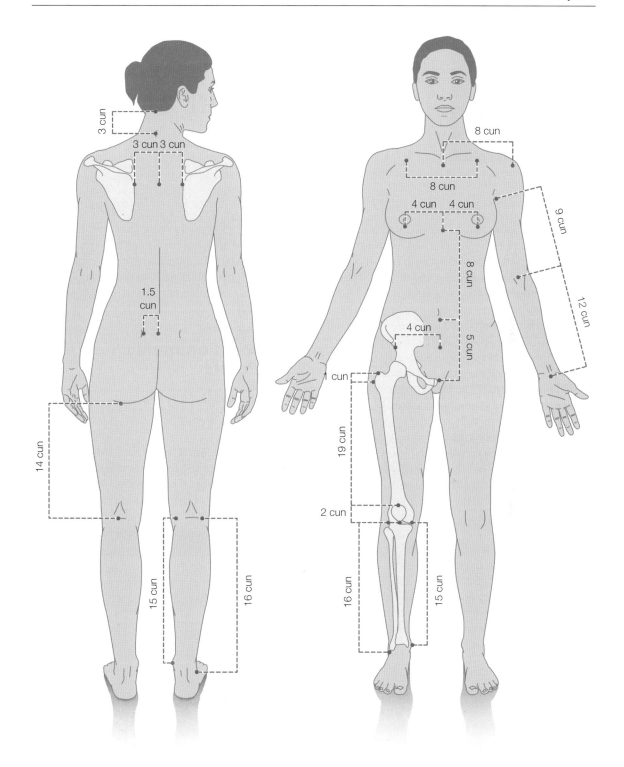

5 Classification of Points

All the body's points may be divided into two broad categories: those whose location and functions have been precisely charted and described, known as *fixed points* or *classified points*, and those that have not been charted, known as *transient points*.

The first broad category includes all the channel and non-channel points. The **channel points** have been grouped into various categories according to their energetic quality and the areas, substances and types of condition they treat. The main categories of these points are discussed later in this chapter.

The **non-channel points** (also known as *extra*, or *miscellaneous points*) include both the traditional extra points, mapped out thousands of years ago, and other more recently discovered ones, called *new points*. They are used in the treatment of specific conditions or body areas.

The second broad category, the **transient points**, are points that can be found anywhere on the body, since their locations vary. They can also appear and disappear because they are an immediate reflection of the particular disharmony and its relationship to the person. The functions and locations of these points are inherently unchartable.

Transient points can be found as reactive points along the channel pathways or other specific areas worked on during a treatment that uses palpatory therapeutic techniques (such as shiatsu). They can also appear anywhere else on the body. Transient points can also be found in the form of pain points, known as *Ashi points* (meaning 'that's it'/'ouch' in Chinese). Ashi points are found anywhere there is pain, tenderness or other abnormal sensation, manifesting either on palpation or spontaneously.

They are generally used to treat pain conditions and their local area, but are also effective in other cases. Pain should be diminished after treatment. All active trigger points are Ashi points, but it is important to realise that not all Ashi points are trigger points.

The Most Commonly Used Points

Here are two informal lists of those points that seem to be used the most often in clinical practice.

The Top Most Commonly Used Points

LI 4 and **ST 36** and **LR 3** seem to rank number one in terms of popularity of use, which is supported by a growing body of research encompassing these particular points.

Major points		Back-shu points	
1	LI 4	1	BL 25
2	ST 36	2	BL 23
3	SP 6	3	BL 18
4	LR 3	4	BL 17
5	KI 3	5	BL 15
6	GB 34	6	BL 13
7	PC 6		
8	HT 7		
9	GV 20		
10	GV 14		
11	GV 4		

Other Commonly Used Points

This list is longer and includes 25 other commonly used points.

1	LU 5	14	KI 6
2	LU 7	15	TE 4
3	LI 11	16	TE 5
4	ST 40	17	GB 21
5	ST 44	18	GB 30
6	SP 3	19	CV 4
7	SP 4	20	CV 6
8	SP 9	21	CV 12
9	SP 10	22	CV 17
10	SI 3	23	Yintang (Ex HN 3)
11	SI 11	24	Xiyan (Ex LE 5)
12	BL 40	25	Huatuojiaji (Ex B 2)
13	BL 60		

The most commonly used points are important for a variety of reasons, including:

- They have a wider range of indications and are therefore used in more cases.
- They are very dynamic and powerful points having stronger therapeutic results than other points of the same channel or category.
- They are also chosen in many cases where the treatment principle and diagnosis are not clarified in detail, so that choosing such a point, even without a diagnosis, is more likely to be of benefit.

The Front-Mu Points

The *front-mu points* (called *mu points* in Chinese and *bo points* in Japanese), also known as *alarm points*, are located on the chest and the abdomen, and are related to their pertaining organs (see Fig. 5.1). It is here that the Qi of each internal organ converges and gathers. The front-mu points have an immediate and direct effect on the internal organs and are therefore used more often in acute conditions to treat the Yang organs.

They are also shown in Table 5.1.

The Back-Shu Points

The *back-shu points* (called *shu points* in Chinese and *yu points* in Japanese), also known as *transporting points*, are located on the back and are closely related anatomically (in the main) to the organ to which they send, or 'transport', Qi directly. They have a direct balancing effect on the internal organs and are used in both acute and chronic conditions, particularly when there is a depletion of the vital substances.

It is worthy of note that, anatomically, the position of these points and their target organ of influence show a considerable overlap with the sympathetic chain in the thoracic spine and extending down to L2. Obviously, when Chinese reasoning was in its infancy, there was no knowledge of the sympathetic chain, and its sphere of influence over the whole of the visceral organ system. This is one of the many examples where Western medicine is falling into line with established Chinese medical definitions.

The back-shu points also treat the orifices that pertain to their associated organ, and are shown in Chapter 14, page 208, and in Table 5.4, page 64.

The *additional shu points* (Table 5.2) are not directly related to the Zang Fu organs and are not traditionally considered to be part of the regular set of shu points. However, they have a special effect on their associated areas, body functions and psycho-emotional aspects and are often used effectively in treatment.

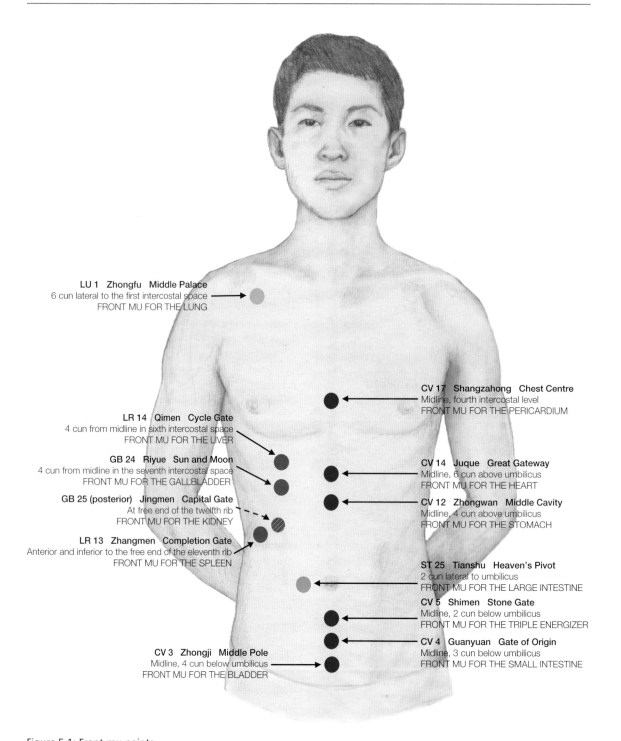

LU 1   Zhongfu   Middle Palace
6 cun lateral to the first intercostal space
FRONT MU FOR THE LUNG

CV 17   Shangzahong   Chest Centre
Midline, fourth intercostal level
FRONT MU FOR THE PERICARDIUM

LR 14   Qimen   Cycle Gate
4 cun from midline in sixth intercostal space
FRONT MU FOR THE LIVER

GB 24   Riyue   Sun and Moon
4 cun from midline in the seventh intercostal space
FRONT MU FOR THE GALLBLADDER

CV 14   Juque   Great Gateway
Midline, 6 cun above umbilicus
FRONT MU FOR THE HEART

GB 25 (posterior)   Jingmen   Capital Gate
At free end of the twelfth rib
FRONT MU FOR THE KIDNEY

CV 12   Zhongwan   Middle Cavity
Midline, 4 cun above umbilicus
FRONT MU FOR THE STOMACH

LR 13   Zhangmen   Completion Gate
Anterior and inferior to the free end of the eleventh rib
FRONT MU FOR THE SPLEEN

ST 25   Tianshu   Heaven's Pivot
2 cun lateral to umbilicus
FRONT MU FOR THE LARGE INTESTINE

CV 5   Shimen   Stone Gate
Midline, 2 cun below umbilicus
FRONT MU FOR THE TRIPLE ENERGIZER

CV 4   Guanyuan   Gate of Origin
Midline, 3 cun below umbilicus
FRONT MU FOR THE SMALL INTESTINE

CV 3   Zhongji   Middle Pole
Midline, 4 cun below umbilicus
FRONT MU FOR THE BLADDER

Figure 5.1: Front-mu points.

Table 5.1: Front-mu points.

Point	Pinyin name	English name	Location	Zang fu organ
LU 1	Zhongfu	Middle Palace	6 cun lateral to CV line, lateral to first intercostal space	LU
CV 17	Shangzhong	Chest Centre	Midline fourth intercostal level	PC
CV 14	Juque	Great Gateway	6 cun above umbilicus	HT
CV 12	Zhongwan	Middle Cavity	4 cun above umbilicus	ST
ST 25	Tianshu	Heaven's Pivot	2 cun lateral to umbilicus	LI
CV 5	Shimen	Stone Gate	2 cun inferior to umbilicus	TE
CV 4	Guanyuan	Gate of Origin	3 cun inferior to umbilicus	SI
CV 3	Zhongji	Middle Pole	4 cun inferior to umbilicus	BL
LR 14	Qimen	Cycle Gate	4 cun from midline, in sixth intercostal space	LR
GB 24	Riyue	Sun and Moon	4 cun from midline in seventh intercostal space	GB
GB 25 (posterior)	Jingmen	Capital Gate	At free end of twelfth rib	KI
LR 13	Zhangmen	Completion Gate	Anterior and inferior to free end of eleventh rib	SP

Table 5.2: Additional shu points.

Governor Vessel Shu point	BL 16
Diaphragm (Blood) Shu point	BL 17
Sea of Qi Shu point	BL 24
Original Qi Gate Shu point	BL 26
Backbone Shu point	BL 29
Perineum (White Ring) Shu point	BL 30
Uterus	BL 32
Vital Region Shu point	BL 43
Upper Arm Shu point	SI 10
Outer Shoulder point	SI 14
Middle Shoulder point	SI 15

The *psycho-emotional back-shu points* (Table 5.3) have a particular relationship to the psycho-emotional aspects of the person.

Table 5.3: Psycho-emotional back-shu points.

Door of the Corporeal Soul	BL 42
Gate of the Ethereal Soul	BL 47
Willpower Room	BL 52
Spirit Hall	BL 44
Abode of Thought	BL 49

The Five Shu Points

On each of the 12 primary channels there are five *shu points* located distal to the elbows and knees, whose quality of Qi can be likened to the flow of water along its course, starting at a well and reaching a distant ocean (Fig. 5.2).

Each of these points (Table 5.5) has an individual energetic character that distinguishes the nature of the Qi flowing through it. This is irrespective of the other categories they may be grouped into. These

Table 5.4: Back-shu points.

Point	Pinyin name	English name	Location	Zang fu organ
BL 13	Feishu	Lung Shu	1.5 cun lateral to tip of spinous process of T3	LU
BL 14	Jueyinshu	Absolute Yin Shu	1.5 cun lateral to tip of spinous process of T4	PC
BL 15	Xinshu	Heart Shu	1.5 cun lateral to tip of spinous process of T5	HT
BL 18	Ganshu	Liver Shu	1.5 cun lateral to tip of spinous process of T9	LR
BL 19	Danshu	Gallbladder Shu	1.5 cun lateral to tip of spinous process of T10	GB
BL 20	Pishu	Spleen Shu	1.5 cun lateral to tip of spinous process of T11	SP
BL 21	Weishu	Stomach Shu	1.5 cun lateral to tip of spinous process of T12	ST
BL 22	Sanjiaoshu	Triple Energizer Shu	1.5 cun lateral to tip of spinous process of L1	TE
BL 23	Shenshu	Kidney Shu	1.5 cun lateral to tip of spinous process of L2	KI
BL 25	Dachangshu	Large Intestine Shu	1.5 cun lateral to tip of spinous process of L4	LI
BL 27	Xiaochangshu	Small Intestine Shu	1.5 cun lateral to midline, level with S1 foramen	SI
BL 28	Pangguangshu	Bladder Shu	1.5 cun lateral to midline, level with S2 foramen	BL

points are also classified in relation to the five phases and are employed in the treatment of imbalances among the elements (Fig. 5.3). This is complex Chinese medical theory and not covered in this book.

The *jing-well points* are located at the distal ends of the 12 regular channels, at the tips of the fingers and toes. At these points, the Qi of the channels is at its most superficial, flowing rapidly in an outward

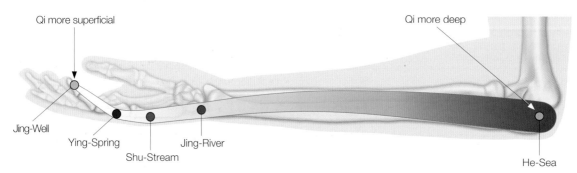

Figure 5.2: Schematic representation of the five shu points. *'Qi circulation is likened to the movement of water: it starts superficially and flows inwards'*, according to the Ling Shu (Spiritual Pivot), first century BCE.

Table 5.5: The 12 primary channels and five shu points.

Primary channel	Five shu points				
	Jing-Well	Ying-Spring	Shu-Stream	Jing-River	He-Sea
Lungs	11	10	9	8	5
Large Intestine	1	2	3	5	11
Stomach	45	44	43	41	36
Spleen	1	2	3	5	9
Heart	9	8	7	4	3
Small Intestine	1	2	3	5	8
Bladder	67	66	65	60	40
Kidney	1		3	7	10
Pericardium	9	8	7	5	3
Triple Energizer	1	2	3	6	10
Gallbladder	44	43	41	8	34
Liver	1	2	3	4	8

direction. It is here that the polarity of Yin/Yang changes as the paired channels flow into one another.

The jing-well points have a powerful effect on the mind and are used for insomnia, anxiety and irritability, and to restore consciousness. They also activate the TM meridians and can be used in cases of pain and other channel disorders. On the Yin channels they are allocated to the Wood element, and on the Yang channels, to the Metal element.

The *ying-spring points*, the second points along the channels, are located at the base of the fingers and toes. The Qi here is likened to a swirling spring where the water gushes outwards. Their function is similar to that of the jing-well points insofar as the Qi here is dynamic and moves rapidly. Thus, the ying-spring points are used to clear pathogenic factors, particularly heat and fire. On the Yin channels they are allocated to the Fire element, and on the Yang channels, to the Water element.

The *shu-stream points*, the third points along the channels, are located on the wrists and ankles on the Yin channels, and on the dorsal aspect of the hands and feet on the Yang channels. The Qi, although still moving quickly, begins to enter a little deeper into the circulation and broadens out.

It is at these points that pathogens penetrate deeper into the channels and where the defensive Qi (Wei Qi) gathers to protect the interior of the body. On the Yin channels, the shu-stream points are primarily used to tonify and nourish the organs, and on the Yang channels, to expel pathogenic factors. On the Yin channels they are also yuan-source points (see below) and are allocated to the Earth element. On the Yang channels they pertain to Wood.

The *jing-river points* are located on the forearm and leg on the Yin channels and are allocated to the Metal element, whereas on the Yang channels they are found at the wrists and ankles and pertain to the Fire element. The Qi at the jing-river points flows

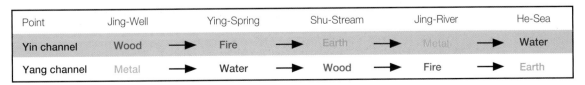

Point	Jing-Well	Ying-Spring	Shu-Stream	Jing-River	He-Sea
Yin channel	Wood →	Fire →	Earth →	Metal →	Water
Yang channel	Metal →	Water →	Wood →	Fire →	Earth

Figure 5.3: Schematic representation of the five phase points. The five phase points correspond to the five shu points.

like a strong current after coming a long way from its source. The Qi at these points is much bigger, wider and deeper, and it is here that pathogens enter into the joints, tendons and bones. The jing-river points are commonly used in the treatment of painful obstruction syndrome and arthritis.

The *he-sea points*, located at the elbows and knees, are where the Qi of the channel becomes deeper and joins the systemic circulation of the body, like a river flowing into the sea ('he' means 'to unite'). The Qi at these points moves slowly inwards towards the pertaining organ. The he-sea points have a deeper but less immediate effect. They are used to harmonise the Qi of the internal organs in both acute and chronic conditions by clearing interior pathogenic factors and regulating the flow of Qi. Some are also important for tonifying the vital substances. On the Yin channels they are allocated to the Water element, and on the Yang channels, to the Earth element.

ST 37, **ST 39** and **BL 39** are three additional he-sea points, known as the *lower he-sea points*, one each for the Large Intestine, Small Intestine and Triple Energizer channels, respectively.

The Yuan-Source Points

The *yuan-source points* for each of the 12 regular channels are located at the wrists and ankles. They have a profound tonifying effect on the underlying energy of the organs and are very important in the treatment of any chronic condition, particularly when there is depletion of the vital substances. In general, they are of increased significance on the Yin channels.

1	LU 9	7	BL 64
2	LI 4	8	KI 3
3	ST 42	9	PC 7
4	SP 3	10	TE 4
5	HT 7	11	GB 40
6	SI 4	12	LR 3

The Xi-Cleft Points

The *xi-cleft points*, also called *accumulation points*, are where the Qi of the channels accumulates, just as water gathers in a crevice or cleft. They are therefore used to treat acute, excess conditions, either of the organ itself or of the channel, particularly when there is pain. On the Yin channels, they also treat disorders of the Blood (including heat and stasis of Blood).

1	LU 6	7	BL 63
2	LI 7	8	KI 5
3	ST 34	9	PC 4
4	SP 8	10	TE 7
5	HT 6	11	GB 36
6	SI 6	12	LR 6

Additionally, there are four xi-cleft points for the eight extraordinary vessels:

Yang Qiao Mai	BL 59
Yang Wei Mai	GB 35
Yin Qiao Mai	KI 8
Yin Wei Mai	KI 9

The Luo-Connecting Points

Each of the 12 primary channels has a luo-connecting channel which diverges from the primary channel at the *luo-connecting point*. There are three additional luo-connecting points.

Each point is employed to harmonise the Qi between the Yin-Yang paired channels via opening their luo-connecting channel. For this reason, they are often used to transfer pathogenic factors from one channel to another (usually from the Yin channel to its Yang pair).

The points are also employed in the treatment of signs and symptoms of disharmony of the 15 luo-connecting channels (12 primary plus three additional), disorders of the five emotions and the five openings (sensory organs).

1	LU 7	7	BL 58
2	LI 6	8	KI 4
3	ST 40	9	PC 6
4	SP 4	10	TE 5
5	HT 5	11	GB 37
6	SI 7	12	LR 5

The three additional luo-connecting points are:

(Great) Spleen	SP 21
Governor Vessel	GV 1
Conception Vessel	CV 15

The Four and Six Command Points

These points are very important and commonly used because they treat any disorder of these areas. The four original command points were:

Face and mouth	LI 4
Head and neck	LU 7
Abdomen	ST 36
Back	BL 40

The four command points later became six when two more points were added.

Chest (thorax)	PC 6
Mind (resuscitation)	GV 26

The Eight Influential Points

The eight *influential points*, or *hui-meeting points*, are points where the energy of certain tissues, vital substances and organs gathers and accumulates. These points have a direct influence on them and are indicated in a wide range of conditions.

Qi	CV 17
Blood	BL 17
Vessels	LU 9
Marrow	GB 39
Bones	BL 11
Sinews	GB 34
Yin organs (Zang)	LR 13
Yang organs (Fu)	CV 12

The 12 Heavenly Star Points of Ma Dan-Yang

Considered the most useful points by the eminent physician Ma Dan-Yang during the 11th century (Song Dynasty, 960–1279 AD).

1	ST 36	7	LR 3
2	ST 44	8	BL 60
3	LI 11	9	GB 30
4	LI 4	10	GB 34
5	BL 40	11	HT 5
6	BL 57	12	LU 7

The Window of the Sky Points

The *window of the sky points*, also known as the *window of heaven points*, were, according to the *Huang Di Nei Jing*, considered to treat the 'Five Regions of the Window of the Sky', i.e. the five sense organs or orifices. The term *tian*, meaning 'sky' or 'heaven', forms part of the Chinese name of seven out of the ten points.

According to the above text, these points are indicated for disorders of the sense organs and neck area, swellings and nodules, psychological disturbances and sudden onset conditions, particularly when there is rebellious Qi. However, there is a great deal of discrepancy as to their functions.

Indications include: headache, dizziness, aphasia, epilepsy, fainting, mental confusion, excessive dreaming, insomnia, diminished memory and concentration, diminished hearing or vision, deafness, tinnitus, eye pain, inability to open the eyes, excessive lacrimation, epistaxis, loss of sense of smell, redness and swelling of the face, dyspnoea, coughing, spitting blood, vomiting, goitre and lymphadenopathy.

The sky window points are located on the upper body, and all but two of them are situated on the neck. Originally, there were five points listed.

1	LU 3
2	ST 9
3	LI 18
4	TE 16
5	BL 10

Five points were subsequently added.

1	CV 22
2	SI 16
3	SI 17
4	GV 16
5	PC 1

However, various sources differ in their opinions on which points are included in this category; for example, it has been suggested that **SI 17** should be replaced by **GB 9**.

The Points of the Four Seas

According to the *Huang Di Nei Jing*, there are four 'seas' in the human body: (1) the Sea of Qi, (2) the Sea of Blood, (3) the Sea of Nourishment, and (4) the Sea of Marrow.

1. The Sea of Qi Points
ST 9, **CV 17**, **GV 14** and **GV 15** are traditionally indicated for both excess and deficiency disorders of Qi, including fullness of the chest, dyspnoea, weak breathing and exhaustion.

2. The Sea of Blood Points
BL 11, **ST 37** and **ST 39** are traditionally indicated for both excess and deficiency disorders of Blood, including heaviness of the body and emaciation.

3. The Sea of Nourishment Points
Also known as the *Sea of Water and Grain points*, **ST 30** and **ST 36** are traditionally indicated for both excess and deficiency disorders of the abdomen, including abdominal fullness and pain, hunger and inability to eat.

4. The Sea of Marrow Points
GV 16 and **GV 20** are traditionally indicated for both excess and deficiency disorders of the marrow, including hyperactivity, excessive libido, dizziness, tinnitus, poor vision and exhaustion. On a psychological level, they are indicated for laziness.

The 13 Ghost Points of Sun Si-Miao

Listed in the *Thousand Ducat Formulas* by the renowned physician Sun Si-Miao in the seventh century (Tang Dynasty, 618–907 AD), and used to treat psychiatric disorders and epilepsy.

1	GV 26	8	CV 24
2	LU 11	9	PC 8
3	SP 1	10	GV 23
4	PC 7	11	CV 1
5	BL 62	12	LI 11
6	GV 16	13	Haiquan (not otherwise referenced due to its inaccessibility below the tongue)
7	ST 6		

6 Segmental, Anatomical and Reference Charts

Head and C1–T1 Segmental Chart

Facial Nerve	Trigeminal Nerve	Accessory Nerve	C1		C2	C3	C4	C5	C6	C7	C8
Orbicularis Oculi		Trapezius									
Zygomaticus		Sternocleidomastoid									
Platysma			Obliquus Capitis Sup. & Inf.								
Buccinator			Rectus Capitis Posterior Maj. & Min.								
Occipitofrontalis			Rectus Capitis Anterior & Lateralis								
Orbicularis Oris			Sternohyoid								
Procerus			Sternothyroid								
Depressor Anguli Oris			Omohyoid								
Corrugator Supercilii							Scalene Group				
Nasalis			Rectus Capitis								
Digastric			Longus Capitis								
Levator Labii Superioris			Spinalis Cervicis								
Depressor Septi Nasi			Splenius Capitis								
Levator Anguli Oris			Splenius Cervicis								
Risorius			Semispinalis Capitis								
Depressor Anguli Oris					Longus Colli						
Mentalis					Semispinalis Cervicis						
	Masseter		Longissimus Capitis								
	Temporalis		Cervical Multifidii								
	Pterygoids		Cervical Rotatores								

Table 6.1 (*Continued*)

Head and C1–T1 Segmental Chart (Continued)

Left panel (columns C3, C4, C5, C6, C7, C8, T1):

Muscle	C3	C4	C5	C6	C7	C8	T1
Levator Scapulae	X	X	X				
Diaphragm	X	X	X				
Supraspinatus		X	X	X			
Infraspinatus		X	X	X			
Teres Minor		X	X	X			
Teres Major		X	X	X			
Latissimus Dorsi				X	X	X	
Subscapularis		X	X	X			
Rhomboids		X	X				
Deltoid		X	X	X			
Coracobrachialis			X	X	X		
Biceps Brachii			X	X			
Brachialis			X	X			
Serratus Anterior			X	X	X		
Pectoralis Major			X	X	X	X	
Triceps Brachii				X	X	X	
Longissimus Capitis			X	X	X	X	
Anconeus				X	X	X	
Extensor Carpi Radialis Longus				X	X		
Extensor Carpi Radialis Brevis				X	X		
Brachioradialis			X	X			
Extensor Carpi Ulnaris				X	X	X	
Extensor Digitorum				X	X	X	
Extensor Digiti Minimi				X	X	X	
Extensor Indicis				X	X	X	

Right panel (columns C5, C6, C7, C8, T1):

Muscle	C5	C6	C7	C8	T1
Supinator	X	X	X		
Palmaris Longus	X	X	X		
Flexor Carpi Radialis		X	X		
Abductor Pollicis Longus		X	X		
Extensor Pollicis Longus		X	X		
Extensor Pollicis Brevis		X	X		
Pronator Teres		X	X		
Flexor Digitorum Superficialis			X	X	X
Pectoralis Minor				X	X
Flexor Carpi Ulnaris				X	X
Flexor Digitorum Profundus				X	X
Flexor Digiti Minimi Brevis				X	X
Opponens Digiti Minimi				X	X
Abductor Digiti Minimi				X	X
Flexor Pollicis Longus			X	X	X
Flexor Pollicis Brevis				X	X
Adductor Pollicis				X	X
Pronator Quadratus			X	X	X
Abductor Pollicis Brevis				X	X
Opponens Pollicis				X	X
Interossei				X	X
Lumbricals				X	X
Palmaris Brevis				X	X
Transversalis Cervicis					X
Sternalis					X

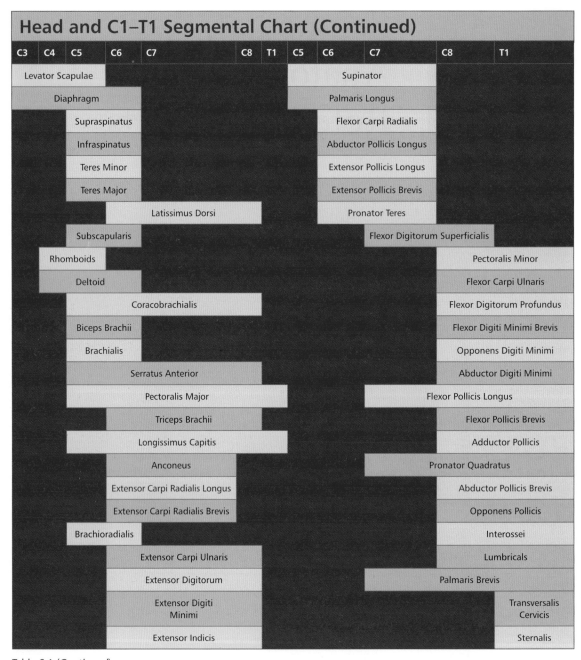

Table 6.1 (*Continued*)

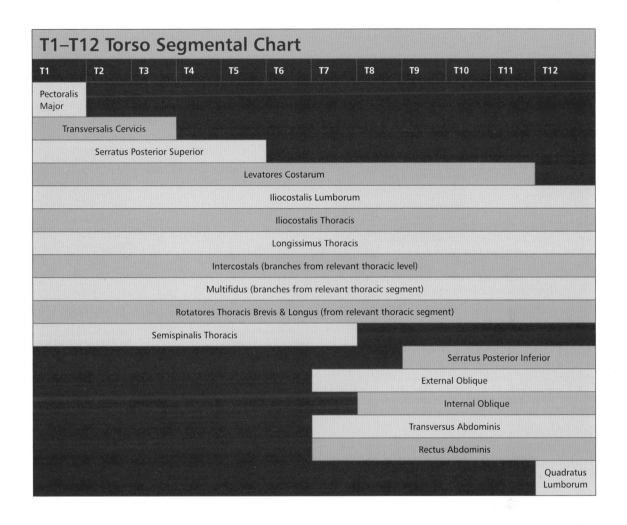

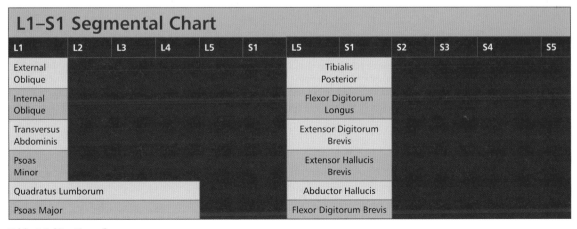

Table 6.1 (Continued)

L2–S5 Segmental Chart (Continued)

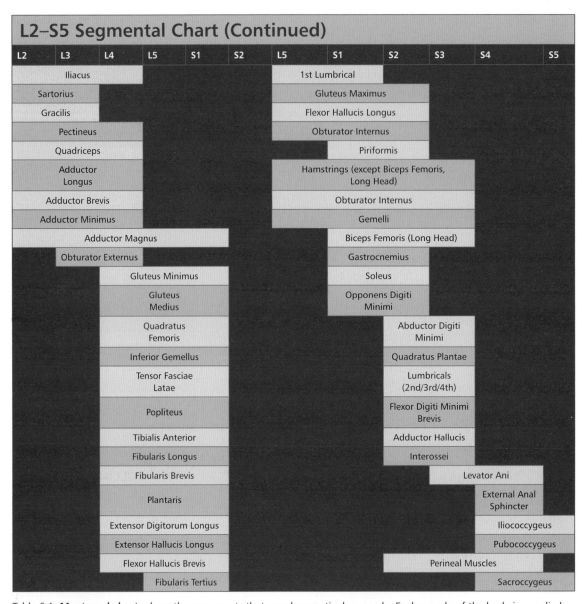

Table 6.1: **Myotomal charts** show the nerve roots that supply a particular muscle. Each muscle of the body is supplied by one nerve root, or a number of them, all of which originate from the spinal column. Some muscles of the neck and face take their motor nerve supply from key cranial nerves (facial nerve and trigeminal nerve). Like spinal nerves, myotomes are organised into segments because they share a common origin.

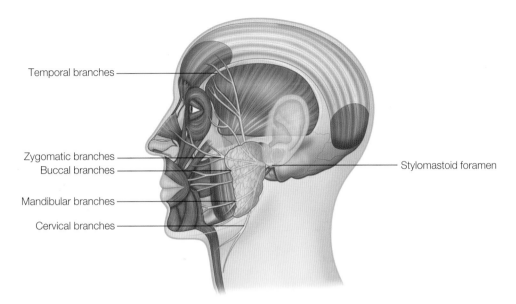

Temporal branches

Zygomatic branches
Buccal branches

Mandibular branches

Cervical branches

Stylomastoid foramen

From the pons of the midbrain, cranial nerve VII, the **facial nerve**, enters the temporal bone through the internal acoustic meatus, and then emerges through the stylomastoid foramen, where it branches into the posterior auricular branch. There are five major branches—temporal, zygomatic, buccal, (marginal) mandibular, and cervical.

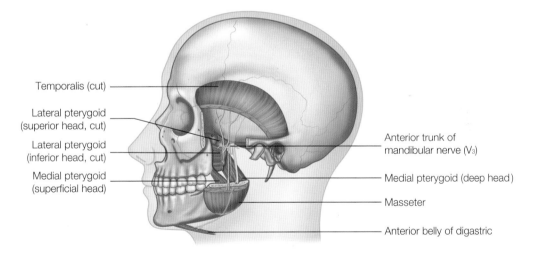

Temporalis (cut)

Lateral pterygoid
(superior head, cut)

Lateral pterygoid
(inferior head, cut)

Medial pterygoid
(superficial head)

Anterior trunk of
mandibular nerve (V₃)

Medial pterygoid (deep head)

Masseter

Anterior belly of digastric

Cranial nerve V, the **trigeminal nerve**, is the largest of the cranial nerves and has three main divisions: ophthalmic (V_1), maxillary (V_2), and mandibular (V_3). The trigeminal nerve is responsible for sensation in the face and for functions such as biting and chewing. Both the ophthalmic division and the maxillary division are purely sensory, while the mandibular division has both sensory and motor functions.

Figure 6.1: There are twelve pairs of cranial nerves, ten which originate from the brain stem and two from inside the brain. They are named according to their distribution or function and numbered according to where they arise in the brain (in order from anterior to posterior). The two most involved with innervation of the facial muscles are shown above.

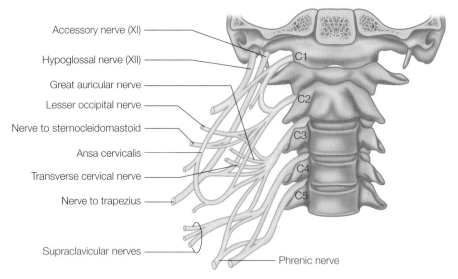

Located in the posterior triangle of the neck and halfway up the SCM, the **cervical plexus** is formed by the anterior rami of C1 to C4.

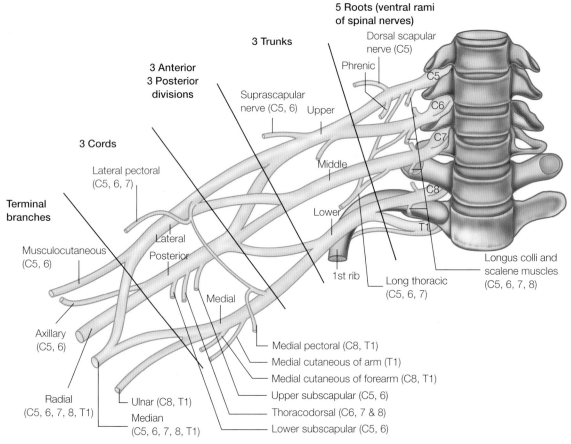

Originating in the neck, the **brachial plexus** passes laterally and inferiorly over rib 1, and enters the axilla. It is formed by the anterior rami of C5 to C8, and most of the anterior ramus of T1.

Figure 6.2: (*Continued*).

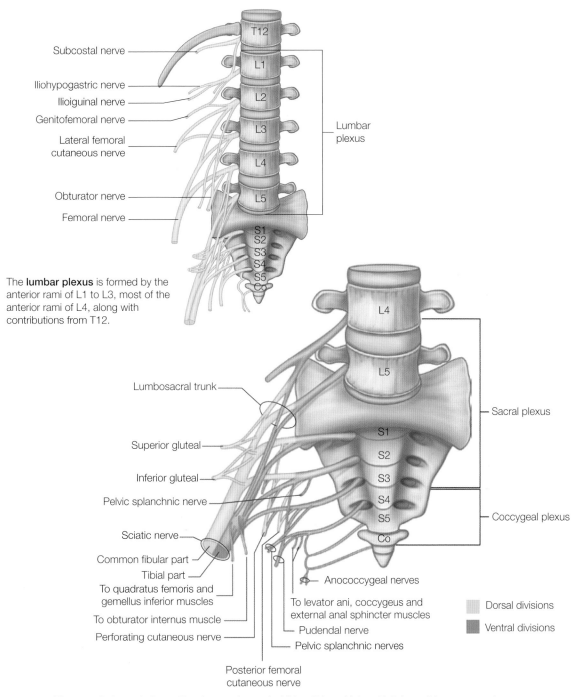

Subcostal nerve

Iliohypogastric nerve
Ilioiguinal nerve
Genitofemoral nerve
Lateral femoral
cutaneous nerve

Obturator nerve
Femoral nerve

T12
L1
L2
L3
L4
L5
S1
S2
S3
S4
S5
Co

Lumbar
plexus

The **lumbar plexus** is formed by the anterior rami of L1 to L3, most of the anterior rami of L4, along with contributions from T12.

Lumbosacral trunk

Superior gluteal

Inferior gluteal

Pelvic splanchnic nerve

Sciatic nerve

Common fibular part
Tibial part
To quadratus femoris and
gemellus inferior muscles
To obturator internus muscle
Perforating cutaneous nerve

L4
L5
S1
S2
S3
S4
S5
Co

Sacral plexus

Coccygeal plexus

Anococcygeal nerves

To levator ani, coccygeus and
external anal sphincter muscles
Pudendal nerve
Pelvic splanchnic nerves

Posterior femoral
cutaneous nerve

Dorsal divisions

Ventral divisions

The **sacral plexus** is formed by the anterior rami of S1 to S4, and L4 and L5. It provides motor and sensory nerves for the posterior thigh, most of the leg and foot, and part of the pelvis. The smaller **coccygeal plexus** has a minor contribution from S4, and is formed mainly by the anterior rami of C5 and C0.

Figure 6.2: A nerve plexus is a branching network of nerves. Here are the primary plexuses. Broadly, the **cervical plexus** serves the head, neck and shoulders; the **brachial plexus** serves the chest, shoulders, arms and hands; the **lumbar plexus** serves the back, abdomen, groin, thighs, knees and calves; and the **coccygeal plexus** serves a small region around the coccyx.

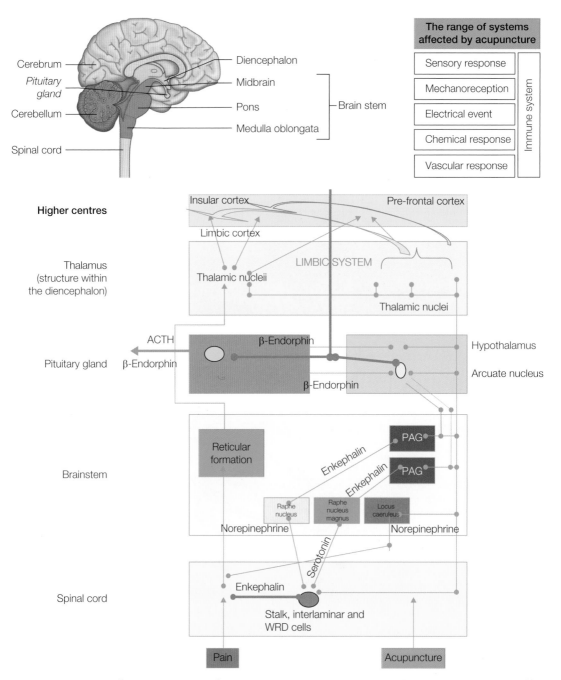

Figure 6.3: Acupuncture effects cover a range of interwoven biological systems. Researching one parameter is a difficulty within the evidence-based approach as a multitude of physical and chemical events occur at the same time. The incoming sensation is registered in the cord and transmitted onwards through the brainstem and into the thalamus, primary sensory cortex and high centres. Switching on of the descending inhibitory pathways involves the hypothalamus (which has a knock-on effect into the pituitary and subsequently hormonal release), arcuate nucleus, periaqueductal grey matter and brainstem nuclei – in particular the Raphe Nucleus Magnus which releases serotonin. The effect of serotonin can be seen during a treatment session with the 'therapeutic sigh' from a client as the sympathetic system steps down and the parasympathetic system becomes more active. Also, pupils become dilated, some sweating on the skin occurs (hands and feet generally) and there may be flushing on the face and ears.

Abbreviations: **PAG** – Periaqueductal grey matter, **ACTH** – Adrenocorticotropic hormone, **WRD** – Wide range dynamic cell (also covers interlaminar cells at spinal cord level)

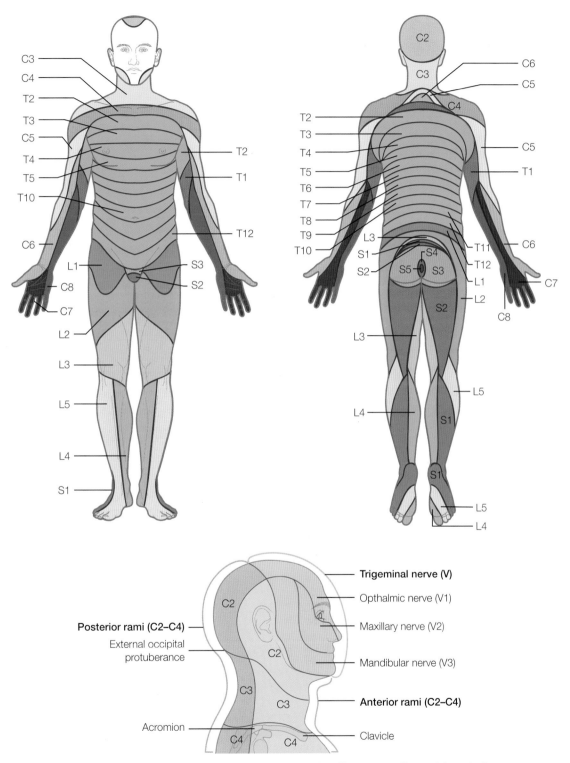

Figure 6.4: **Dermatomal charts** show the neural skin supply from the afferent nerve fibres of the spinal nerves. The trigeminal nerve also supplies a lot of the face in terms of its sensory receptors, and is therefore also represented as a dermatome for ease of reference.

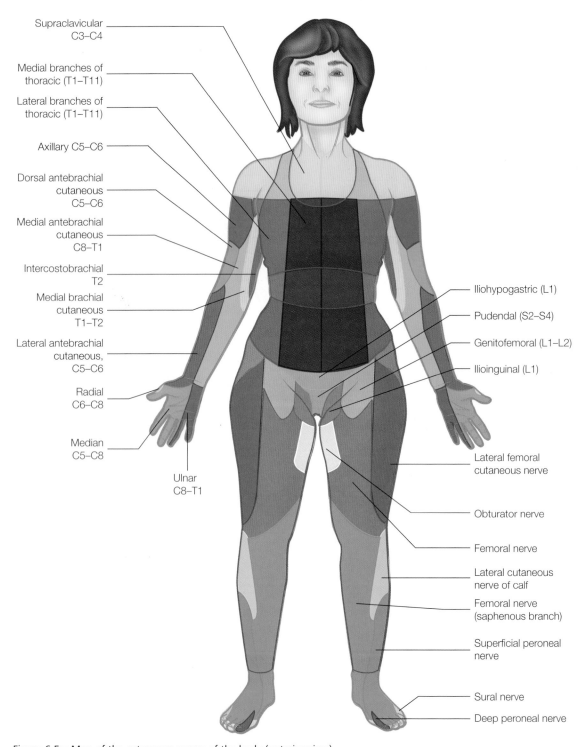

Supraclavicular
C3–C4

Medial branches of
thoracic (T1–T11)

Lateral branches of
thoracic (T1–T11)

Axillary C5–C6

Dorsal antebrachial
cutaneous
C5–C6

Medial antebrachial
cutaneous
C8–T1

Intercostobrachial
T2

Medial brachial
cutaneous
T1–T2

Lateral antebrachial
cutaneous,
C5–C6

Radial
C6–C8

Median
C5–C8

Ulnar
C8–T1

Iliohypogastric (L1)

Pudendal (S2–S4)

Genitofemoral (L1–L2)

Ilioinguinal (L1)

Lateral femoral
cutaneous nerve

Obturator nerve

Femoral nerve

Lateral cutaneous
nerve of calf

Femoral nerve
(saphenous branch)

Superficial peroneal
nerve

Sural nerve

Deep peroneal nerve

Figure 6.5a: Map of the cutaneous nerves of the body (anterior view).

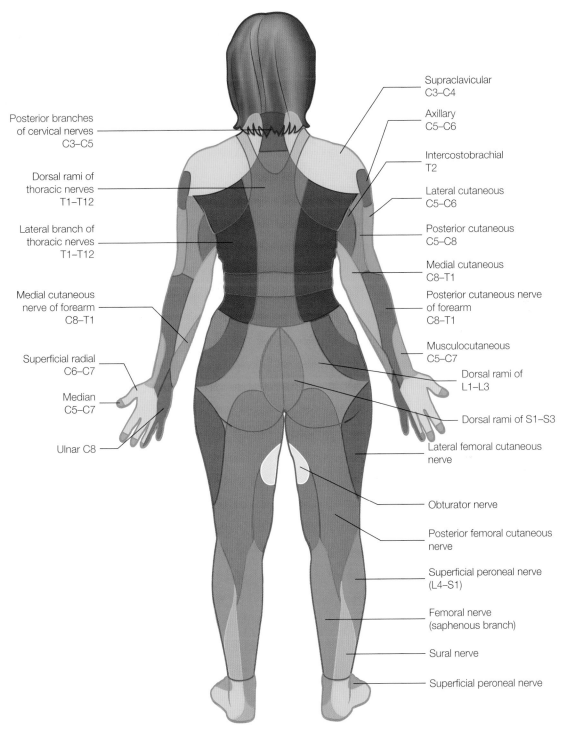

Supraclavicular
C3–C4

Axillary
C5–C6

Intercostobrachial
T2

Lateral cutaneous
C5–C6

Posterior cutaneous
C5–C8

Medial cutaneous
C8–T1

Posterior cutaneous nerve
of forearm
C8–T1

Musculocutaneous
C5–C7

Dorsal rami of
L1–L3

Dorsal rami of S1–S3

Lateral femoral cutaneous
nerve

Obturator nerve

Posterior femoral cutaneous
nerve

Superficial peroneal nerve
(L4–S1)

Femoral nerve
(saphenous branch)

Sural nerve

Superficial peroneal nerve

Posterior branches
of cervical nerves
C3–C5

Dorsal rami of
thoracic nerves
T1–T12

Lateral branch of
thoracic nerves
T1–T12

Medial cutaneous
nerve of forearm
C8–T1

Superficial radial
C6–C7

Median
C5–C7

Ulnar C8

Figure 6.5b: Map of the cutaneous nerves of the body (posterior view).

79

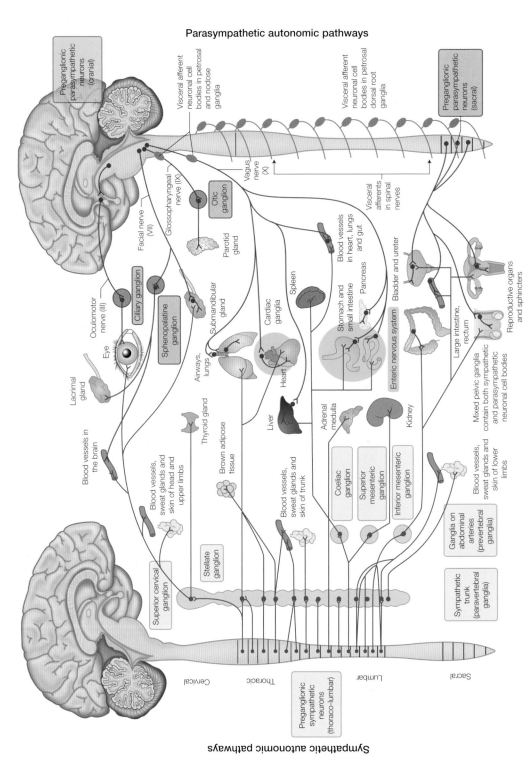

Figure 6.6: **Viscerotomes:** The spinal nerves and the vagus nerve supply the internal organs. In the main, the viscera are under the control of the autonomic nervous system, but the message reaches them via a number of complex ganglia which take their nerve fibres from spinal segments. This can be very relevant when using the back-shu points, for example, as there may be close anatomical connections between an organ and the level you may wish to acupuncture. The autonomic nervous system is divided into sympathetic and parasympathetic components.

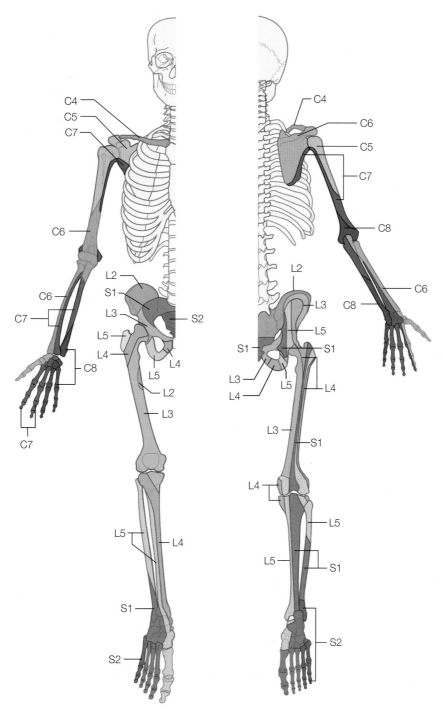

Figure 6.7: **Sclerotomes**: These are the areas of bone that are supplied by single spinal nerves.

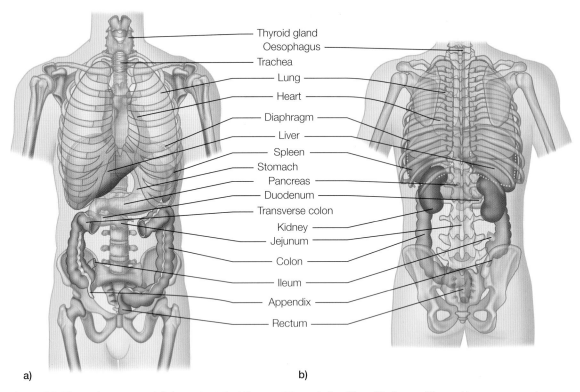

a)   b)

Figure 6.8: **Visceral anatomy**: It is important that the practitioner is familiar with the positions of key organs and landmarks in order to ensure safe practice and to avoid causing internal injury; a) anterior view, b) posterior view.

7 Principles of Point Selection

Chinese Medical Model Ideas

An effective choice of points means that *the points work together to harmoniously treat the whole person at the same time as the specific complaint*. The formation of the points prescription is the cornerstone of acupuncture and other treatment modalities, and requires a thorough understanding of Chinese medicine principles, laid out over the thousands of years of clinical experience gained by all the doctors in the past.

Point qualities and the patient's case history and current symptoms need to be married up. In addition, attention needs to be paid to those environmental, psycho-emotional and physical factors that might play a role in the outcome of the treatment. When all this information has been analysed, a *clear diagnosis* and *principle of treatment* is formulated. The final choice of points and techniques that the practitioner will make is based on this principle, which should outline clearly the *goals and priorities of treatment*. The points reflect internal pathology, so good diagnosis and history taking should lead to a good set of points whereby Qi can be influenced. If there is little response from a point, perhaps that point was inappropriate because not enough investigation went into establishing the root problem.

> An effective treatment includes points to treat the *underlying cause* of the disease, or 'roots' (*ben* in Chinese), and those to treat the *manifestation*, or 'branches' (*biao* in Chinese).

In clinical practice, finding the 'roots' and 'branches' can become rather complex because there is usually a combination of intimately interrelated causes and symptoms. Therefore, in order to devise a 'holistic' treatment rather than a 'symptomatic' one, the practitioner must find the *correct balance for the patient* between working on the roots and branches, and on the causes and symptoms.

Remember, these are your goals as the practitioner and the goals of the patient, and they may not coincide to start with. 'The customer is always right', so it is a case of working with the patient to get them through the short game, and head them towards the long game in due course.

General Principles

In general, if the disorder is primarily due to *deficiency*, the treatment should centre more on the *cause*; if it is more due to *excess*, focus more on the *symptoms*, particularly at the beginning of the course of treatment.

In cases of deficiency, the particular points and techniques that bring the energy inwards, close to the centre of the body and towards the affected area, are chosen. In these circumstances, points directly on the affected site are of most significance, and are known as **local points**. These points can be further divided into **local points** which are *exactly on the affected area* (preferably at its epicentre), and **adjacent points**, which are *close to the affected area* or *surrounding it*.

Conversely, if there are many manifestations of excess and blockage in the form of *pathogenic factors* or *stagnation of Qi and Blood*, the points and techniques that dissipate, expel and move the Qi outwards are chosen. Therefore, points situated away from the problem area, usually towards the extremities, are of most importance. These are known as **distal points**, and many of the most important ones are located on the limbs.

The final selection will most often consist of a combination of local, adjacent and distal points.

Local point selection

Choosing local points is the simplest and oldest method of applying treatment in the world, and is how the *barefoot doctors of classical Chinese practice* were trained to work.

Local points can be considered to work more *locally* than *systemically*; they can be chosen for more *superficial diseases* and are generally thought of as more *symptomatic* in their effects.

> Local and adjacent transient points include:
>
> – **Pain points** and **Ashi points**
> – **Reactive points** on or off the channels
> – Other types of **trigger point**

Points on the back, chest and abdomen can be used as local points to treat internal conditions and diseases of the Zang Fu in cases of either excess or deficiency.

Transient points often form an important part of the treatment, but because they are inherently unchartable, they cannot be listed.

Distal point selection

While a correctly applied treatment of local points is often effective, a holistic treatment focuses on the entire person rather than just the symptom. *Distal points** complement the stimulus at the local point by augmenting the flow of Qi in the affected channels and areas.

---

* In keeping with most textbooks, the term 'distal' has been used throughout this text. However, in reality, the term 'distant', meaning 'far away' or 'somewhere else in relation to the problem area', may be more accurate.

The selection of distal points can be further divided as follows:

- Points on the extremities to treat the centre of the body, and vice versa.
- Distal or proximal points to treat pain and other disorders of the limbs.
- Points on the upper body to treat the lower part, and vice versa.
- Points on the left side of the body to treat the right side, and vice versa (contralateral points).
- Points on the front of the body to treat the back, and vice versa.
- Corresponding points on the Yin-Yang paired channels.
- Corresponding points on the six divisions paired channels.
- Eight Extraordinary Meridians opening and coupled points.
- Points that are related via specific channel connections.
- Symptomatic points, known to treat a specific condition or symptom.
- Special distal points that are beyond the scope of this text, such as ear acupuncture.

Once the area of the problem has been precisely located and the main local and distal points to treat it have been selected, points that also treat the underlying disharmony are chosen. A comprehensive evaluation of all the signs and symptoms and aspects of the person (physical, energetic, emotional, psychological, etc.) is necessary in order to achieve a thorough understanding of the *causes of the problem*, reach a *precise diagnosis*, and form a *clear treatment principle* that will guide the practitioner to devise the *final prescription of points and techniques*.

Depending on which school of thought they belong to and how they work within their traditional practice, and guided by the treatment principle and diagnosis, the practitioner forms a prescription with the most indicated points and techniques. These could be combinations of the following:

- The *eight principles diagnosis*, which is used to determine points and techniques to tonify and nourish or to regulate and disperse.

- The *vital substances diagnosis*, which is used to determine points to influence Qi, Blood, Body fluids, jing and shen.
- The *pathogenic factors (six evils) diagnosis*, which is used to determine points to eliminate exterior or interior dampness, heat, fire, cold, phlegm, wind, etc.
- The *internal organ Zang Fu diagnosis*, which determines the precise disharmony, so that points can be chosen on account of their energetic attributes and the specific relationship that these attributes have to the disharmony.
- The *six divisions differentiation*, which offers a way to ensure that the chosen points have a direct influence on the affected channels and stage of development of the condition.
- The *five phase analysis*, which offers a precise method for selecting points and is applicable in a wide range of cases.

Dan Keown's book, *The Uncharted Body,* is an excellent guide and resource for those wishing to study the complexities of Chinese medicine further.

Western Medical Model Ideas

Acupuncture in the West sometimes gets bad press for its targeted, local, 'treat only the branch' of a problem approach. Certainly, local trigger point work often has a high profile in a Western clinic, sometimes because of time constraints and resource issues of space and staff, but good point choice can also affect the fundamental biology of an individual; in so doing, it can alter mood, stress biology, digestion etc. It can provide as much of a holistic treatment as the full Chinese medical model, but with different reasoning and assessments behind the point choice.

Point choice will be made after a biomedical, scientific and orthodox medical diagnosis such as occurs in the Western medical environment. This could be a GP practice, where acupuncture can be commonly offered for pain conditions, within manual therapist's clinics, right through to consultant level, with increasing numbers of Western-trained doctors and allied health professionals training in acupuncture to augment their existing skills.

Different approaches can be:

- Trigger point needling
- Ashi needling (local/transient points on their own)
- Recipes
- Segmental acupuncture
- Extra-segmental acupuncture
- Points to alter global biology (such as increased endorphin levels/melatonin)
- Sympathetic/parasympathetic autonomic nervous system (ANS) effects
  - Thoracic spine vs craniosacral points
- Electro-acupuncture (see Chapter 3).

Putting the approaches together:

- *Layering a treatment* to affect local to global biology with increasing strengths of points
  - Local biology and physical effects
  - Spinal/segmental biology
  - Central nervous system and biology.

Trigger Point Needling

With the aid of trigger point charts, it is often easy to match a patient's pain picture with a known muscle and the exact location of a known trigger point within it (Figs. 7.1 and 7.2). Needling must then be precise and targeted at that identified spot. Often, if the needle is in the correct place, the patient's pain will be recreated. This is considered good needling.

There are a number of different schools suggesting how a trigger point should be needled. There can be very superficial needling, which may have more of an effect via the ANS. A more common type of needling, however, is to sensitively seek out the centre of the trigger point, possibly find a twitch or spontaneous release in the tissue, and then retain the needle for long enough to alter local biology (blood flow/temperature/muscle fibre relaxation). In the main, trigger points occur in the centre of the muscle bulk. Procuring a set of charts is extremely helpful in order to be accurate with this kind of needling.

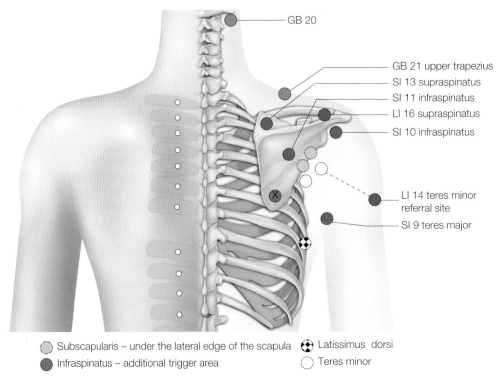

Figure 7.1: Map for shoulder trigger points showing overlap with known acupoints.

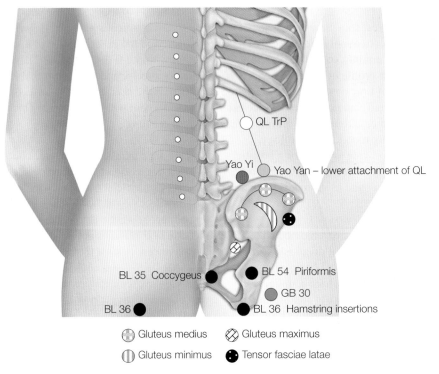

Figure 7.2: Map for lumbar and buttock trigger points showing overlap with known acupoints.

Ashi Needling

Following on from a classical Chinese training concept, Ashi needling is based on simply palpating and finding points of reactivity, which are known as *Ashi points* (see Chapter 1). The practitioner needs to have a good understanding of the course of a meridian if keeping some classical component in their treatment, or, alternatively, these points are located with manual therapy/massage and then needled with the patient helping guide the therapist to the most painful spot.

Note: All active and many non-active trigger points are Ashi points. Non-active trigger points often become active when palpated. Again, the needling type will depend on training, and the necessary depth to evoke a response is variable.

Recipes

There are many books that give recipe suggestions as to which points to use for certain conditions. While this may seem very useful when starting out in acupuncture, it does not encourage full thought and clinical reasoning surrounding a particular patient's condition or their background.

A basic recipe could be considered the 'meat and the pasta' of cooking. Many, many Italian meals start out as meat and pasta! Using this analogy, there are numerous additions, methods and approaches for finalising a way of 'cooking' that would suit the chef and his clientele. Likewise, in acupuncture there are many ways of working, and many different practitioners who will put their own art into their practice and develop technique, point choice and timing in an effort to get the best for the patient.

For some joints, such as the knee, the choice of points around them is limited, and so it is easier to stick to a recipe of points as a baseline. Extra points should then be added in order to help the patient in a more holistic way. Just treating the local problem does not always give the best result, and perpetuating this method of practice unfortunately misses the point of acupuncture and how it can be a whole-person treatment. To simply stick to recipes would make the practitioner something of a technician, which is *not* what good practice can offer.

Segmental Acupuncture

The segmental maps as seen in Chapter 6 provide a reference resource for this section and for enabling point choice. For a full description of the concept behind segmental acupuncture, see Chapter 2. Only the technical application will be dealt with here.

In brief, the concept of segmental acupuncture consists of identifying the aberrant segment, or segmental tissue, on the basis of neuroanatomy and client symptoms, and then bombard it with stimuli from elsewhere in the segment, in an effort to normalise it. This is best reflected in a 'hypothetical' simple case example:

> *'Mrs. A presented with left-sided sciatica, with pain extending through the L5/S1 segment down her thigh, into the calf and foot. She had dug over a large bed at her allotment two days before and had slow onset of back pain, with increasing leg pain subsequent to that. The pain was worse at night, often waking her up at around 2.30–3.30am, with extreme stiffness and difficulty in getting up first thing in the morning.'*

From even this short description, an acupuncture practitioner working with a segmental approach and with Western medical training would think as follows:

Question: *Which points can I use that are local to L5/S1 (suggestion BL 24/25/26).*

The nature and behaviour of this is inflammatory – worse at night/waking at 2.30–3.30am, so some sort of local treatment to the L5/S1 segment would be needed in the recipe. The goal of this would be to improve blood flow, remove inflammatory waste and reduce tone and spasm around the lower back segments. In addition, the aim would be to increase local endorphins and thus reduce pain.

Question: *Where can I place needles so as to reduce activity within the L5/S1 segment but not increase it?*

Using the myotomal chart, the muscles supplied by L5/S1 can be identified, and known acupuncture points applied within those muscles. Because this is an acute problem, and the segment is highly sensitive, a suggestion is to *needle the opposite side to the pain* so as not to increase a sensory input. This is *contralateral needling.*

Suggested points down the right leg, with the patient in a left-side lying or prone position: GB 30, BL 36, BL 37, BL 40 and BL 57. In addition, ST 36 and GB 34 (awkward to needle in the prone position but possible with the lower leg supported on a pillow at the foot) as well as LR 3 give an additional non-channel input.

All these points are within the L5/S1 nerve pathway. Strong stimulation may 'divert' attention to the non-painful leg. You have to *stimulate to achieve sedation,* and so pain problems often need to be treated with strong needle stimulation.

As an additional thought for this person, if there was a lot of bony pain down her anterior shin, suggestive of L5 sclerotomal referral, then *periosteal pecking* on her greater trochanter (also supplied by L5) could provide an equally strong 'bony' sensation. Bony pain can be treated with bony sensory input.

As she improves, bilateral needling could be introduced, as this would enhance the segmental input.

What can be seen here is that the local and distal rule still applies to segmental acupuncture, but the reasoning is purely based on neuroanatomy and not Chinese medical model theories of point function.

Summary of questions to ask when using a segmental approach:

- *Where is the patient's pain?*
- *What nerve supplies that area/structure?*
- *Where shall I place my needles so as to affect that segment locally?*
- *Where shall I place my needles so as to affect that segment distally?*

Extra-Segmental Acupuncture

The idea here is that of diversion. If a client presents with, for example, a painful right shoulder, the use of extra-segmental points with reasonably strong stimulation will divert attention.

However, the method will also fall into the category discussed below of using points that have a global biological effect. This is much like taking a tablet for the shoulder pain: the chemistry of the drug does not just go to the shoulder – it affects the whole body.

If the patient claims that their pain is 5/10 on a visual analogue scale (VAS), see below, then the stimulation from the needle needs to be 6/10 or above in order to have an effect. The whole point of acupuncture is to challenge the body's own systems into action, and so this has to be considered in terms of the level of needle stimulation.

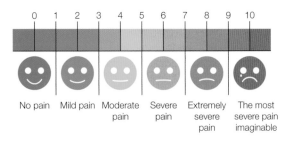

An extra-segmental point could therefore be on the leg and have nothing in common with the nerve supply to the shoulder, which would predominantly be C5/6. It would be best to use one of the known strong points mentioned below in order to enhance a full biological effect.

Points to Alter Global Biology

Increasing scientific research of the effects of acupuncture shows that certain points seem to have a more global biological effect, and that the discussion about point specificity is one that is ongoing. This is in fact the big research question at the moment. It is not *'Does acupuncture work?',* as it used to be, as we have enough evidence to show that it does, but *'Do traditional points work better than sham acupuncture?'*

Sham acupuncture involves needling at a non-meridial point. As well as true acupuncture, or what is called *verum acupuncture,* sham acupuncture has been shown to have an effect on the brain. The brain will *always* register a needle going into the skin. What becomes of interest is which parts of the brain are activated by sham or verum needling, and how that converts into useful information for

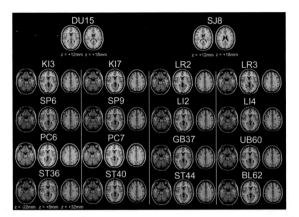

Figure 7.3: Areas in the brain where points become activated or deactivated with acupuncture (from Huang et al. 2012). Note: Du represents the GV meridian, SJ represents the TE meridian, and UB represents the BL meridian.

those actually using acupuncture. This can be seen on fMRI/ blood tests/ measurement of blood flow under ultrasound testing, analysis of heart rate/ gut activity, and more.

Figure 7.3 shows the areas within the brain where points become activated or deactivated with acupuncture. Many more studies are being done into the plasticity and central nervous system effects.

There remains, therefore, the suggestion that *certain points have certain effects* (and so this remains in keeping with the Chinese medical model and point choice for treatments). There are sceptics who refute this idea, however, and say that *acupuncture anywhere will have an effect on the central nervous system* and that the resultant alteration in activity and subsequent neurotransmitter change is what creates the response seen in the patient.

Some of these key points are listed in Table 7.1, but research is ongoing. This list may be extremely small but it provides examples of the 'big' points that send loud messages to the central nervous system via their strong sensory pathways.
These points are also the key strong points that would be chosen in a Chinese medical model reasoning.

Table 7.1: Some of the 'loud' acupuncture points which give a strong sensory input.

Point	Western reasoning	Chinese reasoning
LI 4	■ In the nerve supply of T1, which sends a strong message into the top of the sympathetic chain. Extremely sensory ■ Endorphin, etc. production ■ Affects gut mobility and abdominal pain	■ One of the 'Four Gates' along with LR 3. Opens the body's gates towards heaven, and so, in combination, allows Qi to flow through the whole body, unblocking any stagnation ■ Releases the exterior, thus allowing heat to escape ■ For head and face pain
LR 3	■ In the nerve supply of L5 ■ Very useful for any pain pattern in the lower limb, and back pain in particular from L4/5 area ■ Strongly sensory ■ Endorphin, etc. production	■ One of the 'Four Gates' along with LI 4. Opens the body's gates towards earth, and so, in combination, allows Qi to flow through the whole body, unblocking any stagnation ■ Opens the middle jiao ■ For pain anywhere ■ Clears the head ■ Calms the Liver – involved in stress and anger
ST 36	■ In the nerve supply of L4/5 ■ Strongly sensory ■ Endorphin, etc. production ■ Shown to improve natural killer (NK) cell mobility, thus boosting immune function ■ Alters gut motility	■ Boosts immunity (Wei Qi) ■ Increases power in the lower limbs ■ Aids exhaustion ■ For all emotional disturbances, especially excess (mania and instability) ■ Generates Qi and Blood ■ Harmonises the digestion

(Continued)

Table 7.1: (Continued)

Point	Western reasoning	Chinese reasoning
GB 20	■ In the nerve supply of C1/2 – has a strong parasympathetic effect ■ Endorphin, etc. production ■ Indicated with headache and migraine ■ Alters blood flow in the Circle of Willis	■ Eliminates wind, especially from the head ■ Clears the eyes and all sense organs ■ Relieves pain in the head and neck
GV 20	■ Positioned in the region of the central sulcus of the brain, and so over both motor and sensory cortices ■ Generally stimulating in its effect ■ Endorphin production, but also, in the first instance, adrenaline ■ Tension headaches	■ Head pain and disorder, including dizziness, blood pressure issues, stroke ■ Agitation ■ Lack of memory/cognition ■ Prolapses ■ Brings clear Qi to the head

Sympathetic/Parasympathetic ANS Effects

Points around the cranium and sacrum have parasympathetic effects, while points over the thoracic area – notably the HuatuoJiaji and inner Bladder lines – have sympathetic system effects. In general, if an individual is running on adrenaline, stressed or in pain, then calming the sympathetic system would be the way forwards.

With an effect on the parasympathetic system, the patient will breathe more slowly and deeply, their heart rate slows, and activity is stimulated in the stomach. This is an excellent sign that is anticipated with an acupuncture treatment. A gurgling stomach suggests a direct effect on the gut.

Key points for stimulating parasympathetic activity are: GB 20, BL 10, BL 27 BL 28, BL 31 and BL 32. These are very important in disorders of the urogenital system and gynaecological conditions. By raising the activity in the PSNS, the activity in the SNS must, by nature, come down. Either way, the patient becomes calmer, more rested and less stressed. (See Fig. 6.3 of the nerve supply of the SNS and PSNS.)

To affect the sympathetic tone, the points of the Inner Bladder line or the HuatuoJiaji line are used (Fig. 7.4). This is due to them having direct supply by the dorsal ramus of the relevant spinal level, which also communicates into the sympathetic ganglia at that same level. Nerves from the sympathetic chain will travel out to various groups of ganglia within the abdominal and thoracic cavities and affect organ function by telling them to 'go', where the parasympathetic system will be telling them to 'stop'.

It can be seen that these points can have wide-reaching effects on all kinds of medical condition, such as IBS, Crohn's disease, gynaecological conditions, anxiety disorders, urogenital disorders and asthma.

There is also a strong link between experiencing visceral feelings and emotional distress, with this being an endless loop of one causing the other (Vianna et al. 2006 and the James-Lange Theory). So, by choosing to treat the sympathetic chain for a physical cause, there may well be a knock-on benefit to an emotional state.

Layering

In 2003 Lynley Bradnam, a New Zealand research physiotherapist, proposed a layering concept to enable practitioners to build up a treatment based

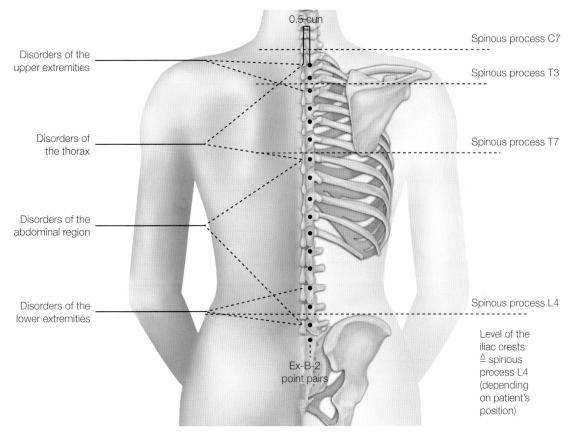

Figure 7.4: The HuatuoJiaji line. Please note that there are two lines running down either side of the spine. For diagrammatic clarity, only the right hand line is shown here.

on point choice of increasing strength and effect through a number of layers of the neural system (Bradnam, 2003). This has proved an excellent model to help those starting out in acupuncture formulate a well clinically reasoned treatment recipe, and has also given them a way to progress their treatments.

The three layers for initial targeted treatment are:

- Local/peripheral effects?
- Spinal/segmental effects?
- Central/supraspinal effects?

On top of these three considerations are the possibilities of affecting the sympathetic system at its outflow in the thoracic spine, and also through central nervous system measures.

Figure 7.5 presents a breakdown of the questions asked during the layering approach, along with suggested acupuncture ideas.

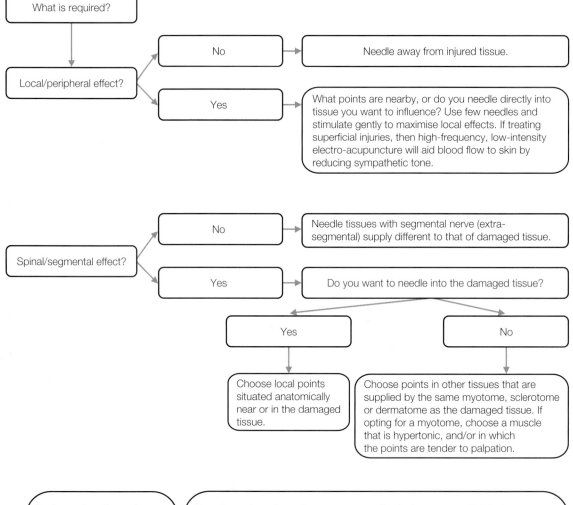

Figure 7.5: *(Continued)*

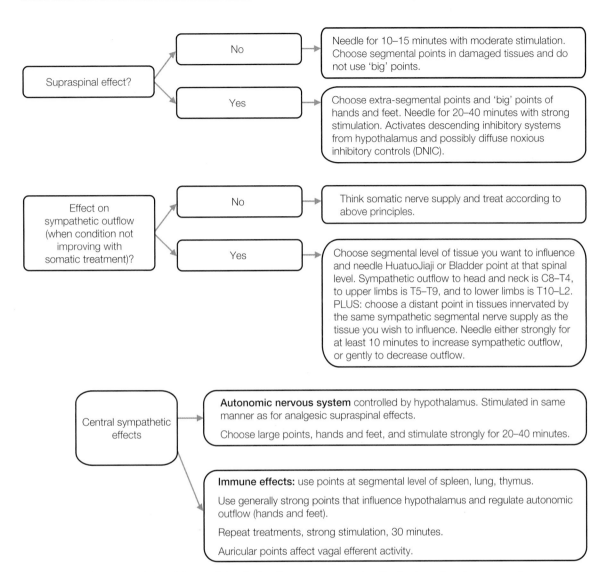

Figure 7.5: A diagrammatic breakdown of the choices in acupuncture using the Bradnam layering approach.

Part II

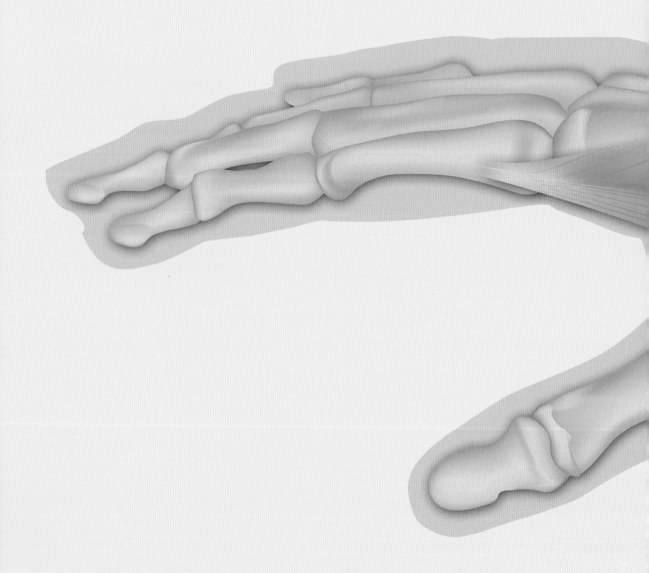

Practice

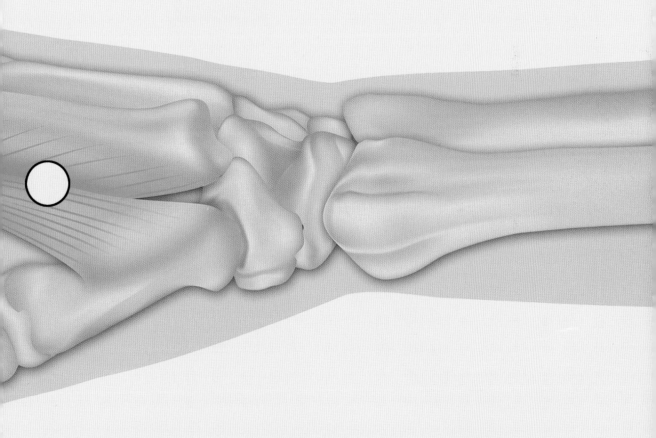

8 Points of the Arm Tai Yin Lung Channel

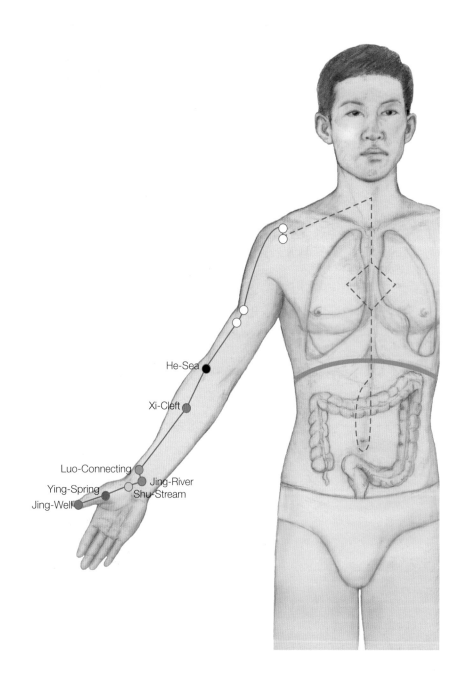

He-Sea

Xi-Cleft

Luo-Connecting

Ying-Spring

Jing-River

Shu-Stream

Jing-Well

手太陰經穴

General	The Lung channel starts on the lateral chest near the coracoid process and travels up the chest slightly, before entering the upper limb. It then descends the anterior aspect of the limb towards the thumb, where it ends on the radial side of the thumbnail. It has 11 points. It is grouped with the Large Intestine under the Metal element in five-element theory.
More specifically	Originating in the Middle Energizer, the channel is said to have links downwards with the Large Intestine (its Yang paired organ), and upwards, through the diaphragm, spreading through the Lungs, trachea and larynx, emerging at Lung 1 just below the lateral end of the clavicle and inferior to the coracoid process. Lung 2 is above the coracoid process and the channel then travels downwards along biceps, through the cubital fossa, and over the flexors and radial deviators of the hand and wrist veering slightly laterally towards the thumb at the radial styloid. It finishes on the radial side of the base of the thumbnail.
Area covered	Chest, Anterior Arm – Antero-Lateral Forearm.
Areas affected with treatment	C4–6 segmental supply, Lungs, chest, Upper Energizer, Throat and larynx, elbow and wrist. Skin conditions (asthma/eczema).
Key points	LU1, LU3, LU5, LU7, LU9, LU10.

LU 1   Zhongfu
Middle Palace

中府

Front-Mu point of the Lungs
Intersection of the Spleen on
the Lung channel

Myotome	C5–C8
Dermatome	C4

Location
On the anterior lateral aspect of the chest, approximately 1 cun inferior and slightly lateral to LU 2, just medial to the coracoid process of the scapula. Situated in the pectoralis major muscle and, more deeply, at the insertion of the pectoralis minor. Also, medially in its deep position, the muscles of the second intercostal space (ICS), or the body of the rib, depending on the individual structure of the rib cage and the shoulder girdle.

To aid location, ask the patient to stretch the arm out forwards (flex the shoulder) to emphasise the pectoralis and anterior deltoid muscles. First, locate LU 2 at the centre of the depression of the deltopectoral triangle, and then, following the

contour of the rib cage, move the tip of the finger inferiorly approximately 1 cun to locate LU 1.

Needling
Remembering the near vicinity of the rib cage to this point, needling should always be oblique and lateral

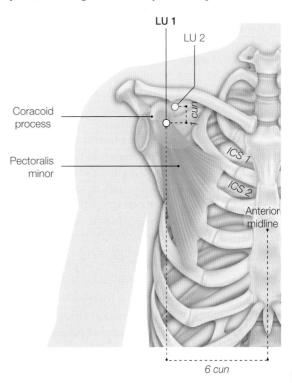

in direction, and depth dependent on the clients build and muscle bulk.

Do NOT needle in a medial direction, because this holds a considerable risk of puncturing the lung and causing pneumothorax. Always take stock of the client's build and framework.

Actions and indications

LU 1 is a *very important and extensively used point* for *many types of respiratory disorders*, particularly *coughing* and *difficulty breathing*.

Its primary functions are to *improve the flow of qi in the chest and benefit respiration by promoting the Lungs' descending and dispersing functions, thus clearing, relaxing and dissipating fullness from the chest.* It effectively *clears heat, stagnation and phlegm from the chest.* It also *releases exterior wind, cold and heat.* LU 1 *strengthens the upper jiao and tonifies Lung qi.*

The breathing rhythm and depth may change or the person may cough or sigh as a reaction to treating this point.

LU 1 is also mentioned as one of the *Eight Points to Clear Heat from the Chest*, alongside ST 12, BL 11 and BL 12.

Main indications of LU 1 include: shortness of breath, chronic weak breathing, dyspnoea, most types of coughing and wheezing (particularly if symptoms are worse when lying down), asthma, bronchitis, pneumonia, and fullness, oppression or pain of the chest, fever and aversion to cold. It has also been extensively employed to treat difficulty swallowing, and pain and swelling of the throat, neck or axilla, in such cases as tonsillitis, laryngitis, pharyngitis, lymphadenopathy and goitre. Furthermore, it has been used for nausea, retching and vomiting (particularly in relation to coughing), gastric flu, haemoptysis, swelling of the face, rhinitis, and nasal obstruction.

LU 1 has also been employed in a variety of other cases, including: respiratory and skin allergies, painful or itchy skin rashes, excessive perspiration, intercostal neuralgia, palpitations, chronic

exhaustion, abdominal distension, hypochondrial pain, and disorders of the gallbladder.

As a *local point*, it is effective in the treatment of *channel disorders*, including: pain of the shoulder, difficulty in abducting and extending the arm, frozen shoulder, pain of the upper arm and upper back, periarthritis of the shoulder, and spasm or shortening of the pectoralis major and minor and the coracobrachialis muscles. It is worth considering in tennis elbow as well as pain in the forearm and carpal tunnel due to potential tension throughout the upper limb fascia.

Main Areas—Chest. Lungs. Nose. Shoulder.
Main Functions—Benefits respiration. Tonifies Lung qi. Regulates chest qi. Dispels stagnation and heat. Releases the exterior.

LU 2   Yunmen
Cloud Gate

Myotome	C5–C8
Dermatome	C4

Location
At the centre of the deltopectoral triangle. This sizeable depression is formed by the clavicle (above), the superior border of the pectoralis major (below) and the anterior border of the deltoid muscle on the lateral side.

To aid location, ask the patient to stretch the arm forwards (flex the shoulder) to emphasise the pectoralis and anterior deltoid muscles.

Needling
Similar to LU 1.

Actions and indications
LU 2 has *similar functions to LU 1*. However, it is not considered as effective for interior Lung disorders and is *preferred for channel complaints*, particularly *pain and stiffness of the shoulder*.

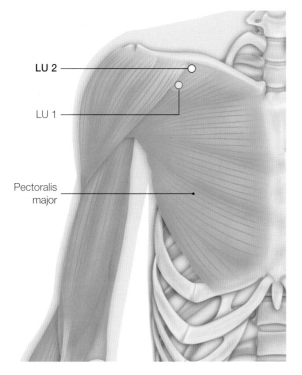

LU 2
LU 1
Pectoralis major

LU 2 is also employed to clear heat, and is mentioned as one of *Seven Points for Draining Heat from the Extremities*. The others are LI 15, BL 40 and GV 2.

> **Main Areas**—Shoulder. Arm. Chest. Lungs.
> **Main Functions**—Regulates qi. Alleviates pain.

LU 3   Tianfu
Upper Arm Assembly

Window of the Sky point

Myotome	C5/C6
Dermatome	C5

Location
Just lateral to the border of the biceps brachii muscle, 3 cun below the end of the axillary crease. Alternatively locate one third of the distance between the axillary crease and LU 5.

To aid location, flex the elbow to palpate the lateral border of the biceps. Also, LU 3 is approximately

level with LI 14, or one hand breadth distal to the axillary fold.

Needling
0.5 to 1 cun perpendicular insertion.
0.5 to 2 cun oblique or transverse insertion, distally along the channel pathway.

Actions and indications
LU 3 is well known for its effect on clearing heat from the Lungs, cooling the Blood and helping the Lungs' descending and dispersing functions. It is also traditionally employed for disorders of the Po (Corporeal Soul). In musculoskeletal medicine it is very useful for shoulder and elbow dysfunctions.

Indications include: nosebleed, cough, asthma, haemoptysis, lymphadenopathy, insomnia, tiredness and a propensity to sadness and grief. Locally, problems involving shoulder forward flexion and abduction may benefit from adding this point into a treatment.

> **Main Areas**—Lungs. Po. Upper arm.
> **Main Functions**—Clears heat. Benefits the Lungs. Calms the Po.

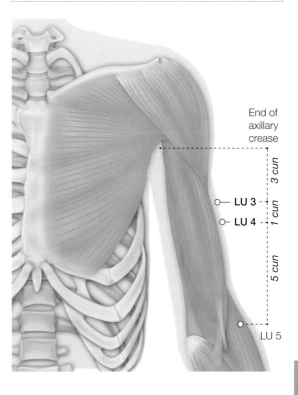

End of axillary crease
3 cun
LU 3
1 cun
LU 4
5 cun
LU 5

LU 4   Xiabai

侠白

Supporting the Lung

Myotome	C5/C6
Dermatome	C5

Location

1 cun distal to LU 3, just lateral to the border of the biceps brachii muscle.

Actions and indications

LU 4 has similar functions to LU 3 in so far as it helps the Lungs' functions. It is also traditionally indicated for disorders of the heart with symptoms such as palpitations, chest pain and shortness of breath as well as other digestive symptoms of anxiety such as belching and feelings of tightness in the chest.

> **Main Areas**—Lungs. Heart. Chest. Arm.
> **Main Functions**—Regulates qi and Blood. Benefits the chest.

LU 5   Chize

尺澤

Cubit Marsh

He-Sea point, Water point

Myotome	C5/C6
Dermatome	C5/C6

Location

On the cubital crease, in the depression on the radial side of the tendon of the biceps brachii and medial to the brachioradialis muscle.

Note: Japanese practitioners use a different location which may be easier and clinically is as effective. The LU 5 (Japan) is situated halfway between the biceps tendon and LI 11. This puts it into a lateral groove by brachioradialis and anatomically gives it greater effect for elbow disorders. Used with LI 11, as a pair, this point helps provide a strong

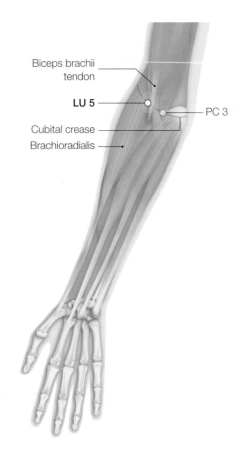

Biceps brachii tendon
LU 5
Cubital crease
Brachioradialis
PC 3

segmental input into C5/6. This can be useful as a distal set of points for shoulder and neck issues.

Needling

0.3 to 1 cun perpendicular insertion, between the tendon of the biceps brachii muscle and the brachioradialis muscle.
Oblique lateral insertion towards LI 11, or vice versa.

Be aware of the cubital fossa anatomy. Avoid deep needling.

For LU 5 (Japan), needling is perpendicular.

Actions and indications

LU 5 *is a major point, used for many disorders of the Lungs*. Its primary functions are to *resolve chronic or acute Lung phlegm conditions, clear heat, nourish yin and moisten the Lungs*. It is particularly indicated for *Lung phlegm heat*. LU 5 can also be employed to *dissipate cold and tonify Lung qi*.

Indications include: acute or chronic productive cough with expectoration of thick, yellow, turbid, brown, dark, green, or bloodstained sputum, chronic dry cough with expectoration of small quantities of dry, sticky, dark or bloodstained sputum, chronic weak cough, profuse white or colourless sputum, gurgling sound in the chest, shortness of breath, dyspnoea, asthma, bronchitis, pneumonia, fullness and heaviness of the chest, thoracic pain, painful or swollen throat, dry throat, tonsillitis, epistaxis, and fever.

LU 5 has also been employed to *open the water passages* and treat cases such as frequent urination, enuresis, urinary retention, oedema, diarrhoea, and swelling of the four limbs.

It has been used to treat a variety of other disorders, including: nausea, vomiting, diarrhoea, abdominal distension, hypochondrial pain, epilepsy, and lower backache.

As a *local point*, LU 5 is important to relax the sinews and alleviate pain at the lateral and anterior aspect of the elbow and arm. Indications include: pain and stiffness of the elbow and arm, lateral epicondylitis, tendinitis, and frozen shoulder.

> **Main Areas**—Lungs. Chest. Upper jiao. Elbow.
> **Main Functions**—Dispels phlegm. Alleviates cough. Clears the Lungs. Opens the water passages.

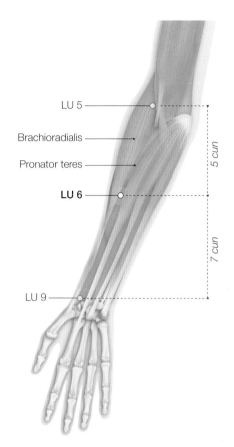

LU 6   Kongzui   孔最
Collection Hole

Xi-Cleft point

Myotome	C5–C8
Dermatome	C6

Location
On the anterior aspect of the forearm, 7 cun above LU 9, on the line joining LU 5 and LU 9. Superficially, in the brachioradialis muscle; more deeply, in the pronator teres, and deeper still, in the flexor pollicis longus.

To aid location, LU 6 is 1 cun above the midpoint of the line connecting LU 5 with LU 9.

Needling
0.3 to 1 cun perpendicular or oblique insertion (insert the needle medial to the margin of the brachioradialis muscle).
0.5 to 1.5 cun oblique insertion proximally or distally along the channel.

Actions and indications
LU 6 is mainly used for *acute, excess conditions of the Lung channel and organ*, of both *interior and exterior origin*. Indications include: *epistaxis, haemoptysis, loss of voice, fever without sweating, acute cough and sore throat, dry throat, asthma, and chest pain*.

It has also been widely employed as a diaphoretic, to treat absence of sweating in febrile diseases because it *augments the Lung function of dispersing qi and controlling the opening and closing of the pores*.

As a *local point*, LU 6 effectively treats pain and stiffness of the arm, elbow and forearm, and difficulty flexing the elbow and fingers.

> **Main Areas**—Nose. Lungs. Skin. Forearm.
> **Main Functions**—Releases the exterior. Diaphoretic. Clears heat from the upper jiao. Arrests bleeding.

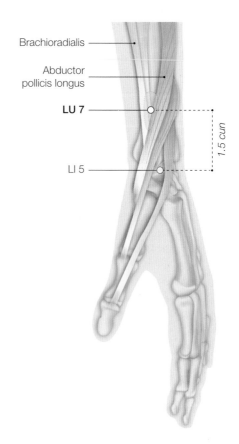

Brachioradialis

Abductor pollicis longus

LU 7

LI 5

1.5 cun

LU 7 Lieque 列 缺
Interrupted Sequence/
Thunder and Lightning

Luo-Connecting point
Opening point of the Conception Vessel
Command point of the head and neck
Heavenly Star point

Myotome	None – superficial tissue
Dermatome	C6

Location
On the most lateral aspect of the radius, at the base of the styloid process, 1.5 cun proximal to the transverse wrist crease. Situated in the narrow V-shaped crevice, between the tendons of the brachioradialis and abductor pollicis longus muscles.

To aid location, slide the tip of the index finger proximally up from LI 5, to slip into the shallow crevice on the distal end of the radius.

Needling
0.3 to 1.5 cun transverse insertion into the crevice, distally or proximally, along the channel pathway.

Traditionally, the former may be more effective to release the exterior, whereas the latter can be considered more effective on the Lungs as opposed to the wrist and thumb.

It can be helpful to lift up (pinch) the skin and subcutaneous tissue to insert the needle.

Actions and indications
LU 7 is a *very important and widely used point* because it is effective in *a large variety of exterior and interior Lung conditions*. Its main functions are to *release the exterior, promote sweating, circulate the defensive qi, stimulate the descending and dispersing of Lung qi, and open the nose*. Also, it effectively *moistens the Lungs, nourishes fluids and yin and tonifies Lung qi*.

LU 7 can release emotional states such as sadness, depression or worry in predisposed patients.

Indications include: dry, tickly, itchy or sore throat due to exterior wind; dryness, heat or yin deficiency; upper respiratory tract infections such as tonsillitis and acute or chronic pharyngitis; acute or chronic asthma and cough due to excess or deficiency, shallow breathing, chronic weak breathing, dyspnoea, and constriction or fullness of the chest. It is also beneficial in such cases as sneezing, itchy nose, nasal discharge or obstruction, rhinitis and loss of smell, and has been used to treat chills and fever in febrile diseases.

LU 7 also *opens the Conception Vessel and nourishes Fluids and Yin throughout the entire body*. It treats general symptoms of *Yin deficiency*, particularly in relation to the Lungs and Kidneys. They include: heat in the five hearts, night sweating, insomnia, malar flush, sensitive skin, scant urination, and weakened sexual or reproductive functions.

LU 7 helps *open the water passages and benefits the urinary system*.

Indications include: oedema and swelling of the face, urinary incontinence (particularly if related to coughing), dysuria, and urinary retention.

LU 7 is the *command point for the back of the head and neck* and is useful in such cases as stiffness of the neck, headache, facial pain or paralysis, and toothache.

Additionally, it has a *strong emotional effect* and can be helpful following bereavement. It helps release stuck or blocked emotional states and is especially indicated for excessive weeping, grief, depression, and melancholy.

It is commonly used in *smoking cessation* treatments and is also helpful in other types of addictions.

As a *local point*, LU 7 can be beneficial to treat pain or impaired movement of the forearm, wrist, thumb or index finger. It is essential for wrist and tendon problems such as De Quervain's tenosynovitis and osteo-arthritis of the carpal bones and CMC joint.

> **Main Areas**—Lungs. Chest. Nose. Throat. Back of the neck. Head. Face. Bladder. Forearm.
> **Main Functions**—Descends and disperses Lung qi. Releases the exterior and dispels wind. Nourishes yin and moistens fluids. Opens the Conception Vessel. Benefits the neck.

LU 8   Jingqu

Channel's Ditch

經渠

Jing-River point, Metal point

Myotome	None – superficial tissue
Dermatome	C6

Location
On the medial margin of the radius, in the depression approximately 1 cun above the transverse wrist crease, level with the high point of the radial styloid process, on the radial side of the radial artery.

Needling
0.1 to 0.3 cun perpendicular insertion.

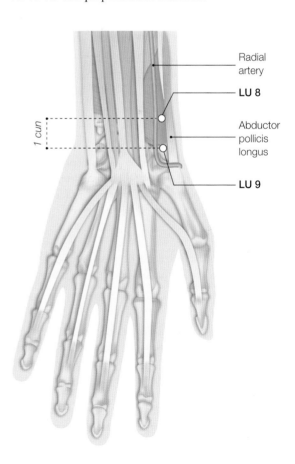

Radial artery

LU 8

Abductor pollicis longus

LU 9

1 cun

Do not puncture the radial artery. LU 8 is listed as one of the potentially dangerous points for needling and anatomical awareness must be used.

Actions and indications

LU 8 is not a very commonly used point, because its effects are not as strong as other Lung channel points. It can, however, be useful to *tonify the Lung qi* and *harmonise the Metal element.*

> **Main Areas**—Lungs. Upper jiao.
> **Main Functions**—Tonifies Lung qi. Harmonises the metal element.

LU 9   Taiyuan
Great Deep Pool

太淵

Yuan-Source point
Shu-Stream point, Earth point
Influential point for the Vessels

Myotome	None – superficial tissue
Dermatome	C6

Location

On the transverse wrist crease, in the depression on the radial (lateral) side of the radial artery. Lateral to the tendon of the flexor carpi radialis and medial to the tendon of the abductor pollicis longus.

To aid location, the sizeable depression of LU 9 is emphasised when the patient abducts the thumb.

Needling

0.2 to 0.5 cun perpendicular insertion between the radius and scaphoid bones into the wrist joint space. 0.2 to 0.5 cun insertion, angled under the abductor pollicis longus tendon towards LI 5.

Do not puncture the radial artery. LU 9 is listed as one of the potentially dangerous points for needling and anatomical awareness must be used.

Actions and indications

LU 9 is a major and *extensively used point to boost the Lung and chest qi, benefit respiration and strengthen the voice.* At the same time, it *resolves phlegm, clears heat, nourishes yin and moistens the Lungs.* It is primarily used in *chronic conditions to strengthen the Lungs and treat cough.*

Indications include: shortness of breath, weak or shallow breathing, dyspnoea, weak or hoarse voice, inability to talk, chronic weak cough, productive cough, dry cough, asthma, chronic bronchitis, emphysema, chronic sore throat, pharyngitis, chronic tiredness, exhaustion, depression, and spontaneous or night sweating.

LU 9 is also effective to *moisten the throat and improve the voice* and is of benefit to professionals such as singers and actors. Moreover, it is used in *smoking cessation* prescriptions.

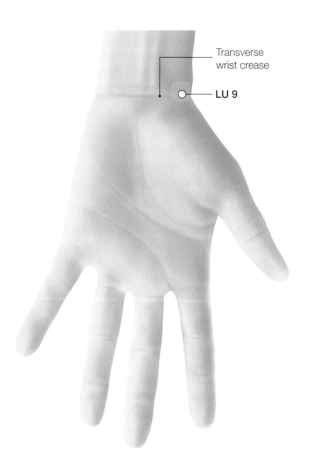

Transverse wrist crease

LU 9

LU 9 is the *influential point for the vessels and pulses* and has been extensively used for *weakness of the circulation and blood vessels*.

Indications include: sluggish circulation, cold extremities, tendency to thread veins and other vessel disorders (including varicose veins, chilblains and Raynaud's); palpitations, weak, irregular or absent pulse; and anaemia, haemoptysis, and chest pain.

As a *local point*, LU 9 can help in the treatment of chronic pain in the wrist, stiffness or inability to move the thumb and weakness of the forearm.

Additionally, LU 9 is located on the distal pulse point (inch point), which is used to determine the condition of the Lungs, Heart and upper jiao functions.

> **Main Areas**—Chest. Lungs. Blood vessels.
> **Main Functions**—Tonifies chest qi. Strengthens the breath and voice. Nourishes Lung yin. Transforms phlegm. Benefits the vessels and improves circulation.

LU 10 Yuji
Fish Border

魚際

Ying-Spring point, Fire point

Myotome	C7/C8
Dermatome	C6/C7

Location
Thenar surface, level with the midpoint of the first metacarpal bone, at the junction of the skin of the palmar and dorsal surfaces.

To aid location, use the fingertip to gently palpate for the small depression between the thenar muscles and metacarpal bone.

Needling
Usually, the best needling site is in the small space between the opponens pollicis and abductor pollicis brevis muscles.

0.3 to 0.8 cun perpendicular insertion.
Prick to bleed. Bleeding LU 10 is effective in cases of severe interior heat or exterior wind heat in the throat.

Actions and indications
LU 10 is an important point for *acute symptoms caused by excessive exterior or interior heat or phlegm-fire in the Lungs*. It is widely used to *soothe and moisten the throat*.

Indications include: acute inflammation of the throat, tonsillitis, pharyngitis, hoarse voice, bronchitis, pneumonia, fever, thirst, cough with chest pain, and thick yellow sticky, dry or bloodstained sputum. Other symptoms include epistaxis, toothache, and headache.

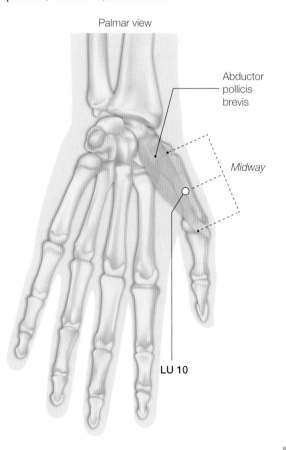

Palmar view

Abductor pollicis brevis

Midway

LU 10

LU 10 has been employed for a variety of other disorders, including: vomiting, abdominal pain and genital itching; and psycho-emotional disturbances such as anger, sadness, fright and restlessness.

> **Main Areas**—Lungs. Throat. Thumb.
> **Main Functions**—Clears exterior heat and phlegm-fire toxins. Benefits the throat.

LU 11   Shaoshang
Lesser Metal

Jing-Well point, Wood point
Second Ghost point

Myotome	None – superficial tissue
Dermatome	C6

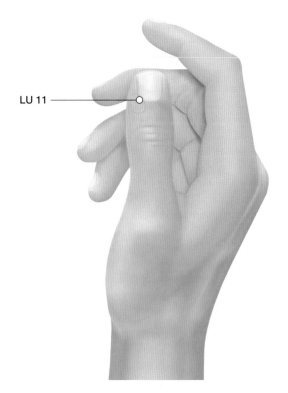

LU 11

Location
On the radial (lateral) side of the thumb, approximately 0.1 cun proximal to the corner of the nail.

To aid location, it is at the intersection of two lines following the radial border of the nail and the base of the nail.

Needling
0.1 to 0.2 cun perpendicular insertion (7 or 13mm needle).
Prick to bleed. Bleeding LU 11 with a three-edged needle is effective in cases of severe interior heat or exterior wind heat causing acute swelling and inflammation of the throat, or acute respiratory problems.

Actions and indications
LU 11 is primarily employed in cases of *inflammation of the throat due to exterior heat.*

Indications include: sore, swollen and painful throat, acute tonsillitis, laryngitis or pharyngitis, goitre, and inflammation of the eyes due to wind heat.

In *common with the other jing-well points*, LU 11 helps *pacify the Heart, calm the mind and restore consciousness* in cases of fainting or coma due to wind stroke.

It also *activates the Lung tendino-muscular meridian* and can treat pain and paralysis or spasticity of the arm following cerebrovascular accident.

> **Main Areas**—Throat. Lung channel. Mind.
> **Main Functions**—Dispels exterior heat and wind. Restores consciousness.

9

Points of the Arm Yang Ming Large Intestine Channel

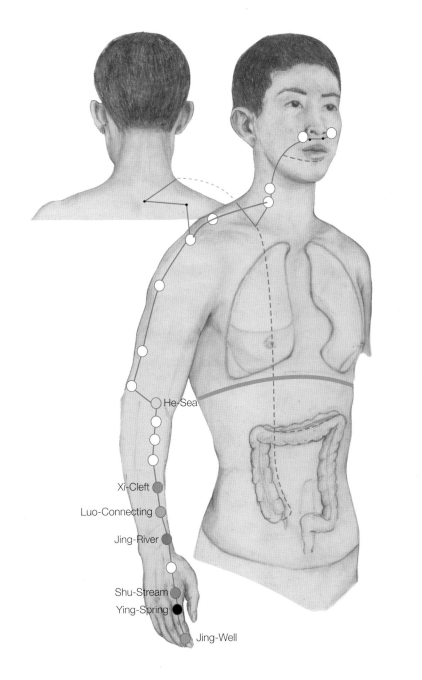

He-Sea

Xi-Cleft

Luo-Connecting

Jing-River

Shu-Stream

Ying-Spring

Jing-Well

手陽明大腸經穴

General	The Large Intestine channel starts at the radial edge of the nail of the index finger, and, crossing the anatomical snuffbox, runs along the lateral forearm to the elbow. It then continues up to the anterior shoulder, across the fibres of the trapezius and SCM into the lower cheek. Crossing the upper jaw, it finishes on the opposite side of the body from its origin, level with the lower edge of the nostril. The channel has 20 points. It is grouped with the Lung under the Metal element in five-element theory.
More specifically	The peripheral pathway is home to one of the most important and well-used points in acupuncture, Hegu LI 4. Having started at the edge of the nail of the index finger, the channel runs up through the junction between the first and second metacarpals in the first interosseous space. From here, it follows the radius up to the lateral elbow crease and then through the middle and anterior deltoid. Crossing the acromioclavicular joint, it picks up the lateral supraspinatus and the lateral edge of the trapezius, before veering slightly more anteriorly towards and crossing the SCM. The internal pathway diverts from LI 16 towards GV 14 and then connects with its paired Yin organ, the Lung. A descending pathway interacts with the Large Intestine. Continuing up into the face, it crosses the mandible and links with the Stomach channel, covering the gums. Midline, it crosses GV 26 and finishes at LI 20, level with the lower edge of the nostril on the *opposite* side of the body.
Area covered	Nose, jaw, anterior and lateral shoulder and arm, elbow and forearm, lateral wrist and carpometacarpal (CMC) joint of the thumb.
Areas affected with treatment	C3–8/T1 segmental supply. Wrist, elbow, anterior and lateral aspects of the shoulder, acromioclavicular area/supraspinatus, SCM and neck, upper jaw and nose. Through internal pathways, abdominal pain and Large Intestine function.
Key points	LI 4, LI 5, LI 10, LI 11, LI 14, LI 15, LI 16, LI 18, LI 20.

LI 1   Shangyang
Metal Yang

商陽

Needling

0.1 cun perpendicular insertion.
Prick to bleed.

Jing-Well point, Metal point

Myotome	None – superficial tissue
Dermatome	C7

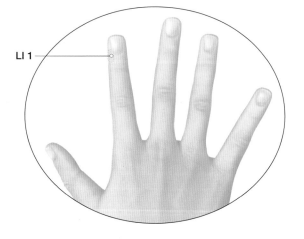

LI 1

Location

On the radial (lateral) side of the index finger, approximately 0.1 cun proximal to the corner of the nail.

To aid location, it is at the intersection of two lines following the radial border and the base of the nail.

Actions and indications

LI 1 clears both interior and exterior heat and wind and is mainly used to treat *acute pain, swelling and inflammation of the throat*. In common with the other jing-well points, LI 1 will *help restore consciousness* in cases of coma or fainting. Additionally, it opens the Large Intestine tendino-muscular meridian and *treats pain along the channel pathway*.

> **Main Areas**—Throat. Large Intestine channel. Mind.
> **Main Functions**—Restores consciousness. Benefits the throat.

LI 2   Erjian
Second Point

二間

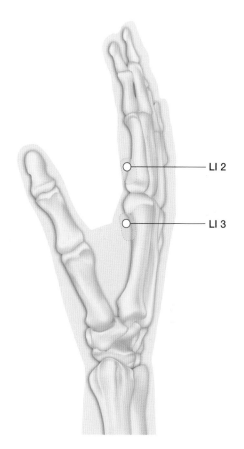

Ying-Spring point, Water point

Myotome	None – superficial tissue
Dermatome	C6

Location

On the radial side of the index finger in the depression distal to the base of second metacarpal, at the junction of the skin of the palmar and dorsal surface of the hand.

To aid location, make a loose fist.

Needling

0.2 to 0.5 cun perpendicular or oblique insertion.

Actions and indications

LI 2 is primarily indicated to *dispel wind, clear heat and reduce swelling*. Symptoms include: sore, swollen throat, inflamed eyes, facial paralysis, toothache, chills and fever and nosebleed.

As a local point it can be used to treat pain and stiffness of the index finger or second MCP joint. It has a beneficial effect on the entire channel and has been traditionally indicated for cold pain of the shoulder manifesting along the Large Intestine channel.

> **Main Areas**—Finger. MCP joint. Throat. Teeth.
> **Main Functions**—Dispels wind and clears heat. Benefits the throat. Alleviates pain and swelling.

LI 3   Sanjian
Third Point

三間

Shu-Stream point, Wood point

Myotome	C8/T1
Dermatome	C6/C7

Location

Just proximal to the radial side of the base of the index finger, in the depression between the muscle

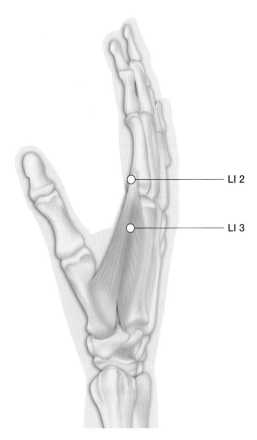

LI 2

LI 3

Main Areas—Throat. Teeth. Finger. Intestines.
Main Functions—Dispels wind and clears heat.
Benefits the face and throat. Alleviates regional
pain.

LI 4   Hegu
Junction Valley

Yuan-Source point
Command point for the face and mouth
Heavenly Star point

Myotome	C8/T1
Dermatome	C6/C7

Location
There are a number of variations of the location of
Hegu since it is a 'large point', as its Chinese name
suggests. It is therefore recommended to palpate the
entire area for the most reactive points.

and the bone. Dorsal to the insertion of the first
dorsal interosseous muscle.

To aid location, make a loose fist.

Needling
0.3 to 1 cun perpendicular insertion.

Actions and indications
LI 3 is primarily indicated to *dispel wind, clear
heat and benefit the face and throat*. Symptoms
include: painful, inflamed and swollen throat or
eyes, toothache, chills and fever, stiffness of the
neck, and epistaxis. It *dispels fullness from the
Large Intestine* and can be used to treat such cases
as diarrhoea and abdominal distension and pain.

As a local point it can be used to treat pain and
stiffness of the index finger or second MCP joint.

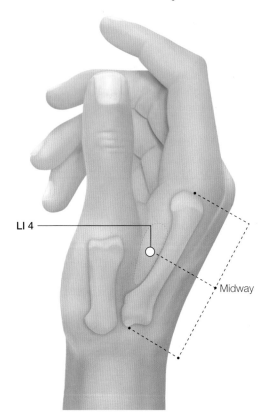

LI 4

Midway

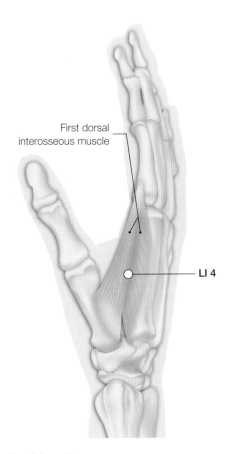

First dorsal
interosseous muscle

LI 4

Standard location

At the centre of the flesh between the first and second metacarpal bones, at the highest point of the bulge of the dorsal interosseous muscle when the thumb is adducted, level with the midpoint of the second metacarpal bone.

Beware the radial artery is situated just distal to the junction of the base of the first and second metacarpal. Do not needle towards the back of the interosseous space.

Contraindications

Contraindicated during pregnancy and heavy menstrual bleeding (can increase flow so patient awareness imperative).

LI 4 is an extremely powerful point, and strong stimulation should be avoided in patients with deficiency conditions. In certain cases even light stimulation can cause sudden sinking of the Qi. It can cause emotional outbursts, hence its familiar

name of 'The Great Eliminator'; elimination of emotional rubbish and physical rubbish in terms of its effect on large intestine activity.

Needling

0.3 to 1 cun perpendicular insertion. The needle should aim to insert into the fascia joining the two bellies of the interosseous muscle. Palpate gently while adducting the thumb to ascertain the small gap. Make sure you are at the highest point of the web. Needling too superficially may well set off a trigger point response across the back of the hand and into the little finger. Whilst this can be effective, it is not as effective as needling deeper into the true bulk of the muscle and attaining deqi sensation of a deep ache.

LI 4 is one of the most common points to cause needle shock. A vaso-vagal response can lead to a sudden drop in Blood Pressure, shaking, and even fainting. ALWAYS treat the client lying down, regardless of the condition being treated.

Actions and indications

Due to its *extremely powerful effect on the body and mind*, LI 4 is *possibly the most commonly used acupoint of the entire body and has been employed in the treatment of most diseases and symptoms. However, beware using it as a panacea for all ills. Cavalier use of this point can mask the usefulness and specificity of other points in a treatment.*

LI 4 *strongly moves stuck Qi and descends excessive Yang, thus alleviating pain and calming the mind.* Due to the powerful effect it has on moving Qi and dispelling stasis, LI 4 is known as the *analgesia point* and is often combined with LR 3 to relax the patient and *alleviate pain of any cause or location.* LI 4 and LR 3 are known as the *Four Gates*, and these points combined have an extremely strong pain-relieving effect.

They are also considered the most important body points in acupuncture anaesthesia (combined with ear points). These two points have similarly powerful Qi-moving qualities (a possible reason for this is that they share the equivalent anatomical location in the largest and strongest muscular areas of the dorsal aspects of the hand and foot).

LI 4 has been extensively used to treat various *acute and chronic pain conditions*, including: pain anywhere in the body, pain following injury, pain of the upper limbs, epigastric pain, acute pain or cramping of the abdomen, painful defecation, tightness, heaviness and pain of the chest, back or neck pain, headaches, and pain of the eyes, ears, nose and throat.

On the *psycho-emotional* level it is effective in cases of anxiety, physical or emotional stress, frequent sighing, constriction of the throat, mental restlessness or agitation, insomnia, irritability, depression, grief, mood swings, psychological shock, extremely introverted or extroverted behaviour, aphasia, palpitations and panic attacks. Furthermore, it is helpful in the *treatment of substance abuse*, bulimia, smoking and addiction-related disorders (see also LR 3) and can help boost the metabolism and detoxify the body in weight loss or other health programmes.

LI 4 strongly *descends Qi and rising Yang, sedates interior wind and treats symptoms of wind stroke*. Indications include: convulsions, loss of consciousness, fainting, dizziness, epilepsy, numbness of the limbs and body, transient ischaemic attack, paralysis or spasticity of the arm following cerebrovascular accident, hemiplegia, and hypertension.

It is a *very important point to dispel exterior wind, cold and heat, induce sweating and regulate the defensive Qi* (wei Qi). It *clears interior heat and Yang Ming heat, transforms phlegm, clears the Lungs, descends rebellious Qi and stops coughing*. It is extensively employed to treat *febrile diseases* and most *exterior and interior Lung disorders*. Indications include: upper and lower respiratory tract infections, fever, aversion to cold, tidal fever, excessive or absent sweating, sneezing, nasal obstruction, runny nose, pain of the nose, sore, swollen or itchy throat, tonsillitis, pharyngitis, coughing, dyspnoea, shortness of breath, asthmatic wheeze, and tightness, pain, heaviness and fullness of the chest.

Additionally, LI 4 helps in cases of *allergies and skin disorders due to wind, heat or toxin accumulation*. Indications include: itchy or red skin rash, acne, boils, eczema, urticaria, nettle rash, insect stings, hay fever, and allergic asthma. Needling LI 4 may also be employed as a medical adjunct in cases of serious allergies or anaphylaxis.

LI 4 is probably the most powerful distal point to treat *disorders of the face, mouth and sense organs*.

Indications include: facial paralysis, facial pain, trigeminal neuralgia, stiffness and pain of the jaw, tinnitus, inflammation of the ears, painful or bleeding gums, mouth abscesses, toothache, swelling of the face, throat or submandibular area, lymphadenopathy, goitre, itchy, painful, red, swollen and inflamed eyes, conjunctivitis, excessive lacrimation, frontal headache, migraine, pain of the whole head, redness of the face, acne, pain or swelling of the nose, epistaxis, allergic rhinitis, and sinusitis.

LI 4 is the yuan-source point of the Large Intestine channel and can be employed to *benefit the intestine* and treat constipation, acute or chronic diarrhoea, gastroenteritis, prolapse of the large intestine and haemorrhoids.

LI 4 is also very important in the treatment of *gynaecological disorders* because it *descends Qi and clears the lower jiao*, thus inducing menstruation, abortion or labour. Indications include: dysmenorrhoea, amenorrhoea, delayed or irregular menstruation, premenstrual syndrome, delayed or prolonged labour, inadequate cervical dilation, and difficulty in expulsion of the placenta.

Furthermore, it is very important in the treatment of *channel disorders* to alleviate pain and treat atrophy or paralysis. Indications include: pain and stiffness along the course of the channel, particularly of the forearm, elbow and shoulder, tendinitis, frozen shoulder, and cramp or spasm, spasticity, atrophy and paralysis of the arms. Also indicated for OA of the CMC joint.

Main Areas—Face. Sense organs. Mouth. Teeth. Eyes. Nose. Chest. Throat. Mind. Lungs. Abdomen. Intestine. Hand.
Main Functions—Moves stuck Qi and dissipates fullness. Relieves pain (analgesic). Descends Yang. Clears heat. Releases the exterior. Alleviates cough.

LI 5   Yangxi
Yang Stream

陽谿

Jing-River point, Fire point

Myotome	None – superficial tissue
Dermatome	C6

Location
On the lateral aspect of the wrist, at the centre of the sizeable depression of the anatomical snuffbox formed by the tendons of the extensor pollicis longus and brevis muscles, between the scaphoid and the radius.

To aid location, extend the thumb to define the anatomical snuffbox.

Needling
0.3 to 1 cun perpendicular insertion, directed into the wrist joint space between the scaphoid and the radius, or oblique needling into the surface tissue – either distally or proximally.

Actions and indications
LI 5 is a very *important point for disorders of the wrist* and thumb, including: pain, swelling, stiffness and inflammation, soft tissue injuries, fracture, arthritis, and tendinitis.

Although it is rarely used for interior complaints, it has traditionally been employed to *clear Yang Ming heat and calm the mind.*

> **Main Areas**—Wrist. Hand. Thumb.
> **Main Function**—Alleviates pain and swelling.

LI 6   Pianli
Diverging Passage

偏歷

Luo-Connecting point

Myotome	None – superficial tissue
Dermatome	C6

Location
On the most lateral (radial) aspect of the forearm, in the shallow depression 3 cun proximal to LI 5, one quarter of the way along the line connecting LI 5 with LI 11.

To aid location, a visible depression appears at LI 6 when the forearm is pronated and the wrist extended.

Needling
0.3 to 0.5 cun perpendicular insertion.
0.5 to 1.5 cun oblique insertion upward or downward along the channel pathway.

Actions and indications
Although it is a luo-connecting point, LI 6 is rarely used for interior complaints. It is *mainly employed*

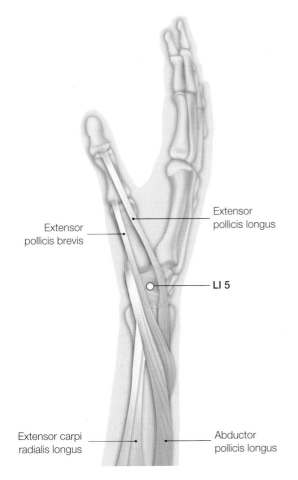

Extensor pollicis longus

Extensor pollicis brevis

LI 5

Extensor carpi radialis longus

Abductor pollicis longus

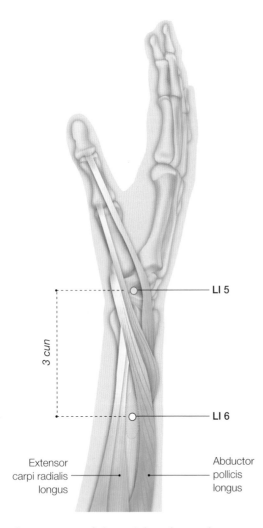

LI 5

3 cun

LI 6

Extensor carpi radialis longus

Abductor pollicis longus

LI 7   Wenliu
Warm Flow

Xi-Cleft point

Myotome	C6/C7
Dermatome	C4

Location
On the most lateral (radial) aspect of the forearm, in the shallow depression 5 cun proximal to LI 5 (2 cun proximal to LI 6), on the line connecting LI 5 with LI 11, over extensor carpi radialis longus.

Needling
0.3 to 1 cun perpendicular insertion.
0.5 to 1.5 cun oblique insertion proximally or distally.

Actions and indications
LI 7 is primarily used in *excess conditions to alleviate pain*, particularly acute pain of the arm. It also *expels exterior pathogenic factors* causing symptoms such as sore, swollen throat, ulceration of the mouth, epistaxis, headache and paralysis, or pain of the face. It *clears Yang Ming heat and calms the mind*, but is rarely used for these purposes.

> **Main Areas**—Forearm.
> **Main Function**—Alleviates pain.

in the treatment of channel disorders and pain of the forearm, although even for this, it is not as commonly used as other points.

It has, however, been *traditionally employed to treat a variety of disorders*, including: sneezing, runny nose, nasal congestion, epistaxis, sore throat, inflammation of the eyes, facial paralysis, deafness, tinnitus, earache, toothache, oedema, swelling of the face and upper body, urine retention, and even madness.

> **Main Areas**—Forearm. Wrist.
> **Main Function**—Alleviates pain.

LI 8   Xialian
Lower Point at the Border

Myotome	C5–C7
Dermatome	C5/C6

Location
On the most lateral (radial) aspect of the forearm, in a depression 4 cun distal to LI 11, one third of the distance along the line connecting LI 11 with LI 5.

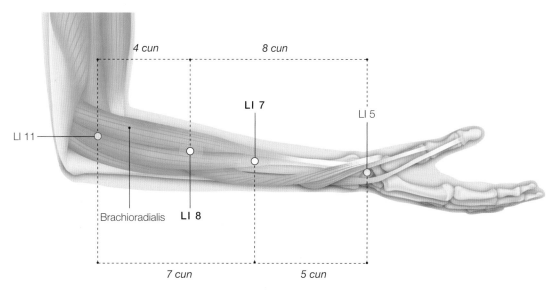

Situated, in a depression between the lateral border of the brachioradialis and the extensor carpi radialis longus.

Needling
0.5 to 1 cun perpendicular insertion.

Actions and indications
LI 8 and LI 9 could be considered as *corresponding to ST 39 and ST 37* which are the lower he-sea points for the *Small Intestine* and *Large Intestine*. Therefore, LI 8 is particularly indicated for disorders of the small intestine. In common with other adjacent points, LI 8 dissipates wind and clears heat, and is also traditionally recommended for Yang Ming heat.

Symptoms include abdominal fullness and pain, weakness of the small intestine, diarrhoea and undigested food in the stool, headache, dizziness, inflammation of the eyes and hemiplegia.

In the modern day practice however, LI 8 is mostly used in channel disorders including weakness, atrophy and regional pain. It is especially indicated for extensor tendinitis, used in combination with other regional points, notably LI 11.

Main Areas—Forearm. Elbow. Intestines.
Main Functions—Regulates Qi and Blood and alleviates pain. Clears heat and dissipates wind. Harmonises the Yang Ming.

LI 9   Shanglian   上 廉
Upper Point at the Border

Myotome	C5–C7
Dermatome	C5/C6

Location
In the depression 3 cun distal to LI 11 on the line joining LI 11 and LI 5. See location note for LI 10.

Needling
0.5 to 1 cun perpendicular insertion.

Actions and indications
LI 9 *corresponds to ST 37*, which is the lower he-sea point for the *Large Intestine* (see also LI 8). Both LI 8 and LI 9 are traditionally indicated for disorders of the intestines. LI 9 has been used for symptoms including abdominal bloating and pain, heat in the intestines and lower jiao and dark urination.

Symptoms include abdominal fullness and pain, weakness of the small intestine, diarrhoea and undigested food in the stool, headache, dizziness, inflammation of the eyes and hemiplegia. However, LI 9 is mostly used in channel disorders and regional pain, and is especially indicated for

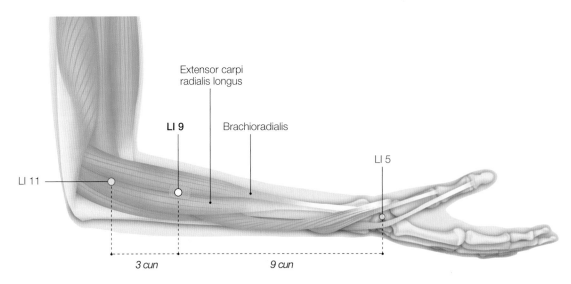

extensor tendinitis, alongside other regional points, notably LI 11.

> **Main Areas**—Forearm. elbow. Intestines.
> **Main Functions**—Regulates Qi and blood and alleviates pain. Clears heat and dissipates wind. Harmonises the Yang Ming.

LI 10   Shousanli
Arm Three Miles

Myotome	C5–C7
Dermatome	C5

Location

In the depression 2 cun distal to LI 11 on the line joining LI 11 and LI 5.

Situated, lateral to the border of the brachioradialis muscle, in the extensor carpi radialis longus, and, more deeply, in the extensor carpi radialis brevis. In its deep position lies the supinator muscle.

To aid location, define the lateral border of the brachioradialis by asking the patient to flex the elbow against resistance given to the lower part of the forearm, which should be in a semi-supine position.

Needling

0.5 to 1.5 cun perpendicular insertion into the extensor carpi radialis longus and brevis muscles, and, more deeply, the supinator muscle.

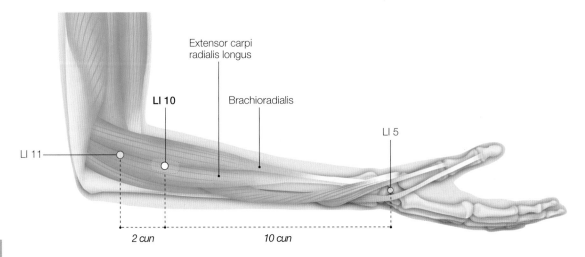

Actions and indications

LI 10 is an *important point to treat pain, stiffness, weakness, motor impairment, atrophy or paralysis of the upper limb* and shoulder.

LI 10, called *Arm Three Miles*, is the corresponding upper limb point to ST 36, or *Leg Three Miles*, and has similar functions, such as *tonifying Qi and Blood and harmonising the Yang Ming*, albeit not as powerfully. Arm and Leg Three Miles are commonly combined in order to *strengthen the four limbs*.

> **Main Areas**—Forearm and elbow. Entire upper limb. Shoulder. Stomach. Intestines.
> **Main Functions**—Strengthens the upper limbs. Alleviates pain. Harmonises the Yang Ming.

LI 11　Quchi
Pond at the Bend

曲池

He-Sea point, Earth point
Heavenly Star point
Twelfth Ghost point

Myotome	C6/C7
Dermatome	C5

Location

At the lateral end of the transverse cubital crease when the elbow is flexed. Approximately midway between LU 5 and the lateral epicondyle of the humerus.

Needling

0.5 to 1.5 cun perpendicular insertion (elbow flexed).

Actions and indications

LI 11 is one of the *most important and powerful points* and has been used to treat a wide range of cases ranging from minor complaints to life-threatening conditions. Its main functions are to *dispel wind and release the exterior, clear heat, transform dampness and damp heat, harmonise the Yang Ming, descend excessive Yang, sedate interior wind* and *dispel stasis via regulating Qi and Blood*. It is important *cool the Blood* and is especially indicated for *skin diseases* and to *alleviate itching*.

Indications include: low or high fever with or without chills and sweating, aching body, headache, inflamed or itchy eyes, nasal obstruction, pain and swelling of the throat, earache, toothache, goitre, phlegm nodules, lymphadenopathy, cough, asthma, dyspnoea, expectoration of yellow sticky phlegm, fullness and heaviness of the chest, upper respiratory tract infections or allergies, abdominal distension and pain, nausea, vomiting, hypochondrial pain and distension, jaundice, hepatitis, liver diseases, diarrhoea, dysentery, gastroenteritis, urinary tract infections, cystitis, dry skin, itchy red skin rash, itching in general, acute or chronic skin diseases, acne, eczema, urticaria, systemic or local inflammatory or allergic conditions, systemic

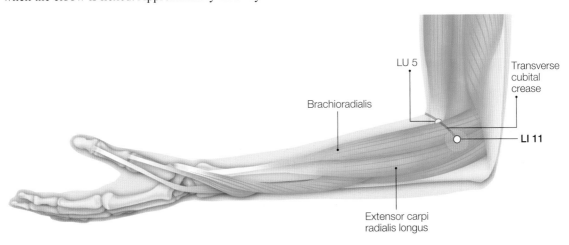

LU 5

Transverse cubital crease

Brachioradialis

LI 11

Extensor carpi radialis longus

swelling or oedema, hypertension, wind stroke, facial paralysis, hemiplegia, and dizziness.

Psychologically, LI 11 helps in cases of depression, mental restlessness and irritability.

LI 11 also *powerfully activates the channel, dispels stasis and alleviates pain* and is one of the most important points for *disorders of the elbow and forearm*.

Indications include: impaired movement and weakness or atrophy of the elbow, arm and forearm, lateral epicondylitis, stiffness of the elbow, pain and stiffness of the shoulder.

> **Main Areas**—Elbow. Forearm. Throat. Face (nose, eyes, mouth, ears). Lungs. Abdomen. Intestines.
> **Main Functions**—Clears heat and damp heat. Descends rising Yang. Regulates Qi. Dispels stasis.

LI 12　Zhouliao　肘髎
Elbow Bone Hole

Myotome	C6/C7
Dermatome	C5

Location
In the large depression just above the lateral epicondyle of the humerus, approximately 1 cun supralateral to LI 11 when the elbow is flexed at 90 degrees. Situated on the lateral aspect of the triceps brachii muscle at the origin of the anconeus muscle.

Needling
0.5 to 1 cun perpendicular insertion (elbow flexed).

Actions and indications
LI 12 is an *important local point* for disorders of the elbow, including: difficulty in flexing and extending the elbow, and pain, atrophy or paralysis of the arm.

> **Main Area**—Elbow.
> **Main Functions**—Regulates Qi and Blood. Alleviates pain.

LI 13　Shouwuli　手五里
Arm Five Miles

Myotome	C5/C6
Dermatome	C5

Location
3 cun proximal to LI 11, just lateral to the border of the biceps brachii muscle. Situated in the brachialis muscle.

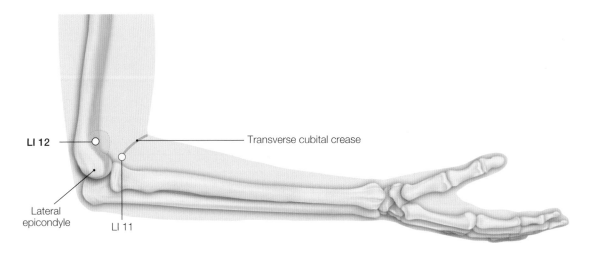

LI 12

Transverse cubital crease

Lateral epicondyle

LI 11

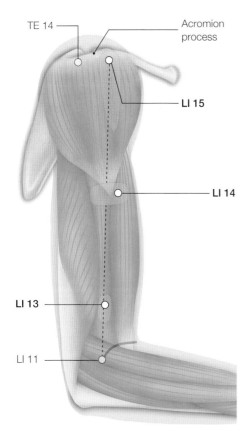

TE 14

Acromion process

LI 15

LI 14

LI 13

LI 11

To aid location, it is one hand width above LI 11. Find the point in a shallow and wide depression that is palpable with the elbow flexed (it shrinks or seems to vanish when the elbow is extended).

Needling
0.5 to 1.5 cun perpendicular insertion.

Actions and indications
LI 13 is not a commonly used point in so far as its internal functions are concerned.

It can however be very helpful as an auxiliary point for problems of the elbow and arm including pain, stiffness and contracture of the elbow and shoulder. Furthermore, it has an effect on the entire upper limb and can be used in cases of atrophy or paralysis. For these purposes it is combined with other major points of the affected area and channel, including: LI 4, LI 10, LI 11, LI 14 and LI 15.

Main Areas—Elbow. Shoulder. Arm. Chest.
Main Functions—Regulates Qi and Blood. Alleviates pain. Benefits the chest and alleviates cough.

LI 14   Binao
Upper Arm Prominence

Intersection of the Small Intestine, Bladder and Yang Wei Mai on the Large Intestine channel

Myotome	C4–C6
Dermatome	C4/C5

Location
On the lateral aspect of the humerus along the line joining LI 11 to LI 15, in the depression slightly anterior and superior to the insertion of the deltoid muscle. Locate with the arm hanging down by the side.

To aid location, ask the patient to lift (abduct) the arm against resistance to contract the deltoid muscle and define its insertion.

Needling
0.3 to 0.7 cun perpendicular insertion.
0.5 to 1.5 cun oblique upward insertion into the muscle.

Actions and indications
LI 14 is used primarily to *treat pain, stiffness, atrophy, paralysis or impaired mobility of the arm and shoulder.* It is particularly indicated for frozen shoulder and difficulty in lifting the arm.

Other symptoms it has been traditionally used for include: pain and inflammation of the eyes, lymphadenopathy in the neck and arm, goitre, and chest pain.

Main Areas—Arm. Shoulder.
Main Functions—Regulates Qi and Blood. Alleviates pain.

LI 15 Jianyu
Shoulder and Clavicle

肩髃

Intersection of the Small Intestine and Yang Qiao Mai on the Large Intestine channel

Myotome	C4–C6
Dermatome	C3

Location
On the anterolateral aspect of the shoulder, in the depression directly inferior to the acromion process, between the anterior and middle fibres of the deltoid muscle, directly anterior to TE 14.

To aid location, it is situated in the anterior of the two distinct depressions formed between the inferior border of the acromion process and the greater tubercle of the humerus. These depressions are usually visible when the patient lifts (abducts) the arm (use resistance if necessary). Define the two depressions as follows: the patient sits with the arm hanging loosely by the side as the therapist gently pulls the arm downward toward the floor, causing the humerus to be drawn away from the scapula, thus defining the two depressions of LI 15 and TE 14.

Needling
With the arm down by the side, 0.5 to 1.5 cun perpendicular insertion. The needle should enter the space between the subacromial bursa inferiorly and the acromion process superiorly.

With the arm down by the side, 0.5 to 2 cun oblique or transverse insertion distally along the channel, between the anterior and medial fibres of the deltoid.

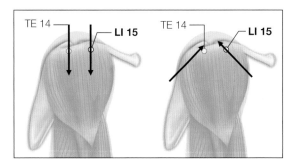

Needling direction

Actions and indications
LI 15 is very useful in *many disorders of the shoulder*. It effectively treats pain and stiffness of the shoulder, particularly if there is *difficulty in lifting (abducting)* the arm and *moving it forwards (flexion of the shoulder)*.

It is particularly indicated for supraspinatus tendinitis, frozen shoulder, periarthritis, heat in the shoulder (inflammation), and atrophy or paralysis of the upper limb.

LI 15 is also mentioned as one of *Seven Points for Draining Heat from the Extremities*, alongside LU 2, GV 2 and BL40.

Other traditional indications include: skin rashes due to exterior wind heat, goitre, toothache, and hypertension.

It is an important fascial connection point from the Bladder tendino-muscular meridian and in anatomy, the most lateral fibres of trapezius blend into this region.

> **Main Area**—Shoulder.
> **Main Functions**—Regulates Qi and Blood. Dispels stasis. Alleviates pain.

LI 16 Jugu
Large Bone (Acromion)

巨骨

Intersection of the Yang Qiao Mai on the Large Intestine channel

Myotome	Accessory nerve, C1–C6
Dermatome	C3

Location
On the superior aspect of the shoulder, at the centre of the large depression formed between the clavicle and the acromion process. Situated in the trapezius and supraspinatus muscles.

LI 16

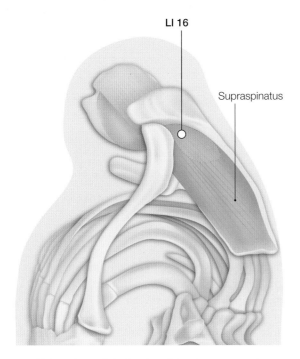

Supraspinatus

To aid location, slide the tip of the finger over the acromion. It should slide into the depression of LI 16.

Needling
0.5 to 1.5 cun perpendicular insertion, directed laterally.

Do not needle deeply in a medial direction, because the apex of the lung may be punctured.

Actions and indications
LI 16 is a powerful point to *regulate Qi and Blood, dispel stasis and alleviate pain*. It is primarily used to treat pain and impaired mobility of the shoulder and arm, especially in chronic cases. Subacromial impingement disorders and anything involving supraspinatus. It is worth checking this point in tennis elbow because the trigger point referral for the lateral end of supraspinatus can refer to the elbow.

LI 16 opens and relaxes the chest, clears phlegm from the upper jiao, and aids the Lungs functions of dispersing and descending. Indications include: pain and swelling of the neck and supraclavicular area, lymphadenopathy, goitre, thyroid disease, heaviness of the chest, dyspnoea, and cough.

LI 16 has also been traditionally employed to treat blood stasis in the chest causing coughing or vomiting blood.

Main Areas—Shoulder. Chest.
Main Functions—Regulates Qi and Blood. Dispels stasis. Alleviates pain. Opens the chest.

LI 17 Tianding
Head's Tripod

Myotome	Accessory nerve, C1–C5
Dermatome	C3

Location
On the lateral aspect of the neck, at the posterior border of the SCM muscle, 1 cun inferior to LI 18.

LI 17 is situated just inferior to the superficial cervical plexus nerve block point.

Needling
0.3 to 0.5 cun perpendicular insertion.

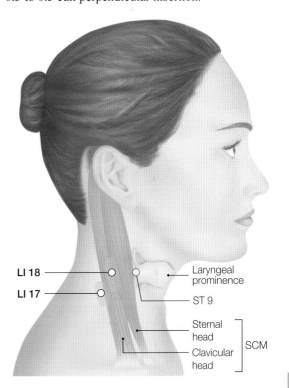

LI 18
LI 17
Laryngeal prominence
ST 9
Sternal head
Clavicular head
SCM

Actions and indications

This point is a delicate point to use, but can aid with *problems with the throat*, including coughing and wheezing. Also issues surrounding loss of voice, hoarseness and persistant cough.

Main Areas—Throat. Ear.
Main Functions—Regulates Qi and Blood. Dispels stasis. Alleviates pain. Opens the chest.

LI 18   Futu

Beside the Prominence

Window of the Sky point

Myotome	Accessory nerve, C1–C6
Dermatome	C3

Location

On the anterolateral aspect of the neck, in the depression between the two heads of the SCM muscle, directly lateral to ST 9, approximately 3 cun lateral to the tip of the laryngeal prominence (Adam's apple).

To aid location, emphasise the SCM border, by asking the patient to turn their head away from the side to be palpated (use resistance if necessary).

Needling

0.3 to 0.5 cun perpendicular insertion.

Do not needle deeply. Do not puncture the external jugular vein.

Actions and indications

LI 18 is primarily used for *disorders of the throat*, including pain, swelling and acute inflammation.

Symptoms include cough, dyspnoea, sore throat, loss of voice and difficulty swallowing caused by exterior wind, phlegm or heat accumulation from febrile or thyroid disease. LI 18 can also be used for paralysis of the throat muscles.

Main Area—Throat.
Main Function—Alleviates swelling and pain.

LI 19   Kouheliao

Mouth Grain Hole

口禾髎

Myotome	Facial nerve (buccal branch)
Dermatome	Trigeminal nerve (maxillary branch)

Location

Directly below the lateral border of the ala nasi, in a small crevice-like depression that feels rather like a grain of rice, level with GV 26.

Note that many texts describe LI 19 as being 0.5 cun lateral to the midline. However, there aren't specific cun measurements for this part of the face and the nostril is used as a guide. It is unclear whether it should be located level with the edge of the nostril or with the centre of it. To avoid confusion, the best way is to use a probe to palpate the small depression

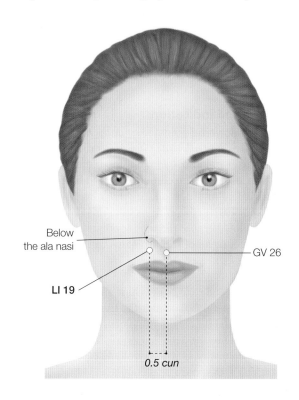

for the most reactive point, which should produce an immediate sensation in the nose or eyes such as tearing, itching or sneezing.

Needling
0.3 to 0.5 cun perpendicular insertion.

Actions and indications
In common with LI 20, LI 19 is used in regional disorders to open nose and clear wind and heat.

LI 19 is effective in cases of facial paralysis with deviation of the mouth, and can also help ease the symptoms of trigeminal neuralgia.

In addition, LI 19 can be used to clear the mind, revive consciousness and treat vertigo and dizziness.

> **Main Area**—Nose. Upper lip. Eyes. Brain.
> **Main Functions**—Opens the nose. Regulates Qi and blood. Clears the brain and dispels wind. Similar to LI 20.

LI 20   Yingxiang
Receiving Fragrance

Intersection of the Stomach on the Large Intestine channel

Myotome	Facial nerve (buccal branch)
Dermatome	Trigeminal nerve (maxillary branch)

Location
In the nasolabial sulcus, level with the midpoint of the lateral border of the ala nasi.

Needling
0.3 to 1 cun transverse insertion, directed upward and medially to join with Bitong.

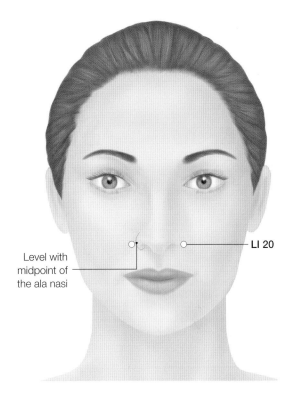

Level with midpoint of the ala nasi

LI 20

Actions and indications
LI 20 is a *major point to open the nose and benefit the breathing*. It is extensively used to treat nasal obstruction, epistaxis, loss of sense of smell and facial pain caused by chronic or acute inflammatory conditions such as rhinitis, nasal polyps and sinusitis.

LI 20 can also treat facial paralysis, acne, swelling or itching of the face, mouth abscesses, toothache, and redness and pain of the eye.

> **Main Areas**—Nose. Eyes. Cheek and mouth.
> **Main Functions**—Improves breathing and smell. Clears heat and dissipates wind. Regulates Qi.

10 Points of the Leg Yang Ming Stomach Channel

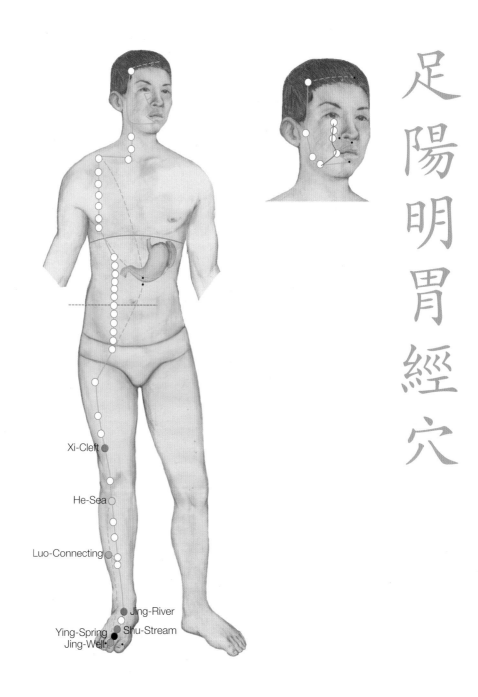

足陽明胃經穴

Xi-Cleft

He-Sea

Luo-Connecting

Jing-River

Ying-Spring
Shu-Stream
Jing-Well

General	The Stomach channel starts immediately below the eye and travels over the face in a 'U' shape, before leaving at the bottom of the jaw and descending the SCM. It crosses the clavicle and continues down the torso, over the breast, then cuts in to run down the edge of the rectus abdominis.
	At the pubis it then veers outwards to cross the hip anteriorly and travels down the anterolateral quadriceps to the patella, through the knee, tibialis anterior. Apart from a small reverse pathway mid-leg, it continues down across the ankle and into the foot, finishing on the lateral edge of the nail on the second toe.
	The channel has 45 points. It is grouped with the Spleen channel under the Earth element in five-element theory.
More specifically	As a continuum from LI 20, the channel emerges onto the face immediately below the orbit of the eye and passes downwards over the zygomatic arch. On the face it unites with the Conception Vessel (CV) channel around the mouth, although it covers primarily the lower jaw, travelling along the mandible and back upwards to cross over the TMJ and at the corner of the hairline.
	From the line on the jaw, near ST 5, the main branch descends across the SCM, into the sternal notch and supraclavicular fossa, and then, crossing the clavicle, runs in a line 4 cun from the midline, over the nipple. It then crosses to a line 2 cun from the midline all the way down the rectus abdominis to the pubic symphysis.
	At ST 12 the internal branch descends to affect the Stomach and Spleen, as well as connecting with a key front-mu point of CV 12. From the pelvis at ST 30, the channel veers laterally over the anterior hip joint and down the lateral quadriceps to the latero-superior border of the patella.
	The point ST 35 is one of the 'eyes' of the knee, and the next point, ST 36, within the tibialis anterior is one of the most widely used acupuncture points for well-being/immune function/stomach disorders and for back pain with or without leg involvement.
	Mid-leg, the channel reverses on itself at ST 39, with another two key points, ST 38 and ST 40, being in line, mid-leg. It continues from here downwards across the ankle, anteriorly, and ends on the lateral edge of the nail of the second toe.
	There are other connections reported with channels such as the tendino-muscular channel of the Stomach, and the Luo and Divergent channels, which show a strong connection of Stomach points on the lower limb continuing to affect the throat and face.
Area covered	All aspects of the trigeminal and facial nerves on the face, jaw, anterior chest and breast, abdomen, pelvis, anterior hip, thigh, knee, ankle and foot.

Areas affected with treatment	Trigeminal nerve on the face. Neurologically, as its path traverses down the body it has points within the nerve supplies of the accessory nerve and C2/3 in the neck, all thoracic nerves (posterior primary rami) and L2–5, S1 in the lower limb. Neck/SCM, anterior chest and abdomen. Stomach and Spleen function. Hip, thigh, knee, ankle and foot. Emotionally there is a Chinese phrase that 'the stomach manifests all the emotions', as many emotional states can lead to symptoms of tightening, 'butterflies', nausea etc. – all of which are witnessed initially in the Stomach.
Key points	ST 3, ST 6, ST 7, ST 8, ST 17 (forbidden point), ST 25, ST 30, ST 31, ST 35, ST 36, ST 38, ST 40, ST 44.

ST 1 Chengqi

Tear Container

Intersection of the Yang Qiao Mai and Conception Vessel on the Stomach channel

Myotome	Facial nerve
Dermatome	Trigeminal nerve

Location

Between the eyeball and the midpoint of the infraorbital ridge, level with the centre of the pupil when the eye is focused straight ahead. Situated in the orbicularis oculi muscle and, in its deep position, the inferior oblique and inferior rectus muscles.

Needling

0.3 to 1 cun perpendicular insertion, angled between the eyeball and the infraorbital ridge.

Support the eyeball with the tip of the finger and insert the needle slowly and carefully while the patient looks upward. Angle the needle slightly downward and then perpendicularly along the inferior orbital wall under the eyeball.

0.3 to 0.5 cun transverse insertion along the orbital ridge, towards the inner or outer canthus.

Use the thinnest needle possible.

Do not manipulate the needle. The patient should keep the eyes as relaxed and still as possible during needle retention and avoid unnecessary blinking. It is best that the eyes remain closed for the duration of the treatment, until after the needle is removed, to avoid the skin being pulled. After removing the needle, apply pressure with a cotton pad for up to one minute.

Needling ST 1 is potentially dangerous and requires special skill and experience. Great care should be taken, as wrongly angled insertion will damage the eye.

ST 1 can bruise easily. If any slight swelling is observed remove the needle immediately and apply pressure and a cold compress. If bruising occurs, apply a cold compress for 2–5 minutes. The bruising should disappear within a week and will not affect the eyesight.

Actions and indications

ST 1 is an important point, used in a *wide variety of eye disorders*. It *clears and brightens the eyes, dispels wind, clears heat and soothes inflammatory reactions* of the eye. Indications include: tired eyes, pain, swelling or redness of the eyes, excessive tearing, itching or dryness of the eyes, migraine, allergies, keratitis, strabismus, deviation of the eye, and spasm or paralysis of the under-eye muscles.

It is also effectively employed to help *improve vision* in a variety of disorders, including: myopia, astigmatism, hypermetropia, retinitis, optic neuritis, glaucoma, night blindness, colour blindness, and cataracts.

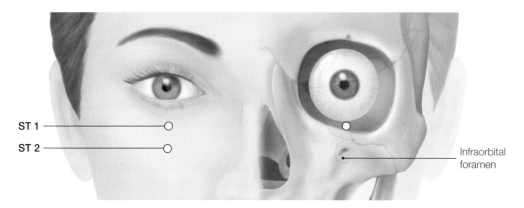

ST 1 is an *important beauty point to improve the appearance of the area under the eyes.* It treats dark circles, bags, puffiness and swelling.

> **Main Areas**—Eyes and area below.
> **Main Functions**—Benefits the eyes and area below. Improves vision. Dispels wind and clears heat. Improves appearance.

ST 2   Sibai
Four Direction Brightness

Myotome	Facial nerve
Dermatome	Trigeminal nerve

Location
In the depression of the infraorbital foramen, in line with ST 1 and ST 3.

To aid location, it is approximately 0.3 cun below ST 1.

Needling
0.1 to 0.3 cun perpendicular insertion into the infraorbital foramen.
0.3 to 0.5 cun transverse insertion upward and outwards.
0.3 cun transverse insertion upward towards ST 1.

0.5 to 1 cun transverse insertion outwards, angled toward SI 18 or other areas of the cheek.
Transverse insertion downward towards ST 3, Bitong, LI 20 or other areas of the cheek.

Actions and indications
ST 2 is an *important point for many eye disorders* and has a general *brightening effect on the eyes. It dissipates wind, clears heat, stops excessive lacrimation and helps to improve the vision.*

Additionally, it *regulates the Qi and Blood circulation,* helping to *alleviate pain of the front of the face, cheeks and eyes.* In comparison to ST 1, ST 2 is less effective for conditions of the eye but more effective for pain, paralysis or spasm of the under-eye and cheek muscles. Also, it is easier to treat than ST 1 and therefore more commonly used.

Indications include: spasm or paralysis of the muscles under the eye, deviation of the eye or cheek, excessive lacrimation due to wind, any acute or chronic inflammatory eye condition, pain, swelling or redness of the eyes, rhinitis, sinusitis, facial pain or paralysis, and trigeminal neuralgia and migraine.

ST 2 is also an *important beauty point for the under-eye area* as it treats puffiness, swelling, bags and dark circles.

> **Main Areas**—Eye. Area below eye. Cheek. Nose.
> **Main Functions**—Dispels wind and clears heat. Stops excessive lacrimation. Improves appearance.

ST 3　　Juliao
Large Bone Hole

Intersection of the Yang Qiao Mai and Large Intestine on the Stomach channel

Myotome	Facial nerve (buccal branch)
Dermatome	Trigeminal nerve

Location

In a palpable depression below the zygomatic arch, directly below ST 1 and ST 2, approximately level with the lower border of the ala nasi. Situated in the zygomatic minor muscle and, more deeply, the levator anguli oris.

To aid location, slide the tip of the finger laterally from the lower border of the ala nasi. It should naturally stop at the depression of ST 3. Alternatively, or additionally, slide the tip of the finger down from ST 1 and ST 2 over the zygomatic arch so that it 'falls' into ST 3.

Needling

0.2 to 0.5 cun perpendicular insertion.
Oblique insertion in various directions, e.g. towards ST 2, ST 4 or LI 20.

Actions and indications

ST 3 is a *primary point for the treatment of nasal obstruction*, sinusitis and pain of the cheek, as it *dispels wind and cold from the face, relieves swelling, promotes Qi and Blood circulation, and alleviates pain*. It also *effectively clears heat and benefits the eyes*.

Indications include: sinusitis, nasal obstruction, epistaxis, allergic rhinitis, allergic swelling of the lips and cheek, frontal headache, toothache, disorders of the upper gums and teeth, facial paralysis, facial pain, trigeminal neuralgia, deviation of the mouth or eye, spasm of the cheek, twitching of the eyelids, excessive lacrimation, inflamed or swollen eyes, conjunctivitis, keratitis, and deteriorating vision.

> **Main Areas**—Cheeks and centre of the face.
> Nose. Sinuses. Eyes. Gums and teeth.
> **Main Functions**—Dispels wind and clears heat.
> Opens the nose. Alleviates pain.

ST 4　　Dicang
Earth Granary

Intersection of the Large Intestine, Yang Qiao Mai and Conception Vessel on the Stomach channel

Myotome	Facial nerve (buccal branch)
Dermatome	Trigeminal nerve

Location

Directly below ST 3, approximately 0.4 cun lateral to the corner of the mouth, at the bottom of the nasolabial sulcus. Situated in the risorius, zygomatic major and, more deeply, the buccinator muscle.

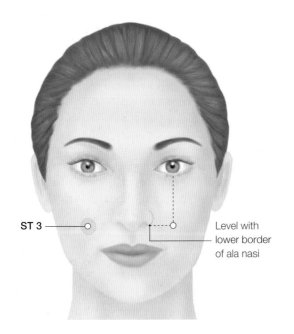

ST 3 —○　　　○····· Level with lower border of ala nasi

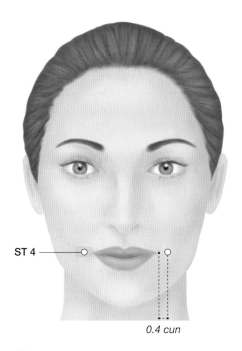

ST 4

0.4 cun

Self-acupressure can be applied regularly throughout the day or when food cravings are experienced.

> **Main Areas**—Mouth. Lips. Front of cheek.
> **Main Function**—Depresses appetite.

ST 5   Daying
Large Receptacle
(Facial Artery)

Myotome	Trigeminal nerve (mandibular branch)
Dermatome	Trigeminal nerve

Needling
0.5 to 2 cun transverse insertion outwards towards ST 5 or ST 6.
0.5 to 1.5 cun transverse insertion upward towards ST 3 or LI 20.
0.2 to 0.3 cun perpendicular insertion into the risorius (also the zygomatic major) and buccinator muscles.

This point can bruise easily. If any slight swelling is observed, remove the needle immediately and apply pressure and a cold compress.

Actions and indications
ST 4 is mainly used to treat *disorders of the mouth and cheek by dissipating wind and cold, relaxing the channels and promoting circulation of Qi and Blood.* Indications include: facial paralysis and pain, trigeminal neuralgia, spasm or tic of the cheek or lips, spasm of the under-eye muscles, excessive salivation, drooling, angular cheilitis, aphasia, inability to eat, bulimia, and excessive hunger.

ST 4 is also commonly employed as a beauty point to release tension of the risorius muscle and to 'lift' the corners of the mouth.

Treatment at ST 4 is also effective to suppress the appetite during weight loss programs.

Location
On the body of the mandible, in the groove-like depression anterior to the border of the masseter muscle.

To aid location, bulge the cheeks out (as if blowing into a wind instrument) or clench the jaw tightly to define the anterior border of the masseter muscle.

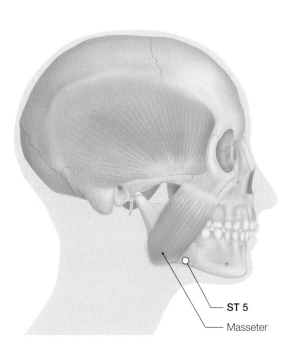

ST 5

Masseter

Needling

0.3 to 0.5 cun perpendicular insertion.
0.3 to 1.3 cun transverse insertion toward ST 6.
0.5 to 1.5 cun transverse insertion toward CV 24
or ST 4.

Actions and indications

ST 5 is primarily employed to *clear the channel, circulate Qi and Blood, and alleviate pain.*

Indications include: pain or swelling of the lower teeth or jaw, caries, periodontitis or other inflammatory conditions of teeth and gums, receding gums, deviation of the mouth, swelling of the cheek, inflammation of the parotid gland, facial paralysis and pain, and clenched jaw.

ST 5 is not as commonly used as ST 6 for jaw problems, because the latter is usually more dynamic.

> **Main Areas**—Cheek. Gums. Jaw. Teeth.
> **Main Functions**—Regulates Qi and Blood.
> Dispels stasis. Alleviates pain.

ST 6   Jiache

Jaw Bone

頰車

Seventh Ghost point

Myotome	Trigeminal nerve (mandibular branch)
Dermatome	Trigeminal nerve

Location

In the depression at the prominence of the masseter muscle, about one finger-width anterosuperior to the tip of the angle of the mandible.

To aid location, clench the jaw (bite) to define the masseter muscle.

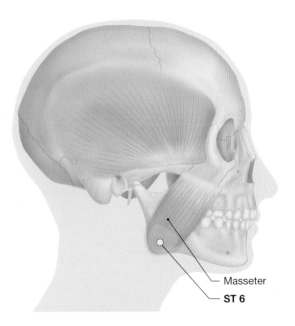

Masseter

ST 6

Needling

0.3 to 0.5 cun perpendicular insertion.
0.5 to 2 cun transverse insertion towards ST 4.
Upward transverse insertion into the masseter.

Actions and indications

ST 6 is *very powerful and commonly used in the treatment of disorders of the jaw and TMJ.* Its primary functions are to *clear the channel, remove obstructions, relax the sinews and alleviate pain.*

Indications include: tightness and pain of the jaw, TMJ syndrome, clenching or grinding of the teeth, tension headache, migraine, toothache, swelling of the cheeks, parotitis, swelling and inflammation of the gums, deviation of the mouth, facial paralysis and pain, and trigeminal neuralgia.

ST 6 can also be used to *calm the mind and relax the head and neck* in cases of mental restlessness causing symptoms such as stress, tension headaches, stiffness and pain of the neck, and insomnia. It has also been traditionally employed to treat excessive salivation.

> **Main Areas**—Jaw. TMJ. Teeth. Cheek.
> Head. Mind.
> **Main Functions**—Benefits the jaw. Dispels stasis.
> Alleviates pain. Calms the mind.

ST 7 Xiaguan 下關
Below the Arch

Intersection of the Gallbladder on the Stomach channel

Myotome	Trigeminal nerve (mandibular branch)
Dermatome	Trigeminal nerve

Location
In the depression of the mandibular notch, anterior to the condyloid process of the mandible, just inferior to the zygomatic arch. Situated in the lateral pterygoid muscle.

To aid location, place a finger on the condyloid process of the mandible with the patient's mouth open. When the mouth is closed, the finger will fall into ST 7. Also, it is directly below GB 3.

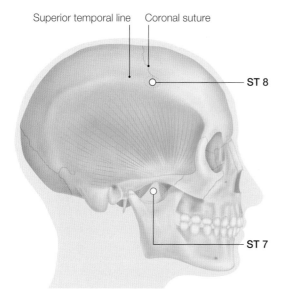

Superior temporal line   Coronal suture

ST 8

ST 7

Treatment note
Needle with the mouth closed and ask client to not speak during session to avoid bending of the needle by muscle action.

Needling
0.3 to 0.5 cun perpendicular insertion, angled slightly downward (in certain cases it can be needled deeper, but this should not be attempted by practitioners without appropriate experience).
1 to 1.5 cun transverse insertion inferiorly towards ST 6, posteriorly towards TE 21, SI 19 or GB 2, or anteriorly along the lower border of the zygomatic arch towards SI 18.

Do not needle deeply, because this holds considerable risk of puncturing any of the vessels located here. Superficially lie the transverse facial artery and vein, and the zygomatic branches of the facial nerve. More deeply, lie the maxillary artery and vein. Also, do not puncture an enlarged parotid gland.

Actions and indications
ST 7 is a *very important point for disorders of the TMJ. It alleviates pain and stiffness of the jaw and benefits the ears, cheeks and teeth.*

Indications include: TMJ pain and stiffness, difficulty opening and closing the mouth, facial paralysis and pain, trigeminal neuralgia, deviation of the eye and mouth, toothache, swelling of the cheek, and parotitis.

It has also been employed to improve hearing and treat deafness, tinnitus, otitis and Ménière's disease.

> **Main Areas**—Jaw. TMJ. Ear. Cheek. Teeth.
> **Main Functions**—Dissipates stasis. Alleviates pain and swelling. Benefits the TMJ.

ST 8 Touwei 頭維
Head Corner

Intersection of the Gallbladder and Yang Wei Mai on the Stomach channel

Myotome	Trigeminal nerve (mandibular branch)
Dermatome	Trigeminal nerve

Location
In the shallow depression at the corner of the forehead, at the superior margin of the temporalis muscle, 0.5 cun within the anterior hairline and 4.5 cun lateral to the anterior midline (GV 24), directly above ST 7 and GB 3.

To aid location, clench the jaw to define the border of the temporalis muscle and slide the tip of the finger directly upward from ST 7 and GB 3. The fingertip should slip into the shallow depression formed by the bony cleft of the superior temporal line and the superior border of the temporalis muscle, along the coronal suture. On light palpation, the pulse of the temporal artery can be perceived.

Needling
0.5 to 1 cun transverse insertion downward towards GB 4, or posteriorly.
Pick up the cutaneous tissue of the scalp (pinch the scalp) and insert the needle subcutaneously, under the epicranial aponeurosis parallel to the bone.

Actions and indications
ST 8 is an important point to *clear the head and brighten the eyes*. It helps *resolve dampness, dissipate wind and stop excessive lacrimation.*

Common indications include: headache, migraine, muzzy or heavy feeling in the head, dizziness, vertigo, poor concentration, depression, mental and psycho-emotional disorders, facial paralysis, eye disorders, excessive lacrimation, twitching or spasm of the eye muscles, and diminishing or blurred vision.

> **Main Areas**—Head. Eyes. Mind.
> **Main Functions**—Dispels wind and dampness. Benefits the head, brain and eyes. Stops lacrimation.

ST 9   Renying   人迎
Man's Prognosis
(Carotid Artery)

Intersection of the Gallbladder on the Stomach channel
Sea of Qi point
Window of the Sky point

Myotome	C1/C2
Dermatome	C3

Location
In the carotid triangle, anterior to the border of the SCM muscle, between the common carotid artery and the thyroid cartilage, approximately 1.5 cun lateral to the tip of the laryngeal prominence (Adam's apple). Situated at the lateral border of the omohyoid muscle. In its deep position lie the longus capitis and the anterior scalene muscles.

Contraindications
Ensure that the client does not suffer from carotid sinus hypersensitivity syndrome before applying any form of treatment to the throat area.

If the person feels dizzy or faint during or after the treatment, it could mean that the blood pressure has dropped below normal. Lie the patient down with the legs raised. Having a sweet drink (such as fruit juice) may also help. It is also possible that the person may feel nauseous or cold due to excessive sympathetic nerve stimulation. Allow the person to rest for at least 20 minutes, or, in severe cases, call an ambulance.

If the superficial fascia of the throat is very tight, the head should be raised at the back using cushion(s)

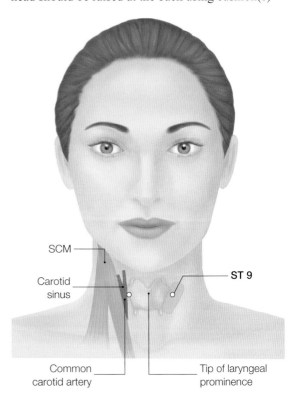

SCM
Carotid sinus
ST 9
Common carotid artery
Tip of laryngeal prominence

so that it is tilted forwards slightly. This position relaxes the fascia, making needling much easier (needling should not be applied if the fascia is taut).

Needling

0.3 to 1.2 cun perpendicular insertion, medial to the artery. Push the artery laterally towards the SCM with the fingers of one hand and insert the needle into the space between the thyroid cartilage and the artery with the other hand.

Depending on the depth and exact angle of insertion, different results will be achieved.

This point is one of the most dangerous points and requires special skill in needling. Do not needle deeply and do not apply any manipulation other than very small rotation.

Do not puncture any of the numerous vessels and nerves lying in the vicinity of this location: superficially, the anterior jugular vein and transverse cervical nerve, and deeper, branches of the superior thyroid artery and vein, the superior laryngeal nerve and the superior root of the ansa cervicalis. Slightly laterally, lies the vagus nerve, not to mention the carotid artery and internal jugular vein.

Do not puncture an enlarged thyroid gland.

Actions and indications

ST 9 is a *very important point to clear heat, subdue excessive Yang and descend rising Qi.* It also *effectively regulates Qi and Blood circulation and alleviates pain.* Furthermore, it is *important to moisten and open the throat, stop swelling and benefit the Lungs and breath.*

Indications include: redness of the face and eyes, hot flushes, headache, fever, sweating, palpitations, tachycardia, dizziness, mental restlessness, fright, panic attack, high or low blood pressure, insomnia, pain in the lower back or anywhere in the body, pain or constriction of the chest, asthma, speech impairment, diseases of the thyroid, oesophageal constriction, plum stone throat, difficulty swallowing, tonsillitis, goitre, and swelling or pain in the throat due to interior or exterior heat, wind or dampness.

ST 9 is also *useful for menopausal symptoms* such as hot flushes, hypertension, anxiety and insomnia.

Stimulation at ST 9 *increases parasympathetic activity* while *decreasing that of the SNS.* Carotid artery massage causes *vasodilation and reduction in heart rate and output,* thus causing a *decrease in blood pressure.* It has a *powerful calming and relaxing effect* on the entire body and mind. Therefore, it is more effective to apply manual pressure directly to the artery rather than needling the exact ST 9 acupuncture location.

Manual pressure of the ST 9 area is one of the most important *first aid manipulations* to be used in cases of symptoms due to excessive rising of Yang Qi, including: hot flushes, palpitations, dizziness, hypertension, emotional upset, fright, and panic.

Acupuncture may be considered more effective in the treatment of local disorders of the throat, including inflammation of the larynx and thyroid disease.

> **Main Areas**—Throat. Thyroid gland. Face. Head. Brain. Heart. Blood vessels.
> **Main Functions**—Descends rising Yang. Clears heat. Calms the mind and body. Increases PSNS activity. Lowers heart rate and output. Lowers blood pressure. Benefits the throat and thyroid.

ST 10   Shuitu
Liquid Passage

Myotome	Accessory nerve, C1–C5
Dermatome	C3

Location

On the anterior border of the SCM muscle, midway between ST 9 and ST 11.

Needling

0.3 to 0.8 cun perpendicular insertion.

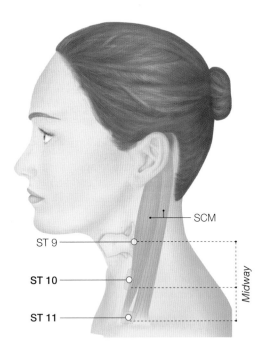

Neither insert deeply nor puncture any of the numerous vessels of this region (see ST 9).

Actions and indications

Although ST 10 is not a commonly used point, it can be effective in cases of *sore, swollen throat, disorders of the thyroid gland*, goitre, disorders of the vocal chords, difficulty breathing or swallowing, and asthma.

> **Main Areas**—Throat. Thyroid gland.
> **Main Function**—Benefits the throat.

ST 11   Qishe
Residence of the Breath Qi

Myotome	Accessory nerve, C1–C5
Dermatome	C3

Location

Above the medial end of the clavicle, between the clavicular and sternal heads of the SCM muscle.

To aid location, it is level with CV 22.

Needling

0.3 to 0.5 cun perpendicular insertion.

Situated above major vessels and the apex of the lung; deep insertion may cause a pneumothorax.

Actions and indications

ST 11 is mainly used for *respiratory disorders* due to Lung Qi counterflow and *diseases of the throat*.

> **Main Areas**—Throat. Thyroid gland.
> **Main Function**—Benefits the throat.

ST 12   Quepen
Empty Basin

Intersection of the Large Intestine, Small Intestine, Triple Energizer, Gallbladder and Yin Qiao Mai on the Stomach channel

Myotome	None
Dermatome	C3

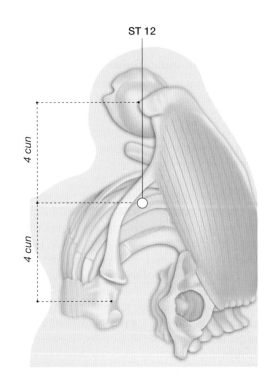

Location
At the midpoint of the supraclavicular fossa, 4 cun lateral to the midline (approximately level with CV 22).

To aid location, hook the tip of the index finger over the clavicle to find its posterior border.

Contraindications
All forms of treatment are contraindicated during pregnancy and heavy menstruation.

Needling
0.3 to 0.5 cun perpendicular insertion, directly behind the clavicle to avoid the needle tip going too far posteriorly and puncturing the apex of the lung.

Needling this location is potentially dangerous. Avoid deep insertion because there is considerable risk of puncturing the apex of the lung or the subclavian vessels. Superficially, do not puncture branches of the supraclavicular nerve.

Actions and indications
ST 12, similarly to ST 9, is an important point for *descending excessive upward rising of Qi. It also effectively opens and relaxes the chest, benefiting the lungs and respiration.*

It has been widely employed to treat: hypertension, hot flushes, redness of the face, dizziness, fullness of the chest, dyspnoea, cough, asthma, hiccup, swelling of the throat, lymphadenopathy, intercostal neuralgia, and pain in the shoulder and neck.

ST 12 is mentioned as one of the *Eight Points to Clear Heat from the Chest,* alongside LU 1, BL 11 and BL 12, and is considered important to *clear heat from the upper jiao.*

> **Main Areas**—Chest. Lungs. Shoulder.
> **Main Functions**—Descends rising Qi. Lowers blood pressure. Clears heat.

ST 13   Qihu
Door of the Breath

Myotome	C5–C8
Dermatome	C4

Location
In the depression directly below ST 12, just under the inferior border of the clavicle, on the mid-mamillary line, 4 cun lateral to the midline. Situated in the clavicular head of the pectoralis major, and deeper, the subclavius muscle.

To aid location, it is directly below ST 12 and approximately level with CV 21 and KI 27.

Needling
0.3 to 1 cun transverse insertion medially, laterally or downward along the Stomach channel.
0.2 to 0.5 cun perpendicular insertion.
1 to 2 cun subcutaneously towards LU 2 or CV 21.

Do not needle deeply, because this poses considerable risk of puncturing the lung.

Actions and indications
Treatment at ST 13 is rarely employed, although it is applicable for *disorders of the chest and respiratory system* including: heaviness and pain of the chest, dyspnoea, cough, and hiccup.

It can also be effectively employed to *treat pain and stiffness of the infraclavicular region and shoulder* and disorders of the breasts.

> **Main Areas**—Clavicle. Shoulder. Chest.
> **Main Functions**—Alleviates pain and stiffness. Benefits the breathing.

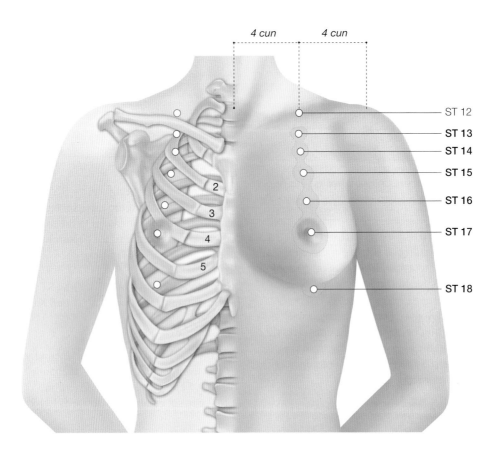

4 cun *4 cun*

ST 12
ST 13
ST 14
ST 15
ST 16
ST 17
ST 18

ST 14   Kufang
Breath Storeroom

Myotome	C5–C8
Dermatome	T2

Location
In the first intercostal space, in the depression directly below ST 13, on the infra-mammary line, 4 cun lateral to the anterior midline.

To aid location, it is approximately level with CV 20 and KI 26.

Needling
0.4 to 0.8 cun transverse insertion medially, laterally or downward along the Stomach channel.
0.2 to 0.5 cun perpendicular insertion.

Do not needle deeply, because this poses considerable risk of puncturing the lung.

Actions and indications
Treatment at *ST 14, ST 15 and ST 16 helps expand and relax the chest and descend counterflow Qi.*

Indications include: respiratory disorders, fullness and constriction of the chest, dyspnoea, intercostal neuralgia, regional stiffness or pain of the chest and ribs, swelling and pain of the mammary glands, and mastitis. Choose between these points, depending on which are more sensitive to pressure palpation.

> **Main Areas**—Chest. Breast.
> **Main Functions**—Alleviates pain and swelling. Benefits the breast and Lungs.

ST 15   Wuyi
Hiding the Breath

Myotome	None – superficial tissue
Dermatome	T2/T3

Location
Directly below ST 14, in the second intercostal space, on the infra-mammary line, 4 cun lateral to the midline (approximately level with CV 19 and KI 25). The location of ST 15 and ST 16 may vary, depending on the individual structure of the mammary glands.

Needling
0.4 to 0.8 cun transverse insertion medially, laterally or downward along the Stomach channel.
0.2 to 0.5 cun perpendicular insertion.

Do not needle deeply, because this poses considerable risk of puncturing the lung.

Actions and indications
Treatment at *ST 14, ST 15 and ST 16 helps expand and relax the chest and descend counterflow Qi.*

Indications include: respiratory disorders, fullness and constriction of the chest, dyspnoea, intercostal neuralgia, regional stiffness or pain of the chest and ribs, swelling and pain of the mammary glands, and mastitis. Choose between these points, depending on which are more sensitive to pressure palpation.

> **Main Areas**—Chest. Lungs. Breast.
> **Main Functions**—Alleviates pain and swelling. Benefits the breast and Lungs.

ST 16   Yingchuang
Breast Window

Myotome	None at surface
Dermatome	T3

Location
Situated directly below ST 15, in the third intercostal space, on the infra-mammary line, 4 cun lateral to the midline (approximately level with CV 18 and KI 24). See also location note for ST 15.

Needling
0.4 to 0.8 cun transverse insertion medially, laterally or downward along the Stomach channel.
0.2 to 0.5 cun perpendicular insertion.

Do not needle deeply, because this poses considerable risk of puncturing the lung.

Actions and indications
Treatment at *ST 14, ST 15 and ST 16 helps expand and relax the chest and descend counterflow Qi.*

Indications include: respiratory disorders, fullness and constriction of the chest, dyspnoea, intercostal neuralgia, regional stiffness or pain of the chest and ribs, swelling and pain of the mammary glands, and mastitis. Choose between these points, depending on which are more sensitive to pressure palpation.

> **Main Area**—Breast.
> **Main Function**—Alleviates pain and swelling.

ST 17   Ruzhong
Breast Centre (Nipple)

Myotome	None at surface
Dermatome	T4

Location
At the centre of the nipple.

Note: The male nipple should be level with the fourth intercostal space and 4 cun lateral to the anterior midline; however, in the female it varies, depending on the individual structure of the mammary glands.

Contraindications
Needling and moxibustion is contraindicated. This is a reference point and is not generally used for actual treatment.

Soreness, pain, swelling and redness of the nipples are *signs that may be used diagnostically*. These signs point to Liver Qi stagnation, Liver heat, Blood stasis and/or phlegm accumulation in the breast, which can be caused by hormonal imbalances, breast disease or pregnancy.

> **Main Areas**—Nipple. Breast. Uterus. Mind.
> **Main Functions**—Lifts sinking Qi. Resuscitates consciousness. Increases libido.

ST 18   Rugen
Breast Root

Myotome	None at surface
Dermatome	T4/T5

Location
In the fifth intercostal space, on the infra-mammary line, 4 cun lateral to the anterior midline.

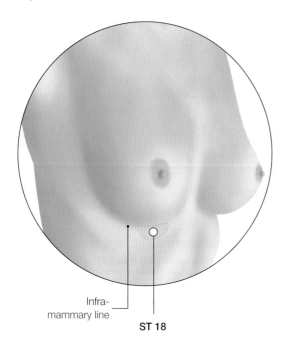

Infra-mammary line

ST 18

To aid location, it is at the base of the breast, in line with the nipple.

Needling
0.3 to 0.7 cun perpendicular insertion.
0.5 to 1.5 cun transverse medial or lateral insertion.

Do not needle deeply, because this poses considerable risk of puncturing the lung.

Actions and indications
ST 18 is an *important point to expand and relax the chest* and is a *major point for many disorders of the breast*.

Indications include: pain, swelling, fibrosis and many disorders of the mammary glands, insufficient lactation, mastitis, pain or tightness of the chest, hypochondrial distension and pain, asthma, bronchitis, and cough.

> **Main Areas**—Breasts. Lungs. Chest. Liver.
> **Main Functions**—Dispels stasis. Benefits the breasts.

ST 19   Burong
Not Contained

Myotome	T7–12 rectus abdominis edge
Dermatome	T6/T7

Location
Just below the costal margin, 6 cun above the level of the umbilicus and 2 cun lateral to the midline.

To aid location, it is level with CV 14 and KI 21.

Note: In persons who have a narrow costal angle, a location of 2 cun lateral to the midline may fall on the costal cartilage. Therefore, the 2 cun distance must be decreased, so that the point will be located closer to the midline. In some such cases, the first point below the rib cage is ST 20 (level with CV 13 and KI 20) or even ST 21 (level with CV 12).

Consequently, it could be considered either that ST 19 and ST 20 and/or ST 21 fall at the same location, or that ST 19 and/or ST 20 are in fact inside the rib cage and cannot be accessed for treatment (in effect they do not 'exist'). This means that needling and massage at ST 20 or ST 21 would be the same as for ST 19, and not the same as that for a normal ST 20 or ST 21 location further down.

The simplest way to overcome this problem is to consider that treatment at this 'multiple point' would combine the functions of all these points.

Needling
0.5 to 1 cun perpendicular insertion.

Do not needle deeply, particularly if there is enlargement of the liver or heart, or if the patient is very thin. Needling deeply will puncture the peritoneum.

Actions and indications
ST 19 is not a very commonly used point, because other points are more effective in the treatment of interior complaints (such as ST 21, CV 12 and ST 25). It can, however, be employed to *harmonise the Stomach and ease stagnation in the middle jiao*.

Indications include: epigastric fullness and pain, vomiting, hypochondrial pain, gallstones, inflammation of the gallbladder, indigestion, poor appetite, abdominal distension, abdominal rumbling, intercostal neuralgia, dyspnoea, cough, and chest pain.

Main Areas—Stomach. Abdomen. Heart.
Main Function—Harmonises the middle jiao.

ST 20 Chengman
Receiving Fullness

承滿

Myotome	T7–T12 rectus abdominis edge
Dermatome	T8

Location
1 cun below ST 19, 5 cun above the level of the umbilicus, 2 cun lateral to CV 13. See note for ST 19.

Needling
0.5 to 1 cun perpendicular insertion.

Do not needle deeply, particularly if there is enlargement of the liver or heart, or if the patient is very thin. Needling deeply will puncture the peritoneum.

Actions and indications
ST 20 is not a very commonly used point, because other points are more effective in the treatment of interior complaints (such as ST 21, CV 12 and ST 25). It can, however, be employed to *harmonise the Stomach and ease stagnation in the middle jiao*.

Indications include: epigastric fullness and pain, vomiting, hypochondrial pain, gallstones, inflammation of the gallbladder, indigestion, poor appetite, abdominal distension, abdominal rumbling, intercostal neuralgia, dyspnoea, cough, and chest pain.

Main Areas—Stomach. Abdomen. Heart.
Main Function—Harmonises the middle jiao.

ST 21 Liangmen
Grain Gate (Epigastrium)

梁門

Myotome	T7–T12 rectus abdominis edge
Dermatome	T9

Location
2 cun lateral to CV 12, 4 cun above the level of the umbilicus.

To aid location, see note for ST 19.

Needling
0.5 to 1.5 cun perpendicular insertion.

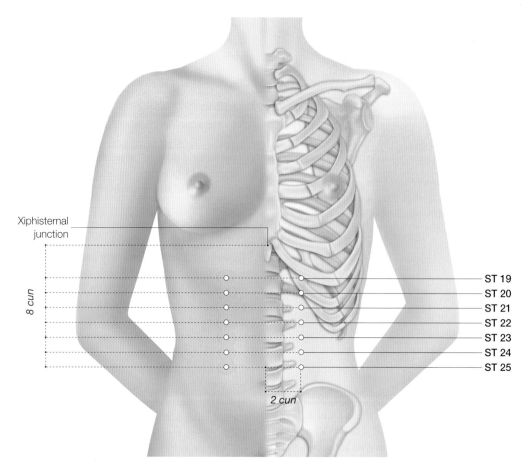

Xiphisternal junction

8 cun

ST 19
ST 20
ST 21
ST 22
ST 23
ST 24
ST 25

2 cun

Do not needle deeply, particularly if there is enlargement of the liver or heart, or if the patient is very thin. Needling deeply will puncture the peritoneum.

Actions and indications

ST 21 has similar functions to ST 19 and ST 20, but is much more commonly used. It *may be considered as a front-mu point for the Stomach but more for excess conditions when compared to CV 12*. It is especially useful in cases of *rebellious Stomach Qi*. ST 21 is an important point to *harmonise the Stomach, ease stagnation from the middle jiao and descend rebellious Qi*.

Indications include: epigastric fullness, heaviness, tightness and hardness, stomach pain, indigestion, heartburn, gastritis, gastric ulceration, hiatus hernia, nausea, vomiting, hypochondrial distension and pain, abdominal distension, loose stools, diarrhoea, undigested food in the stools, poor appetite, and abdominal rumbling.

Main Areas—Epigastrium. Abdomen. Heart.
Main Functions—Descends rebellious Qi. Relieves stagnation. Harmonises the Stomach.

ST 22 Guanmen

Shutting the Gate (Pylorus)

關門

Myotome	T7–T12 rectus abdominis edge
Dermatome	T9/T10

Location

1 cun below ST 21, 3 cun above the level of the umbilicus.

To aid location, it is 2 cun lateral to CV 11.

Needling
0.5 to 1.5 cun perpendicular insertion.

Do not needle deeply, particularly in thin patients because this will puncture the peritoneum.

Actions and indications
ST 22 is not a very commonly used point but it can be employed in similar situations as adjacent Stomach channel points such as ST 21, ST 23 and ST 24.

> **Main Areas**—Epigastrium. Abdomen. Chest.
> **Main Function**—Regulates Stomach Qi.

ST 23 Taiyi
Great Unity

太乙

Myotome	T7–T12 rectus abdominis edge
Dermatome	T9/T10

Location
1 cun below ST 22, 2 cun above the level of the umbilicus, 2 cun lateral to CV 10 and KI 17.

Needling
0.5 to 1.5 cun perpendicular insertion. See also ST 21 and ST 25.

Actions and indications
See also ST 21 and ST 25.

> **Main Areas**—Stomach. Heart.
> **Main Functions**—Harmonises the middle jiao.
> Soothes the Heart and calms the mind.

ST 24 Huaroumen
Chime Gate

滑肉門

Myotome	T7–T12 rectus abdominis edge
Dermatome	T10

Location
1 cun below ST 22, 1 cun above the level of the umbilicus, 2 cun lateral to CV 9.

Needling
0.5 to 1.5 cun perpendicular insertion. See also ST 21 and ST 25.

Actions and indications
See also ST 21 and ST 25.

> **Main Areas**—Stomach. Abdomen. Heart.
> **Main Functions**—Harmonises the Stomach and intestines. Calms the mind.

ST 25 Tianshu
Heaven's Pivot

天樞

Front-Mu point of the Large Intestine

Myotome	T7–T12 rectus abdominis edge
Dermatome	T10

Location
2 cun lateral to the centre of the umbilicus (CV 8), on the rectus abdominis muscle.

Needling
0.5 to 1.5 cun perpendicular insertion.

Do not needle deeply, particularly in thin patients, because this will puncture the peritoneum.

Actions and indications
ST 25 is a *very important point and is widely used to alleviate abdominal pain and regulate the lower jiao*. It helps *clear dampness and heat and regulate the intestines*, as well as *promote the descending of Stomach Qi and relieve food retention*.

Indications include: disorders of the intestines, abdominal rumbling, distension, swelling and pain, gastroenteritis, diarrhoea, dysentery, foul smelling stools, mucus or blood in the stools, appendicitis,

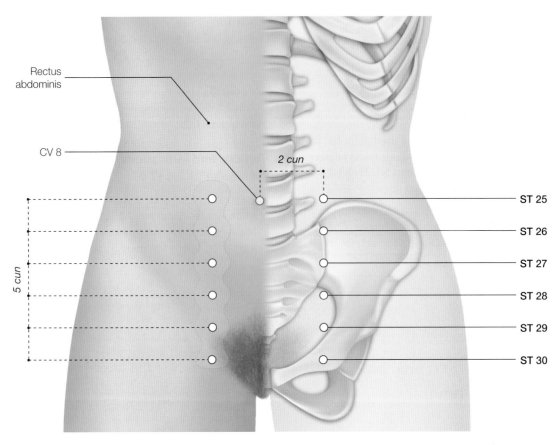

Rectus abdominis

CV 8

2 cun

5 cun

ST 25
ST 26
ST 27
ST 28
ST 29
ST 30

Crohn's disease, dry stools, constipation, obstruction of the intestines, retching, nausea and vomiting, dysuria, leucorrhoea, irregular menstruation, and dysmenorrhoea.

Main Areas—Intestines. Umbilicus. Abdomen. Uterus.
Main Functions—Clears dampness and heat. Regulates Qi in the lower jiao. Benefits the intestines.

ST 26   Wailing
Outer Mound

Myotome	T7–T12 rectus abdominis edge
Dermatome	T10/T11

Location
On the rectus abdominis muscle, 1 cun below the umbilicus, 2 cun lateral to the midline.

To aid location, it is level with CV 7.

Needling
0.5 to 1.5 cun perpendicular insertion.

Actions and indications
ST 26 is not a very commonly used point although it can be employed in similar situations as adjacent Stomach channel points such as ST 25, ST 27 and ST 28. All these points have an effect on the *lower abdomen, intestines, urinary bladder and uterus* and are indicated in cases of: distension, heaviness, swelling or pain of the abdomen; abdominal rumbling, diarrhoea, constipation, hernia, dysuria, cystitis, dysmenorrhoea, menstrual irregularities, infertility, and spermatorrhoea.

> **Main Areas**—Intestines. Abdomen.
> **Main Function**—Regulates the lower jiao.

ST 27   Daju
Great Bulge

Myotome	T7–T12 rectus abdominis edge
Dermatome	T11

Location
2 cun below the umbilicus, 2 cun lateral to the anterior midline.

To aid location, it is level with CV 5.

Needling
0.5 to 1.5 cun perpendicular insertion.

Do not needle deeply, particularly if the patient is very thin. Do not puncture the peritoneum or a full bladder.

Actions and indications
ST 25, ST 27 and ST 28 all have an effect on the *lower abdomen, intestines, urinary bladder and uterus* and are indicated in cases of: distension, heaviness, swelling or pain of the abdomen; abdominal rumbling, diarrhoea, constipation, hernia, dysuria, cystitis, dysmenorrhoea, menstrual irregularities, infertility, and spermatorrhoea.

> **Main Area**—Abdomen.
> **Main Function**—Regulates the lower jiao.

ST 28   Shuidao
Waterway

Myotome	T7–T12 rectus abdominis edge
Dermatome	T11

Location
3 cun below the umbilicus, 2 cun lateral to the anterior midline.

To aid location, it is level with CV 4.

Needling
0.5 to 1.5 cun perpendicular insertion.

Do not needle deeply, particularly if the patient is very thin. Do not puncture the peritoneum or a full bladder.

Actions and indications
ST 28 *benefits the whole of the lower abdomen* and is particularly useful in the *treatment of urogenital disorders* and *problems of the reproductive organs and uterus*.

Indications include: distension, heaviness and swelling or pain of the lower abdomen, hernia pain, dysuria, haematuria, cystitis, urinary tract infections, dysmenorrhoea, menstrual irregularities, prolapse of the uterus, pelvic inflammatory disease, frigidity and infertility, and spermatorrhoea, prostatitis and erectile dysfunction.

> **Main Areas**—Urogenital system. Uterus.
> **Main Functions**—Clears dampness and heat. Regulates Qi in the lower jiao. Benefits menstruation. Increases libido and fertility.

ST 29   Guilai
Restoring Position

Myotome	T7–T12 rectus abdominis edge
Dermatome	T12

Location
4 cun below the umbilicus, 2 cun lateral to the anterior midline. To aid location, it is level with CV 3.

Needling

0.5 to 1 cun perpendicular insertion.

Do not needle deeply, particularly if the patient is very thin. Do not puncture the peritoneum or a full bladder.

Actions and indications

ST 29 has similar actions to ST 28 and ST 30. It has been widely employed to treat *disorders of the reproductive and urogenital system*.

It is particularly indicated for amenorrhoea, dysmenorrhoea and lower abdominal pain, cold in the lower abdomen, infertility, uterine prolapse, diminished libido, impotence and testicular swelling or pain.

> **Main Areas**—Lower Abdomen. Uterus. Genitals.
> **Main Function**—Regulates the lower jiao.

ST 30 Qichong
Qi Surge

Intersection of the Chong Mai on the Stomach channel
Sea of Nourishment point

Myotome	T7–T12 rectus abdominis edge
Dermatome	T12

Location

2 cun lateral to the anterior midline (CV 2), superior and slightly lateral to the pubic tubercle, on the medial side of the femoral artery and vein.

Needling

0.5 to 1 cun perpendicular insertion.

Do not needle deeply, particularly if the patient is very thin. Do not puncture the anterior cutaneous branch of the iliohypogastric nerve or branches of the superficial epigastric artery and vein. More deeply and slightly laterally, avoid the femoral vein or artery.

Actions and indications

ST 30 is considered one of the most *important points to promote fertility and regulate menstruation*. It helps *regulate Qi and Blood in the lower jiao and dispels stasis*.

Indications include: infertility, amenorrhoea, irregular menstruation, abnormal uterine bleeding, dysmenorrhoea, frequent miscarriage, leucorrhoea, prolapse of the uterus or rectum, haemorrhoids, pain of the external genitals, impotence, spermatorrhoea, frequent urination, lower abdominal pain, twisting abdominal pain, inguinal hernia, and testicular retraction and pain. Additionally, it has been employed to treat difficulty in delivering the placenta and insufficient lactation.

According to classical texts, the Chong Mai emerges at the point where the femoral artery pulse is perceived at ST 30. Treatment is applied here in order to *regulate the Chong Mai and descend rebellious Stomach Qi*.

Additionally, ST 30 has been extensively used as a *mental focus point during Qigong practice*.

> **Main Areas**—Reproductive organs. Uterus. Testicles. Bladder. Intestines. Lower abdomen.
> **Main Functions**—Benefits the lower jiao. Regulates Qi and Blood. Benefits menstruation. Improves sexual function. Increases fertility.

ST 31 Biguan
Thigh Gate

Myotome	L2/L3
Dermatome	L1

Location

On the anterolateral aspect of the thigh, below the hip, in the prominent depression appearing when the thigh is flexed, between the sartorius and tensor fasciae latae muscles. Situated approximately level with the lower border of the pubic symphysis and directly below the ASIS.

To aid location, slide the tip of the finger directly downward from the tip of the ASIS, with the patient's hip in flexion. The finger will naturally slide into the large depression of ST 31.

This is a large point and may be accessed from a slightly wider area, extending both superiorly toward the ASIS, and inferiorly, on the lateral side of the sartorius muscle.

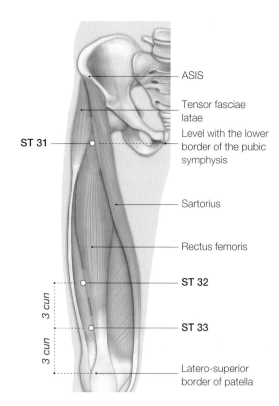

ASIS

Tensor fasciae latae

Level with the lower border of the pubic symphysis

Sartorius

Rectus femoris

ST 32

ST 33

Latero-superior border of patella

Needling
1 to 2.5 cun perpendicular insertion.

Actions and indications
ST 31 is a *very powerful point to benefit the hips and improve flow of Qi and Blood to the entire lower extremity*. It *dispels wind and dampness from the hips and lower limbs* and is commonly employed to treat restricted movement, stiffness, contraction, atrophy, paralysis, numbness and pain of the hips, knees and entire lower limb.

It can also be effectively employed to alleviate lumbar and abdominal pain.

> **Main Areas**—Hips. Lower limbs.
> **Main Functions**—Dissipates stasis and alleviates pain and stiffness. Dispels wind and dampness.

ST 32　　Futu
Crouching Rabbit

Myotome	L2–L4
Dermatome	L2

Location
6 cun above the latero-superior border of the patella, on the line joining the lateral border of the patella with the ASIS. To aid location, it is approximately two hand-widths above the latero-superior border of the patella.

Needling
1 to 2 cun perpendicular insertion.

Actions and indications
ST 32 is primarily used as a *local point to clear dampness, wind and cold from the channel and to alleviate pain*.

> **Main Area**—Thigh.
> **Main Functions**—Dispels wind, dampness and cold. Alleviates pain.

ST 33　　Yinshi
Yin Market

Myotome	L2–L4
Dermatome	L2/L3

Location
3 cun above the latero-superior border of the patella, on the line joining the lateral border of the patella with the ASIS.

To aid location, it is approximately one hand-width above the latero-superior border of the patella.

Needling

1 to 2 cun perpendicular insertion.

Actions and indications

ST 33 is primarily used as a *local point to clear dampness, wind and cold from the channel and to alleviate pain.*

> **Main Area**—Thigh.
> **Main Functions**—Dispels wind, dampness and cold. Alleviates pain.

ST 34   Liangqiu   梁丘
Ridge Mound

Xi-Cleft point

Myotome	L2–L4
Dermatome	L3

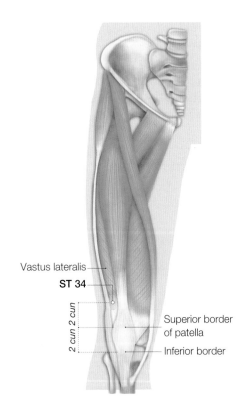

Vastus lateralis

ST 34

2 cun 2 cun

Superior border of patella

Inferior border

Location

In the depression 2 cun proximal to the latero-superior border of the patella, between the rectus femoris and vastus lateralis muscles, on the line connecting the ASIS to the lateral border of the patella.

To aid location, a visible depression appears at ST 34 when the leg is extended.

Needling

0.5 to 1.5 cun perpendicular insertion.
1 to 2 cun horizontal insertion towards SP 10.

Actions and indications

ST 34 is frequently treated in excess disorders to pacify the stomach, alleviate pain and descend rebellious Qi.

Indications include: acute stomach ache, spasm of the stomach, gastritis, heartburn, bitter taste, nausea, and vomiting.

ST 34 is also important to clear channel obstructions and benefit the knees. Symptoms include: pain, swelling, stiffness and restricted movement of the knee, thigh and leg.

It has also been employed to treat a variety of other symptoms, including diarrhoea, mastitis and palpitations.

> **Main Areas**—Stomach. Epigastrium. Lower limbs. Knees.
> **Main Functions**—Pacifies the Stomach. Descends rebellious Qi. Alleviates pain.

ST 35   Dubi (Wai Xiyan)   犢鼻
Calf's Nose (Lateral Eye of the Knee)
外膝眼

Myotome	None – within lateral fat pad of knee
Dermatome	L3

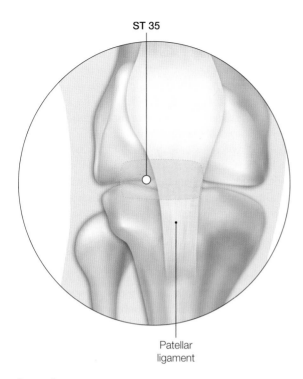

ST 35

Patellar
ligament

Location
Lateral to the patellar ligament, in the large
depression appearing when the knee is flexed.
In its deep position, situated in the knee joint space
between the articular surfaces of the femur and tibia.

Treatment note

A flexed knee to 90 degrees offers the best angle for
needling this point.

Needling
1 to 2 cun perpendicular insertion, angled slightly
medially, towards the centre of the knee joint,
or BL40.
1 to 1.5 cun horizontal insertion, through or under
the patellar ligament to connect with the Nei Xiyan
(Ex LE 4).
1 to 2 cun oblique superior medial insertion under
the patella.

Actions and indications
This is a very *important point for the treatment
of disorders of the knee* including: pain, stiffness,
swelling and restricted movement. It can be used
in such conditions as chronic degenerative or

rheumatoid arthritis of the knee, articular cartilage
degeneration, chondropathy and lateral meniscus
injury. Combine it with Nei Xiyan (Ex LE 4) – the
two points are known as the 'Eyes of the Knee'.

Main Area—Knees.
Main Functions—Alleviates pain, stiffness and
swelling. Strengthens the knees.

ST 36 Zusanli 足三里
Leg Three Miles

He-Sea point, Earth point
Command point of the abdomen
Sea of Nourishment point
Heavenly Star point

Myotome	L5/S1
Dermatome	L5

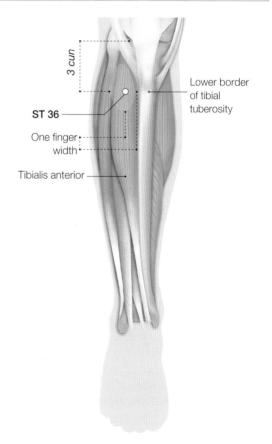

3 cun

ST 36

One finger
width

Tibialis anterior

Lower border
of tibial
tuberosity

Location

On the tibialis anterior muscle, approximately one finger-width lateral to the tibial crest, level with the lower border of the tibial tuberosity, 3 cun below the knee crease. Approximately 1 cun anterior and inferior to GB 34.

To aid location, it is approximately one hand-width below ST 35. Locate it in a small opening between the fibres, on the high point of the tibialis anterior muscle belly.

Needling

0.5 to 1.5 cun perpendicular insertion.
1 to 3 cun oblique insertion, directed distally along the channel.

Actions and indications

ST 36 is one of the most *dynamic and widely used points and has been employed in almost every disorder*. It *strengthens the middle jiao Qi and boosts the vital substances: Qi, Blood, fluids, Yin and Yang*. Treatment applied to ST 36 is *important in most chronic disorders where there is weakness of the Stomach, Spleen and other organs*.

There is an extremely wide range of both actions and indications for ST 36. However, it is impossible to list every symptom here, or attribute the listed symptoms to only a single syndrome because many of them overlap and many symptoms appear in different syndromes. Therefore *understanding the underlying actions* of ST 36, rather than its indications only, is the *cornerstone* to using it effectively in treatment.

The main functions of ST 36 can be listed as follows:

Strengthens the body and boosts Qi, Blood, Yin and Yang. Tonifies Stomach and Spleen Qi, strengthens the digestion and benefits the entire abdomen. Strengthens the central Qi and raises sinking Qi. Regulates nutritive and defensive Qi and strengthens the immune system whilst helping to expel exterior pathogenic factors. Warms and tonifies Yang and restores collapsed Yang (with moxa). Descends rebellious Stomach Qi. Regulates

the intestines. Resolves dampness. Clears heat and cools the body. Nourishes Yin and generates fluids. Dispels stagnation from the chest. Benefits the Heart and Lungs. Calms the mind and soothes stress. Strengthens the legs and benefits the knees. It is a key distal point for lumbosacral back pain and sciatica due to its innervation being L5.

General symptoms of insufficient Qi for which ST 36 has been extensively employed, include a feeling of lack of vitality, general tiredness and weakness, debility, flaccidity of the flesh and muscles, prolapse of organs, atrophy and paralysis; spontaneous sweating, breathlessness, dyspnoea, asthma, weak immunity, allergies and recurrent infections.

Common symptoms of *deficiency, heat or rebellious Qi in the Stomach, intestines or anywhere else in digestive system* include: abdominal distension, poor appetite, indigestion, food cravings, compulsive overeating, nausea, vomiting, morning sickness, abdominal rumbling, flatulence, loose stools, diarrhoea, undigested food in the stools, constipation, thirst, dry mouth and tongue, difficulty swallowing, heartburn, abdominal or epigastric pain, belching, hiccup, acid stomach, gastritis, oesophagitis, gastric ulceration and hiatus hernia.

Common symptoms of *Blood and Yin deficiency* that ST 36 is indicated for include: dry skin and hair, premature ageing or excessive wrinkling of the skin, weakness of the tendons and muscles, general musculo-skeletal stiffness, floaters in the eyes, dry eyes, inflammation of the eyes, blurred vision, dizziness, anaemia, depression, mood swings, scanty menstruation, infertility, postpartum dizziness, backache, dry mouth and feelings of heat.

ST 36 is also very important in many *disorders of the breasts* including pain, palpabable nodules, fibrocystic breast disease, mastitis and insufficient lactation. ST 36 has a *powerful effect on the entire chest* and can be used for tightness, heaviness or pain of the chest, angina, palpitations and other disorders of the heart.

ST 36 also has a *very powerful effect on the brain and nervous system*. It has been shown to elicit reduced neural activity in the limbic system, which is why it is traditionally indicated for *calming the mind* in cases of emotional imbalances including anxiety, fear, anger, sadness and even manic behaviour or madness. Also, it has been traditionally indicated for a variety of other symptoms and disorders that we can associate with the limbic system. These include seizures, epilepsy, loss of consciousness, tics, reduced sense of smell, excessive or reduced hunger, thirst or sweating. Other symptoms include difficulty with learning, concentrating and speaking, poor memory, insomnia, drug or alcohol addiction and imbalanced libido.

It is also traditionally indicated for other neurological problems including wind stroke, spasms, tics and tremors, cramps, aphasia, mental disorientation and loss of consciousness. ST 36 stimulation can cause vasodilation in areas of the brain affected by ischaemia in stroke patients. Furthermore, it regulates blood pressure and helps with both hypotension and hypertension.

ST 36 is extensively employed in *most disorders of the lower limbs* including stiffness, tiredness, weakness and atrophy or paralysis. It is also particularly indicated for disorders of the knees, including degeneration the cartilage, meniscus problems, arthritis and pain, stiffness or swelling.

Moreover, ST 36 is used in weight loss programs to *harmonise the Stomach and increase metabolism.*

ST 36 can be stimulated on *athletes before and after exercising*, in order to strengthen the lower limbs.

ST 36 is effective to boost *beauty treatments* in combination with other points that lift the Qi (such as GV 20 and CV 6) together with local points on the face.

ST 36 has also been traditionally employed to treat a variety of other symptoms and disorders, including stiffness and tightness of the jaw muscles, TMJ disorders, tetany, chills and fever, headache, unclear or diminishing eyesight, sore throat, and tinnitus.

Main Areas—Entire body. Abdomen. Chest. Mind. Stomach and Spleen. Digestive system. Lower limb. Knee.
Main Functions—Tonifies and lifts Qi and Yang. Nourishes Blood, fluids and Yin. Boosts the immune system. Benefits the Stomach and Spleen. Regulates Qi. Calms the mind.

ST 37   Shangjuxu
Upper Large Hollow

Lower He-Sea point of the Large Intestine channel
Sea of Blood point

Myotome	L5/S1
Dermatome	L5

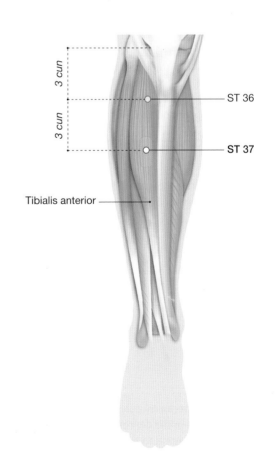

3 cun

3 cun

ST 36

ST 37

Tibialis anterior

149

Location

On the tibialis anterior muscle, 3 cun below ST 36 or 6 cun below the knee crease and one finger-width lateral to the tibial crest.

To aid location, it is two hand-widths below the knee crease.

Needling

1 to 1.5 cun perpendicular insertion.

Actions and indications

ST 37 is an *important point to clear dampness and heat from the Large Intestine, alleviate diarrhoea and regulate Spleen and Stomach Qi*. It is useful in any *acute or chronic disorder affecting the intestines*.

Symptoms include: loose stools, diarrhoea, undigested food in the stools, abdominal rumbling, constipation, abdominal distension and pain, and umbilical pain.

Additionally, ST 37 *clears the channel* and alleviates pain and stiffness of the leg.

ST 37 has also been traditionally employed to treat a variety of other symptoms such as fullness and pain of the chest, dyspnoea, shortness of breath, flank pain, stomach pain and swelling of the face.

> **Main Areas**—Large Intestine. Digestive system. Abdomen.
> **Main Functions**—Regulates the Large Intestine. Dispels dampness. Alleviates pain and diarrhoea.

ST 38   Tiaokou
Ribbon Opening

條口

Myotome	L5/S1
Dermatome	L5

Location

On the tibialis anterior muscle, 8 cun above the lateral malleolus, in the depression approximately one finger-width lateral to the tibial crest.

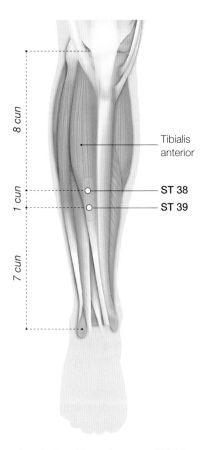

Tibialis anterior

ST 38

ST 39

8 cun

1 cun

7 cun

To aid location, it is midway between ST 35 and ST 41.

Needling

1 to 1.5 cun perpendicular insertion.

Actions and indications

ST 38 has *similar functions to ST 37 and ST 39. Additionally, it expels wind, cold and dampness from the Stomach channel, alleviates pain and benefits the shoulder*.

Indications include: pain or numbness of the leg or knee, stomach ache, and pain and stiffness of the shoulder. For best results when treating shoulder problems, mobilise the joint at the same time as stimulating ST 38.

> **Main Areas**—Shoulder. Digestive system.
> **Main Functions**—Dispels wind, dampness and cold. Alleviates pain. Benefits the shoulder.

ST 39　Xiajuxu
Lower Large Hollow

Lower He-Sea point of the Small Intestine channel
Sea of Blood point

Myotome	L5/S1
Dermatome	L5

Location
1 cun below ST 38 (9 cun below the knee crease), one finger-width lateral to the tibial crest.

Needling
1 to 1.5 cun perpendicular insertion.

Treatment and applications
The functions and treatment of ST 39 are *similar to ST 37 and ST 38* although it has a greater effect on the *Small Intestine*. It is mainly used for symptoms such as abdominal distension and pain, abdominal rumbling, diarrhoea and pain or stiffness of the lower limbs.

> **Main Areas**—Small Intestine. Digestive system. Abdomen.
> **Main Functions**—Regulates the intestines. Alleviates pain.

ST 40　Fenglong
Abundant Bulge

Luo-Connecting point

Myotome	L5,S1
Dermatome	L5

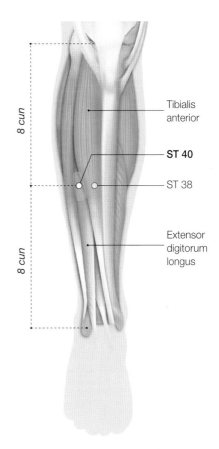

8 cun

8 cun

Tibialis anterior

ST 40

ST 38

Extensor digitorum longus

Location
On the anterolateral aspect of the leg, 8 cun below the knee crease, two finger-widths lateral to the tibial crest.

To aid location, it is one finger-width lateral to ST 38. Palpate gently with the fingertip to find the depression on the lateral border of the extensor digitorum longus. If this point is indicated it will often feel as a bump rather than a hollow – hence its Chinese name.

Needling
0.5 to 1.5 cun perpendicular insertion.

Actions and indications
ST 40 is *possibly the most important point used to resolve phlegm* from any part of the body and is particularly important for the *digestive and*

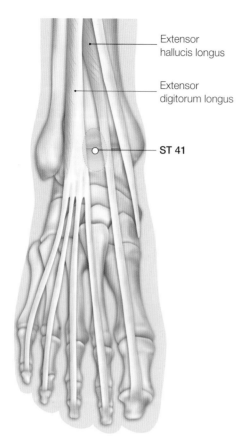

Extensor
hallucis longus

Extensor
digitorum longus

ST 41

respiratory systems. It effectively *transforms dampness, opens and relaxes the chest and alleviates cough, clears heat* and *calms and clears the mind*.

Indications include: tightness, heaviness and pain of the chest, productive cough, dyspnoea, asthmatic wheezing, bronchitis, pneumonia and other diseases accompanied by heavy phlegm build-up, nausea, vomiting and epigastric pain, mental restlessness, anxiety, insomnia, depression and other psychological disturbances, palpitations, epilepsy, Ménière's disease, feeling of muzziness and heaviness, vertigo, dizziness and headache, numbness of the legs and body, and lipomas, lumps, cysts and tumours.

Main Areas—Chest. Head. Mind. Lungs. Stomach. Heart.
Main Functions—Resolves phlegm and transforms dampness. Opens the chest. Relieves cough. Calms and clears the mind. Benefits the digestive system.

ST 41　Jiexi
Dividing Cleft

解谿

Jing-River point, Fire point

Myotome	None – in superficial tissue
Dermatome	L5

Location
On the front of the ankle, at the junction of the dorsum of the foot and the leg, in the depression between the tendons of the extensor digitorum longus and extensor hallucis longus muscles.

To aid location, it is level with the prominence of the lateral malleolus, when the foot is flexed at right angles to the leg. Extend the toes against resistance to define the tendons.

Needling
0.5 to 1.5 cun perpendicular insertion.
Oblique insertion medially under the tendon of extensor hallucis longus towards SP 5.
Oblique insertion laterally under the tendon of extensor digitorum longus towards GB 40.

Actions and indications
ST 41 is an important point for many disorders of the ankle. Furthermore, it clears Stomach heat, dispels wind, clears the head, brightens the eyes and calms the mind.

Indications include: swelling and pain of the ankle and dorsum of the foot, weakness of the lower limbs, burning pain in the stomach, thirst, constipation and abdominal distension, headache, redness and pain of the eyes, and vertigo, dizziness, mental restlessness and insomnia.

This location is very important because it is where the gravity line passes through the ankle. As such, it is a reference point for ensuring vertical alignment in standing Qigong practice.

Main Areas—Ankle. Foot. Stomach. Head.
Main Functions—Alleviates pain. Clears heat.

ST 42   Chongyang
Surging Yang

衝陽

Yuan-Source point

Myotome	None – in superficial tissue
Dermatome	L5

Location
On the highest point of the dorsum of the foot at the pulse of the dorsalis pedis artery, approximately midway between the tuberosity of the navicular bone and the base of the fifth metatarsal bone. Situated in the small depression between the bases of the second and third metatarsal bones and the lateral and intermediate cuneiform bones, just lateral to the tendon of the extensor digitorum communis that attaches to the second toe.

To aid location, palpate softly with the fingertip to ascertain the gentle pulse of the dorsalis pedis artery.

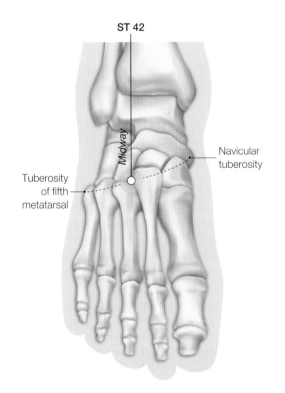

ST 42

Midway

Navicular tuberosity

Tuberosity of fifth metatarsal

The dorsalis pedis artery causes this location to be sensitive to all forms of treatment.

Needling
0.2 to 0.5 cun perpendicular insertion. The needle tip should enter the small gap between the bones.

Actions and indications
Although ST 42 is the yuan-source point and therefore tonifies the Stomach and Spleen Qi, it is not as commonly employed for this purpose as other points (such as ST 36, SP 6 and SP 3). It can, however, be useful in such cases to treat a variety of *digestive symptoms* such as poor appetite, vomiting, loose stools and epigastric pain.

ST 42 can also be used to *calm the mind and treat poor concentration, tiredness, weakness, exhaustion, mental restlessness and fright*. As a local point, ST 42 also helps *relieve channel blockages and alleviate pain*. Symptoms include: deviation of the mouth, facial pain, toothache, and atrophy, swelling or pain of the dorsum of the foot and toes.

Traditionally, the *strength and quality of the pulse* at ST 42 (dorsalis pedis artery) is considered to indicate the state of the body's Yang Qi, whereas the ST 8 pulse (temporal artery) is related to the state of the jing. The pulse at Renying ST 9 (carotid artery) discloses the general prognosis. Also, the pulses at the wrist (radial artery at LU 9 and LU 8), neck (common carotid at ST 9) and dorsum of the foot (dorsalis pedis artery at ST 42) are known as the Heaven, Earth and Man pulses.

> **Main Areas**—Stomach. Middle jiao. Foot. Mind.
> **Main Functions**—Tonifies Qi and Yang. Alleviates swelling and pain.

ST 43   Xiangu
Sunken Valley

陷谷

Shu-Stream point, Wood point

Myotome	S2/S3
Dermatome	L5

Location
On the dorsum of the foot, in the depression just proximal to the MTP joint, between the second and third metatarsal bones.

Alternative location
In some cases a stronger reaction can be achieved at a more proximal location, further up the channel. Also, in the case of swelling of the joint, it can't be treated at the classic location and using a more proximal site can be very helpful in alleviating these symptoms.

Needling
0.3 to 0.5 cun perpendicular insertion.

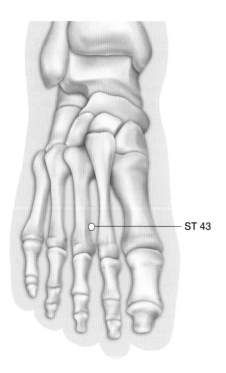

ST 43

Actions and indications
ST 43 is rarely used for interior Stomach disorders, because other Stomach channel points are more effective. It is, however, useful for *regional disorders* such as injury and pain of the dorsum of the foot and metatarsals.

> **Main Area**—Foot.
> **Main Functions**—Regulates Qi and Blood. Alleviates swelling and pain.

ST 44   Neiting
Inner Court

內庭

Ying-Spring point, Water point
Heavenly Star point

Myotome	None – in superficial tissue
Dermatome	L5

Location
Between the second and third toes, proximal to the margin of the web (at the end of the crease), between the MTP joints.

This is a strong point and care should be taken not to over-stimulate it in deficient patients.

Needling
0.3 to 0.5 cun perpendicular insertion between the second and third MTP joints.

Actions and indications
ST 44 is a *dynamic and widely employed point*. Its primary functions are to *clear heat from the Stomach, dispel wind, clear heat from the face and head, and calm the mind*. It also clears damp heat from the Stomach and eliminates food stagnation.

Indications include: various digestive disorders, burning epigastric pain, abdominal distension and pain, diarrhoea, dysentery, enteritis, constipation, abdominal rumbling, gastritis and heartburn, halitosis, bleeding gums, mouth abscesses,

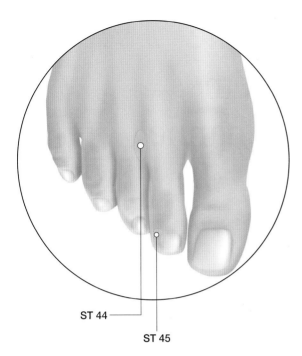

ST 44 ———

ST 45

ST 45 Lidui
Running Point

厲兑

Jing-Well point, Metal point

Myotome	None – in superficial tissue
Dermatome	L5

Location
On the lateral side of the second toe, 0.1 cun proximal to the corner of the nail. At the intersection of two lines following the lateral border of the nail and the base of the nail.

Needling
0.1 cun perpendicular insertion.

Actions and indications
ST 45 has *similar functions to the other jing-well points as it calms the mind and resuscitates consciousness.* Additionally, it is employed to *clear heat from the Yang Ming and Stomach channel* and to *clear the eyes and head.*

Indications include: facial paralysis, deviation of the mouth and swelling of the face, sinusitis, epistaxis, toothache, tonsillitis and pharyngitis, abdominal distension and fullness, and mental restlessness, agitation, insomnia, epilepsy, fainting and coma.

periodontitis, dental caries and toothache, headache due to Stomach heat (particularly frontal headache), epistaxis, conjunctivitis and red, swollen or painful eyes, chills and fever, febrile diseases, thirst, facial pain or paralysis, trigeminal neuralgia and deviation of the mouth, and pain along the course of the channel.

As a local point, *ST 44 helps* alleviate swelling, stiffness and pain of the dorsum of the foot, MTP joints and toes.

> **Main Areas**—Stomach. Digestive system. Face. Mouth. Eyes. Head. MTP joints and toes.
> **Main Functions**—Clears heat and damp heat. Benefits the digestive system. Alleviates swelling and pain.

> **Main Areas**—Face. Eyes. Mouth. Stomach. Stomach channel. Mind.
> **Main Function**—Resuscitates.

155

11 Points of the Leg Tai Yin Spleen Channel

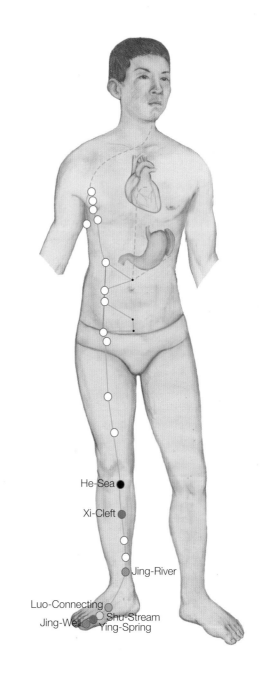

足太陰脾經穴

He-Sea
Xi-Cleft
Jing-River
Luo-Connecting
Jing-Well
Shu-Stream
Ying-Spring

General	Beginning at the medial edge of the nail of the hallux, the Spleen channel runs upwards across the medial longitudinal arch, around the medial malleolus and up through the medial aspect of the tibia to cross the knee. Ascending the medial quadriceps, at the upper thigh it continues up the anterior aspect of the lower trunk, in the line of the ASIS, veering laterally as it reaches the anterior chest, with SP 20 lying just below LU 1.
	It then has an important *descent* into the sixth or seventh intercostal space, mid-axillary line, thus finishing on the lateral rib cage.
	The channel has 21 points. It is grouped with the Stomach under the Earth in five-element theory.
More specifically	SP 1 is situated on the medial edge of the nail of the hallux, and the channel runs medially backwards across the foot, following the longitudinal arch. Ascending just in front of the medial malleolus (SP 5 being the medial eye of the ankle joint), it then moves behind the tibia to follow the flexor digitorum longus along the medial border.
	It travels upwards to the pes anserinus on the medial tibial condyle and crosses the knee, heading into the vastus medialis. Continuing up the medial quadriceps, SP 12 and SP 13 are anterior to the anatomical hip, and the channel then meets and sends a branch to the Conception Vessel (at CV3, CV 4 and then also CV 10). Branches from these points travel upwards to connect with the Spleen and Stomach (the Yin-Yang pair).
	SP 14–16 lie on the lateral aspect of the abdomen, under the rib cage, with SP 17–20 lateral to the nipple and sitting across the pectoralis major as a marker. SP 20 is just below LU 1 on the chest, but, importantly, the channel descends to the mid-axillary line within the sixth and seventh intercostal space, finishing at SP 21, which is a point of note.
Area covered	Medial foot, ankle, knee. Hip joint. Lateral abdomen. Lateral chest.
Areas affected with treatment	Stomach and Spleen digestive function. Emotional states causing digestive upset. Gynaecological conditions. Lower limb issues with ankle, knee and hip.
Key points	SP 3, SP 4, SP 5, SP 6, SP 9, SP 10, SP 21.

SP 1   Yinbai

隱白

Hidden White

Jing-Well point, Wood point
Third Ghost point

Myotome	None – superficial tissue
Dermatome	L5

Location
On the medial dorsal aspect of the big toe, approximately 0.1 cun proximal to the corner of the nail.

To aid location, it is the intersection of two lines following the medial border and the base of the nail.

Needling
0.1 cun perpendicular insertion.

Actions and indications
SP 1 is possibly the most important point to *arrest bleeding* anywhere in the body because it aids the Spleen function of *holding Blood* and *raising Qi*. It also *invigorates Blood* and *dispels stasis*.

It is particularly useful in the treatment of *disorders of the lower jiao*, including: excessive or abnormal uterine bleeding, dysmenorrhoea,

157

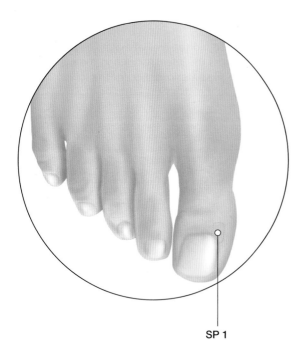

SP 1

threatened miscarriage, postpartum haemorrhage, chronic leucorrhoea, prolapse of the uterus or rectum, haemorrhoids, blood in the stools or urine, abdominal distension, and varicose veins. For all the above disorders, SP 1 is usually treated with moxibustion.

Moxibustion at SP 1 has also been employed as a first aid procedure to arrest haemorrhage anywhere in the body.

SP 1 *clears the Heart and calms the mind*, in common with the other jing-well points, and can be

used in such cases as: dizziness, vertigo, fainting, loss of consciousness, depression, and insomnia.

> **Main Areas**—Uterus. Blood vessels. Mind.
> **Main Functions**—Arrests bleeding. Lifts Qi. Calms and clears the mind.

SP 2   Dadu

Great Pool

Ying-Spring point, Fire point

Myotome	None – superficial tissue
Dermatome	L5

Location
Located on the medial aspect of the big toe, in the small depression distal and inferior to the first MTP joint.

To aid location, it is at the junction of the skin of the plantar and dorsal surface, between the flesh and bone.

Needling
0.3 to 0.5 cun perpendicular insertion.

Actions and indications
Although SP 2 is not as commonly used as other Spleen points, it can be effective to *harmonise the*

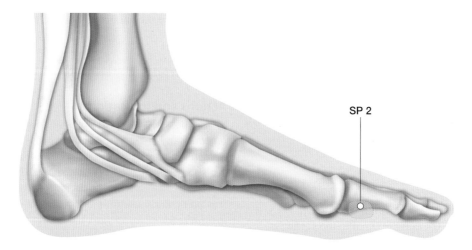

SP 2

Spleen and Stomach and resolve dampness and clear heat, particularly from the digestive system. Symptoms include: chills and fever, stomach ache, vomiting, diarrhoea, abdominal distension, chest pain, and insomnia.

Additionally, moxibustion helps *warm Yang* and *lift sinking Qi.*

As a local point, SP 2 is useful in cases of swelling, pain, arthritis, gout, deformity or injury of the first MTP joint.

> **Main Areas**—MTP joint. Toe. Digestive system.
> **Main Functions**—Clears dampness and heat.

SP 3   Taibai
Great White

Shu-Stream point, Earth point
Yuan-Source point

Myotome	L5/S1
Dermatome	L5

Location
On the medial aspect of the foot, in the small depression proximal and inferior to the head of the first metatarsal bone, at the junction of the skin of the plantar and dorsal surface. Between the abductor hallucis tendon and first metatarsal bone. In its deep position lies the flexor hallucis brevis muscle.

To aid location, slide your fingertip proximally over the medial aspect of the first MTP joint into the depression formed between the flesh and bone.

Needling
0.3 to 1 cun perpendicular insertion under the bone.

Actions and indications
SP 3 is a major point to *fortify the Spleen* and *Earth element*. It *boosts transformation and movement*, *regulates the middle jiao* and *benefits the digestive system*. It is one of the most important points to *resolve dampness, reduce swelling* and *clear damp heat*, and *promotes Qi and Blood circulation*, *relieves stasis* and *alleviates pain.*

Common indications include: tiredness, weakness and heaviness of the limbs and body, sweet cravings and tendency to weight gain and obesity, fluid retention, cellulite, and oedema, hypothyroidism, diabetes, abdominal distension, pain or rumbling, stomach ache, heartburn, indigestion, poor appetite, nausea and vomiting, loose stools, diarrhoea, gastroenteritis, dysentery, candidiasis, blood in the stools, constipation and haemorrhoids, leucorrhoea, vaginitis, frequent urination, dysuria and cystitis, headache, productive cough, and fluid in the lungs.

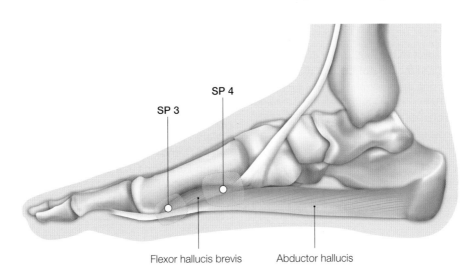

SP 4

SP 3

Flexor hallucis brevis   Abductor hallucis

Additionally, SP 3 helps the *Spleen 'House Thought' (Yi)* and improves mental functions and concentration in such cases as: poor memory, sleepiness, feeling of heaviness and muzziness, depression, mental confusion, arteriosclerosis, and declining mental faculties.

Another usage of SP 3 is to strengthen the muscles, limbs and spine and treat chronic lower backache, spinal disorders and weakness, atrophy or paralysis of the limbs.

As a local point, it may be used to treat gout, arthritis or injury of the big toe and first MTP joint.

> **Main Areas**—Digestive system. Intestines. Urinary system. Muscles. Mind.
> **Main Functions**—Transforms dampness. Tonifies Spleen Qi and Yang.

SP 4   Gongsun
Grandfather Grandson
(Yellow Emperor)

Luo-Connecting point
Opening point of the Chong Mai

Myotome	L5/S1
Dermatome	L5

Location
On the medial aspect of the foot, in the depression distal and inferior to the base of the first metatarsal bone, at the junction of the skin of the plantar and dorsal surface. Between the abductor hallucis tendon and the first metatarsal bone. In its deep position lies the flexor hallucis brevis muscle.

To aid location, slide your fingertip proximally from SP 3 along the shaft of the first metatarsal, into the depression formed between the muscle and the bone.

Needling
0.3 to 1.5 cun perpendicular insertion, under the bone.

Actions and indications
SP 4 is a very important and widely used point for a variety of therapeutic purposes. Its primary functions are to *regulate the Chong Mai* and *dispel stasis* from the three jiao. Additionally, it is extensively employed to *regulate the middle jiao, boost the Stomach and Spleen* and *augment Blood production*, and helps *transform dampness* and *dispel swelling*.

In relation to the *digestive system*, SP 4 has been widely employed in the treatment of: chronic or acute abdominal pain, distension, fullness or heaviness, abdominal rumbling, flatulence, constipation, irritable bowel syndrome, Crohn's disease, gastroenteritis, dysentery, epigastric pain, gastritis, hiatus hernia, heartburn, oesophagitis, nausea, vomiting, and morning sickness during pregnancy. SP 4 can also be useful to *alleviate nausea* and digestive symptoms caused by heavy medication, including chemotherapy, particularly in combination with PC 6 and ST 36.

SP 4 is very *important in gynaecology* because it regulates menstruation and benefits the uterus.

Indications include: irregular menstruation, premenstrual syndrome, dysmenorrhoea, endometriosis, polycystic ovarian syndrome, amenorrhoea, excessive menstrual bleeding, and infertility.

SP 4 is very important to *relieve stasis from the chest, regulate the Heart and calm the mind*. It has been extensively employed to treat: chronic or acute pain and heaviness of the chest, angina pectoris, vascular disease, anaemia and psychosomatic disorders including insomnia and depression.

> **Main Areas**—Stomach. Abdomen. Uterus. Heart. Mind.
> **Main Functions**—Opens the Chong Mai. Tonifies the Spleen and Stomach. Nourishes Blood. Regulates Qi. Dispels Blood stasis. Benefits menstruation.

SP 5   Shangqiu
Metal Hill

Jing-River point, Metal point

Myotome	None – in muscle space
Dermatome	L4/L5

Location
In the depression anterior and inferior to the medial malleolus, midway between the navicular tuberosity and the prominence of the medial malleolus.

Needling
0.3 to 0.5 cun perpendicular insertion.
1 to 1.5 cun oblique insertion toward ST 41.

Actions and indications
SP 5 is mainly used for *disorders of the ankle and foot* as well as the leg and knee in combination with other local and adjacent points.

However, it also effectively treats interior conditions by virtue of its functions of *boosting the Spleen and Stomach, drying dampness* and *regulating Qi and Blood.*

Symptoms include: abdominal distension and pain, diarrhoea, abdominal rumbling, stomach ache, indigestion, heartburn, vomiting, constipation, haemorrhoids, heaviness of the limbs, oedema, breast pain, infertility, dysmenorrhoea, and endometriosis.

SP 5 has also been traditionally used to treat a variety of other disorders, including: tiredness and lethargy, depression, insomnia, excessive thinking, chills and fever, jaundice, stiffness of the tongue, convulsions, and swelling of the throat.

> **Main Areas**—Ankle. Abdomen.
> **Main Functions**—Regulates Qi and Blood. Dries dampness. Benefits the lower jiao.

SP 6   Sanyinjiao
Three Yin Intersection

Intersection of the Liver and Kidney on the Spleen channel

Myotome	L5/S1/S2
Dermatome	L4

Location
In the soft depression 3 cun superior to the prominence of the medial malleolus, posterior to the medial tibial border. Situated in the flexor digitorum longus muscle and more deeply, in the tibialis

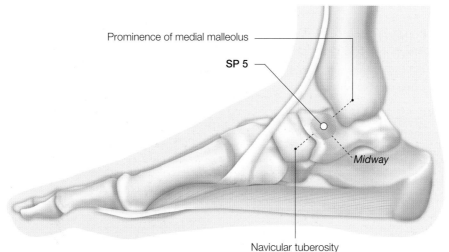

Prominence of medial malleolus

SP 5

Midway

Navicular tuberosity

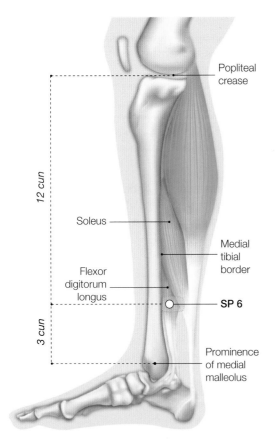

Popliteal crease

12 cun

Soleus

Flexor digitorum longus

3 cun

Medial tibial border

SP 6

Prominence of medial malleolus

Needling

0.5 to 2 cun perpendicular insertion.
2 to 3 cun perpendicular insertion to join with GB 39.
0.3 to 1.5 cun insertion in a slightly posterior or proximal direction.

Actions and indications

SP 6 is one of the top most commonly used points and is of utmost importance in any treatment aiming to *nourish Blood and Yin, calm and cool the body and mind and strengthen the Spleen, Liver* and *Kidneys*, whose channels converge here.

Additionally, SP 6 is important to *regulate Qi and Blood, dispel stasis* and *alleviate pain*.

SP 6 is an important point to benefit the *digestive system* and is widely employed to *resolve dampness* and *damp heat*, particularly from the middle and lower jiao. It is extensively employed in cases of: poor appetite and digestion, stomach ache, abdominal rumbling, abdominal distension and pain, loose or unformed stools, diarrhoea, gastroenteritis, constipation, and irritable bowel syndrome.

It is also of primary importance in gynaecology because it *regulates the uterus and menstruation* and *induces labour*.

Indications include: dysmenorrhoea, amenorrhoea, irregular or delayed menstruation, delayed and difficult labour, difficulty in discharging the placenta, infertility, frigidity, leucorrhoea, genital itching or pain, dysuria, frequent urination, cystitis, urethritis, and incontinence.

SP 6 *cools and nourishes Yin and calms the mind* and is beneficial in such cases as: dizziness, tinnitus and vertigo, headache, feeling of heat, skin diseases, dry mouth and throat and night sweats, hypertension, palpitations, and restlessness, insomnia and depression.

SP 6 has also been widely employed in a variety of other disorders, including: chronic tiredness and exhaustion, blurred vision, tinnitus, emaciation, obesity, bulimia, swelling, oedema, diabetes, and liver disease.

posterior muscle. In its deep position, it is situated in the flexor hallucis longus muscle.

To aid location, SP 6 is approximately one hand-width (the patient's, not the clinician's) proximal to the medial malleolus. Palpate the large, trench-like depression (often larger and softer in women) gently and carefully to ascertain the most reactive point(s).

Alternative locations

It could be considered that a slightly more anterior location affects the Liver more, a posterior one the Kidney, and a central one the Spleen.

SP 6 can be extremely sensitive and painful, particularly during the premenstrual phase, so not treat during pregnancy and heavy menstrual bleeding; strong stimulation can bring on menstruation early, particularly in Spleen-deficient patients.

As a *local point* it effectively treats weakness, atrophy or paralysis of the lower limb and oedema or pain of the ankle or foot.

> **Main Areas**—Entire body. Abdomen. Uterus. Liver. Spleen. Kidney.
> **Main Functions**—Boosts the Spleen and Stomach. Transforms dampness. Nourishes Blood and Yin. Calms the mind. Dispels stasis. Benefits menstruation. Promotes labour.

SP 7   Lougu
Leaking Valley

Myotome	L5/S1
Dermatome	L4

Location
3 cun proximal to SP 6, in a depression immediately posterior to the medial tibial border.

Needling
0.5 to 1.5 cun perpendicular insertion.

Actions and indications
SP 7 is not a very commonly used point, although it has been traditionally employed to *fortify the Spleen, promote urination, resolve dampness* and *reduce swelling*.

Symptoms include: abdominal distension, abdominal rumbling, dysuria, urinary retention, arthritis, and swelling and cold pain of the leg and knee.

SP 8   Diji
Earth's Cure

Xi-Cleft point

Myotome	L4/L5/S1
Dermatome	L4

Location
5 cun inferior to the knee crease, in the depression posterior to the medial tibial border. Between the soleus muscle and the tibia.

The depression of SP 8 is formed between the medial tibial border (just superior to the medial end of the soleal line), the soleus muscle (inferiorly), and the insertion of the popliteus muscle (superiorly).

To aid location, SP 8 is one third of the distance between the popliteal (knee) crease and the prominence of the medial malleolus, or 3 cun (one hand-width) distal to SP 9.

SP 8 is a very powerful point and should be stimulated lightly in deficient patients. Also, strong treatment at this location can bring on early menstruation, particularly in Spleen-deficient patients.

Needling
0.5 to 2 cun perpendicular insertion.

Actions and indications
SP 8 is an important and powerful point to *resolve stasis, alleviate pain* and *regulate the flow of Qi and Blood* in the abdomen and along the entire course of the Spleen channel. In common with the other xi-cleft points, it helps to *moderate acute conditions* and *arrest bleeding*.

It is also very important to *regulate the uterus and menstruation*. Common indications include: abdominal distension and pain, diarrhoea, dysmenorrhoea, excessive or abnormal uterine bleeding, irregular menstruation, ovarian cysts, uterine fibroids, and endometriosis.

SP 8 has been employed to *harmonise the Spleen* and *resolve dampness* from the middle and lower jiao. Symptoms include: abdominal distension and pain, poor appetite, diarrhoea, rectal bleeding, haemorrhoids, spermatorrhoea, retention of urine, and oedema.

In addition, SP 8 treats *acute pain* anywhere along the channel, especially in the knees and legs.

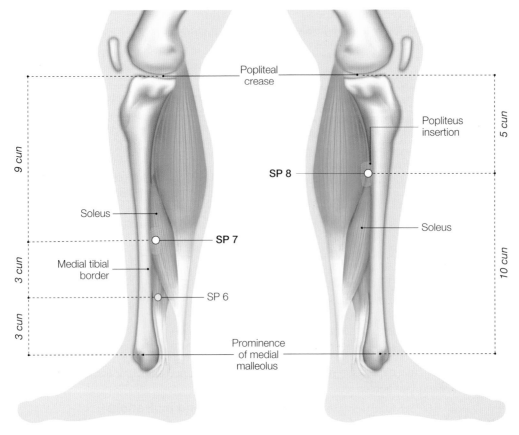

Main Areas—Uterus. Abdomen. Knee.
Main Functions—Invigorates Blood.
Dispels stasis. Regulates menstruation.

SP 9   Yinlingquan   陰陵泉
Yin Mound Spring

He-Sea point, Water point

Myotome	L4/L5/S1
Dermatome	L5

Location
In the depression below the medial tibial
condyle, between the medial tibial border and the
gastrocnemius muscle. The popliteus muscle is
situated in its deep position. Locate with the knee
flexed.

To aid location, run your fingertip upward along the
groove posterior to the medial border of the tibia
until it naturally comes to a halt at the lower border
of the medial tibial condyle.

Needling
0.5 to 1 cun perpendicular insertion along the
posterior tibial border towards, or deeper, to join
with GB 34.

Actions and indications
SP 9 is one of the most powerful points to *open the
water passages, drain dampness* and *regulate the
lower jiao*, particularly in relation to the *intestines*
and the *urogenital systems*.

Its main indications include: dysuria, cystitis,
urethritis, urinary retention, incontinence,
leucorrhoea, irregular menstruation, abdominal
distension, abdominal pain, diarrhoea, undigested
food in the stools, mucus in the stools, dysentery,
enteritis, oedema, and swelling of the lower limbs
and abdomen.

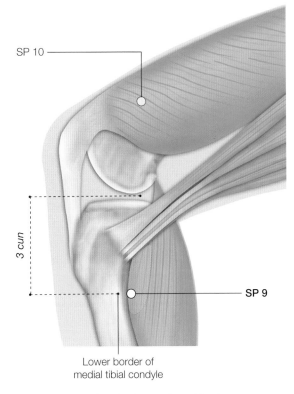

SP 10

3 cun

SP 9

Lower border of
medial tibial condyle

and level with ST 34. Locate and treat with the knee flexed.

To aid location, place the (left) palm over the (right) knee so that the fingers are on the lateral side and point upward. The tip of the thumb will lie on SP 10 (approximately).

Needling
0.5 to 1.5 cun perpendicular insertion.

Actions and indications
SP 10 is a major point for *many disorders of the Blood*. It *regulates and cools Blood, removes stasis* and *arrests bleeding*, with its broadest application in *gynaecological and skin diseases*. It helps *regulate menstruation* and dispel stasis from the uterus, as well as having a powerful soothing effect on the skin, particularly if there is inflammation and itching.

Common indications include: abnormal uterine bleeding, irregular menstruation, excessive

It is also very effectively employed in the treatment of *channel disorders*, including: pain or swelling at the medial aspect of the knee, pain of the thigh and lumbago.

> **Main Areas**—Lower jiao. Urogenital system.
> Intestines. Abdomen. Knee.
> **Main Functions**—Drains dampness. Regulates the lower jiao. Alleviates pain.

SP 10 Xuehai
Sea of Blood

血海

Myotome	L2–L4
Dermatome	L3

Location
In the depression on the protuberance of the vastus medialis muscle, 2 cun proximal to the medial superior border of the patella. Directly above SP 9

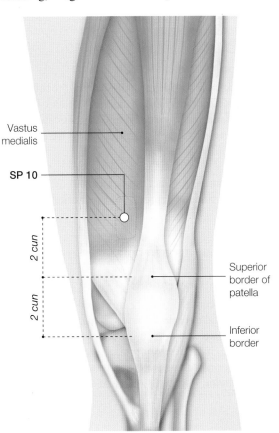

Vastus
medialis

SP 10

2 cun

2 cun

Superior
border of
patella

Inferior
border

menstruation, dysmenorrhoea, amenorrhoea, haematuria, genital sores, dermatitis, inflamed or itchy skin, ulceration, eczema, psoriasis, urticaria, herpes zoster, allergies, and other skin disorders.

Additionally, SP 10 can be employed to *dispel dampness* and treat symptoms such as dysuria, leucorrhoea and nausea.

As a *local point*, SP 10 can be used to treat pain of the medial side of the knee and thigh.

> **Main Areas**—Skin. Gynaecological system. Genitals.
> **Main Functions**—Invigorates and cools Blood. Alleviates itching. Dispels dampness.

SP 11　Jimen
Separation Gate

箕門

Myotome	L2–L4
Dermatome	L2/L3

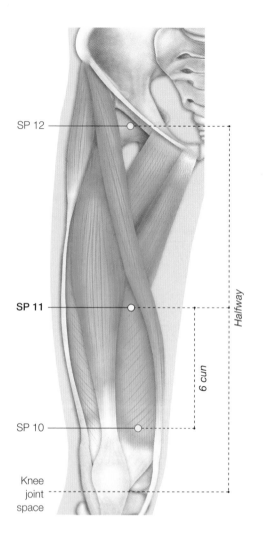

Location
At the midpoint of the medial aspect of the thigh, in a depression between the anterior border of the sartorius and vastus medialis muscles. Locate 6 cun proximal to SP 10, or 8 cun proximal to the upper medial border of the patella.

To aid location, contract the sartorius to define its border and find the depression just anterior to it.

Needling
0.5 to 1.5 cun perpendicular insertion.

Actions and indications
SP 11 has been traditionally employed for urinary disorders and to drain dampness and clear heat from the lower jiao. Although it is not a very commonly used point, it can be useful for genitourinary problems since it opens the energy toward the genital region and lower abdomen, either as a

supplementary point or as an alternative, when other points have not been effective.

Nevertheless, SP 11 can be very useful to regulate Qi and blood and activate the channel in cases of weakness, atrophy, paralysis and other disorders such as medial thigh pain, meralgia paraesthetica, anteromedial knee pain, buckling knee, and as a distal point for problems of the inguinal region or anterior hip.

> **Main Areas**—Medial thigh. Knee. Inguinal area. Genitourinary system. Lower abdomen.
> **Main Functions**—Activates the channel and strengthens the lower limbs. Alleviates pain. Opens the genitourinary area. Drains dampness and clears heat.

SP 12 Chongmen
Surging Gate

衝門

Intersection of the Liver and Yin Wei Mai on the Spleen channel

Myotome	None
Dermatome	L1

Location
On the inguinal groove, in the depression of the saphenous hiatus, just lateral to the femoral artery, approximately 3.5 cun lateral to CV 2.

To aid location, SP 12 is slightly more than one hand-width lateral to the anterior midline. It is about one finger-width lateral to the palpable femoral artery and approximately 1 cun lateral to LR 12.

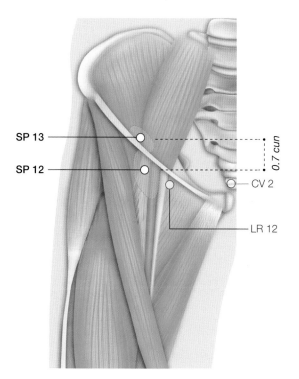

SP 13
SP 12
0.7 cun
CV 2
LR 12

Important note
Traditionally, SP 12 was treated by moxibustion rather than needling, because the latter was considered dangerous. However, moxibustion is not recommended at SP 12, except in very rare cases, and direct moxibustion is contraindicated. Pressure techniques are easier to employ and are therefore more readily recommended.

Needling
0.5 to 1.2 cun perpendicular insertion, on the lateral side of the femoral artery. See also LR 12.

For other regional anatomy, see LR 12.

Actions and indications
Although SP 12 is not very commonly used due to its sensitive location, it is a *very effective point to regulate Qi and Blood circulation, dispel stasis* and *alleviate pain*, and in common with LR 12, it *has a very powerful effect on the entire lower limb*.

Both these points have similar effects on the entire blood circulation and are indicated for *disorders of the lower limbs, groin and lower abdomen*. Indications include: poor circulation, vascular disorders, cold legs and feet, hernia, testicular pain or swelling, impotence, dysmenorrhoea, and uterine prolapse.

SP 12 also helps *drain dampness* and *regulate urination* and has been used to treat: dysuria, urinary retention, or pain, swelling and cold in the lower abdomen.

As a *local point*, SP 12 can be used to treat muscle strain and sciatica. It is also especially indicated for meralgia paraesthetica since it is situated exactly along the course of the femoral nerve.

> **Main Areas**—Lower limbs. Groin. Blood Vessels.
> **Main Functions**—Improves Qi and Blood circulation. Dispels cold from the channels. Alleviates pain.

SP 13 Fushe
Bowel Abode

府舍

Intersection of the Liver and Yin Wei Mai on the Spleen channel

Myotome	T7–L1
Dermatome	T12

Location
Approximately 0.7 cun superior and slightly lateral to SP 12, 4 cun lateral to the anterior midline.

Needling
0.5 to 1 cun perpendicular insertion.

Actions and indications
Although SP 13 is not a very commonly employed point, it can be useful in cases of lower abdominal or groin pain, tightness and hernia. Its primary function is to regulate and relax the intestines.

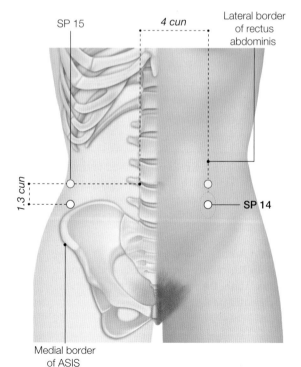

SP 15
4 cun
Lateral border of rectus abdominis
1.3 cun
SP 14
Medial border of ASIS

> **Main Areas**—Lower abdomen. Groin. Intestine.
> **Main Function**—Regulates Qi in the intestines.

SP 14 Fujie
Abdominal Stagnation

腹結

Myotome	T7–L1
Dermatome	T10/T11

Location
Approximately 1.3 cun inferior to SP 15 and 4 cun lateral to the anterior midline.

SP 15 may also be located slightly further laterally, at a distance of 4.5 cun from the anterior midline.

Needling
1 to 1.5 cun perpendicular insertion.

Actions and indications
SP 14 is not very commonly used, although treatment can be successfully applied here for *similar purposes to SP 15*. Its primary functions are to *regulate the intestines, dispel cold* from the lower jiao and *descend rebellious Qi* from the chest. It is particularly indicated for diarrhoea and abdominal tightness and pain.

> **Main Areas**—Intestines. Abdomen.
> **Main Functions**—Regulates Qi in the intestines. Descends rebellious Qi.

SP 15 Daheng
Great Horizontal

大橫

Intersection of the Yin Wei Mai on the Spleen channel

Myotome	T7–L1
Dermatome	T10

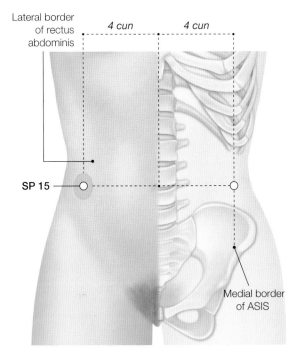

Lateral border of rectus abdominis

4 cun   4 cun

SP 15

Medial border of ASIS

SP 15 has also been used for an assortment of other symptoms and disorders, including: weakness and heaviness of the limbs and body, chronic tiredness, heat or cold in the abdomen, and depression.

> **Main Areas**—Intestines. Abdomen.
> **Main Functions**—Tonifies the Spleen. Regulates the intestines. Treats constipation.

SP 16   Fuai
Abdominal Suffering

Intersection of the Yin Wei Mai on the Spleen channel

Myotome	T7–L1
Dermatome	T8/T9

Location

In the large depression directly below the costal arch, lateral to the margin of the rectus abdominis muscle. Approximately 4 cun lateral to the midline, 3 cun above SP 15, level with CV 11 and ST 22.

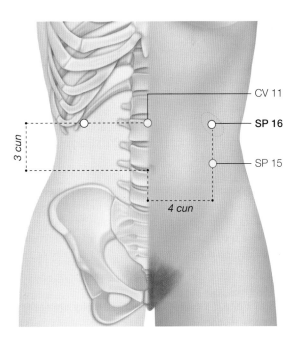

CV 11
SP 16
SP 15
3 cun
4 cun

Location

4 cun lateral to the centre of the umbilicus, in a large and soft shallow depression lateral to the margin of the rectus abdominis muscle.

To aid location, the 4 cun can be measured from the medial border of the ASIS. SP 15 is usually situated on the long crease crossing the centre of the abdomen horizontally.

Needling

0.5 to 1.5 cun perpendicular insertion.

Actions and indications

SP 15 is a very useful point for the treatment of many *disorders of the intestines and abdomen*. Its functions are similar to those of ST 25 (the front-mu point of the Large Intestine), although it is used more often in the treatment of *chronic deficiency conditions*, particularly *constipation*.

It has been extensively employed to treat a variety of *digestive disorders*, including irritable bowel syndrome, flatulence, loose stools, chronic diarrhoea, dysentery, abdominal distension, and lower abdominal pain due to weakness of the Spleen.

SP 16 is located slightly more medially, and/or inferiorly, in patients who have a narrow costal angle.

SP 16 may also be located slightly further laterally, at a distance of 4.5 cun from the anterior midline.

Needling

0.5 to 1.5 cun perpendicular insertion.

Actions and indications

SP 16 has been traditionally employed in the treatment of digestive disorders caused by *disharmony of the Spleen and Large Intestine.*

Symptoms include: indigestion, abdominal distension and pain, periumbilical pain, abdominal rumbling, diarrhoea, dysentery, and constipation.

> **Main Areas**—Hypochondrium. Abdomen.
> **Main Function**—Harmonises the Spleen and Large Intestine.

SP 17   Shidou
Food Cavity

 食竇

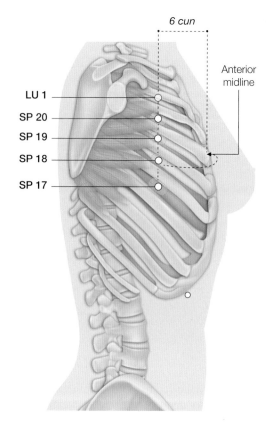

Myotome	L5/S1
Dermatome	L5

Location

Approximately 6 cun lateral to the anterior midline, three intercostal spaces below SP 20, lateral to the mammary glands.

To aid location, it is level with the sixth rib or intercostal space, depending on the individual structure of the rib cage. Most acupuncture texts describe the location of SP 17 in the fifth intercostal space, which can be misleading.

Needling

0.4 to 1 cun transverse insertion, laterally along the intercostal space.

For disorders of the breast, needle under the glands medially towards the nipple, 0.5 to 1.5 cun.

Do not needle into the mammary glands, nor deeply, because this poses a considerable risk of puncturing the lung and inducing a pneumothorax.

Actions and indications

SP 17 was traditionally considered an important point to treat a variety of ailments, including postpartum abdominal distension, insufficient lactation, ascites, jaundice, malaria, and urinary retention.

Its indications emphasise *digestive disorders* and *food retention* caused by *dysfunction of the Spleen.* Symptoms include: indigestion, nausea, vomiting, inability to eat, fullness of the chest and abdomen, heartburn, difficulty swallowing, and stomach ache.

Additionally, moxibustion at this location was considered to *cure life-threatening conditions.*

In the modern-day practice, however, it is seldom used for these purposes and is mainly indicated for *disorders of the ribs and mammary glands*, including: rib pain, intercostal neuralgia, mastitis, and fibrocystic breast disease.

Main Areas—Chest. Ribs. Breast.
Main Function—Regulates Qi and Blood.

SP 18   Tianxi
Celestial Cleft

Myotome	C5–T1
Dermatome	T4

Location
Approximately 2 cun lateral to the nipple, two intercostal spaces below SP 20, lateral to the mammary glands.

To aid location, it is approximately level with the nipple. Depending on the size and shape of the mammary glands, SP 18 may have to be located further laterally. Most acupuncture texts describe the location of SP 18 in the fourth intercostal space.

Needling
0.4 to 1 cun transverse insertion laterally, following the contour of the rib cage.
For breast pain and fibrocystic breast disease, needle medially under the mammary glands, towards the nipple, 0.5 to 1.5 cun.

Do not needle into the mammary glands, nor deeply, because this poses a considerable risk of puncturing the lung.

Actions and indications
SP 18 is not very commonly employed, although it can be useful in the treatment of *disorders of the breast, ribs and thoracic cage*. It helps stimulate lactation and treats tightness, pain and constriction of the chest.

Main Areas—Chest. Ribs. Breast.
Main Function—Regulates Qi and Blood.

SP 19   Xiongxiang
Chest Village

Myotome	C5–T1
Dermatome	T3

Location
Lateral and superior to the nipple, one intercostal space below SP 20, lateral to the mammary glands.

Needling
0.4 to 1 cun transverse insertion laterally, following the contour of the rib cage.

Actions and indications
SP 19 can be useful in the treatment of *disorders of the breast, ribs and thoracic cage*. It helps stimulate lactation and treats tightness, pain and constriction of the chest.

Main Areas—Chest. Ribs. Breast.
Main Function—Regulates Qi and Blood.

SP 20   Zhourong
Complete Nourishment

Myotome	C5–T1
Dermatome	T2

Location
On the chest, one intercostal space below LU 1, approximately 6 cun lateral to the anterior midline.

To aid location, it is inferior to the insertion of the pectoralis minor muscle, depending on the individual structure of the thoracic cage. Most acupuncture texts describe the location of SP 20 in the second intercostal space.

Needling

0.4 to 1 cun oblique or transverse insertion laterally, following the contour of the rib cage.

Do not needle deeply, because this poses a considerable risk of puncturing the lung.

Actions and indications

SP 20 is not a very commonly used point, although it can be useful to treat *disorders of the chest and ribs*, including: intercostal neuralgia, lymphadenopathy, swelling and pain of the breasts, dyspnoea, cough, and lung diseases.

> **Main Areas**—Chest. Ribs. Breast.
> **Main Function**—Regulates Qi and Blood.

SP 21 Dabao 大包
Great Embrace

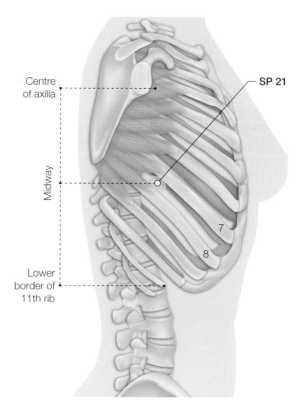

Centre of axilla

Midway

SP 21

7

8

Lower border of 11th rib

Great Luo-Connecting point of the Spleen

Myotome	C5–C8
Dermatome	T6

Location

On the mid-axillary line, midway between the centre of the axilla and the lower border of the eleventh rib. SP 21 usually falls in the seventh intercostal space, but in some cases it may be in the sixth.

To aid location, it is approximately one hand-width below the axilla.

Needling

0.3 to 0.5 cun oblique insertion laterally, following the contour of the thorax.

Do not needle deeply. This poses a considerable risk of puncturing the lung and inducing a pneumothorax.

Actions and indications

Although SP 21 is not a very commonly used point, it can be very effective to *invigorate Blood* and *dispel stasis* and is specifically indicated to *treat pain, of any cause or location*, which does not respond to any other treatment.

It is also indicated for a variety of *disorders of the chest, Heart, Lungs and Spleen*, including: thoracic fullness and pain, intercostal neuralgia, rib pain, coughing, dyspnoea, circulation disorders, exhaustion, cold body and limbs, shivering, pain or flaccidity of the joints, and weakness of the limbs and body.

> **Main Areas**—Ribs. Thorax. Breast. Entire body.
> **Main Functions**—Invigorates Blood and dispels stasis. Dispels cold and warms the body. Alleviates pain.

12 Points of the Arm Shao Yin Heart Channel

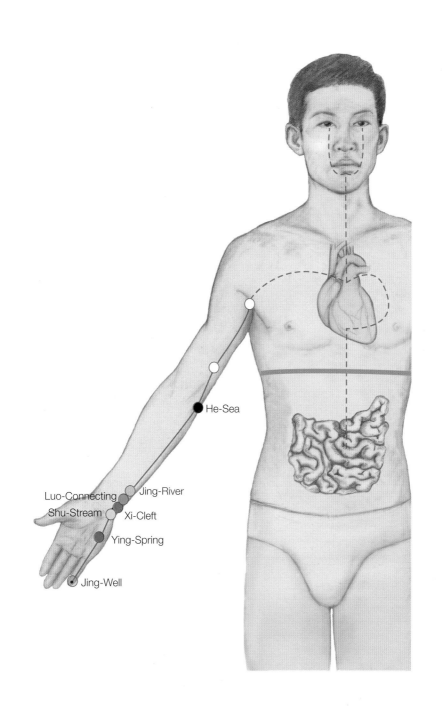

He-Sea

Luo-Connecting
Jing-River
Shu-Stream
Xi-Cleft
Ying-Spring
Jing-Well

手少陰心經穴

General	The Heart channel originates in the chest but for treatment purposes emerges at the axilla and travels down the medial aspect of the arm, all the way to the tip of the little finger. Its pathway is seen clearly in cases of angina, with the spread of pain down the course of the channel. The channel has 9 points. It is grouped with the Small Intestine under the Fire element in five-element theory.
More specifically	Starting in the chest, centrally in the heart and surrounding area, it has a branch that descends to affect the Small Intestine (its Yang partner). Another branch moves upwards towards the face and can affect the oesophagus/face and cheek. It is interesting that in emotional states, to which the Heart as an organ is vulnerable, physical manifestations can often be seen with difficulty in the throat/swallowing, and also in skin conditions on the face/cheek. It is also interesting that the Chinese written character for the Heart does not give it a root in its pictogram, for 'flesh', which is found with all of the other organs. The Heart, therefore, is not considered of the flesh but more of the Spirit, and is thus treated in all mental health/emotional states. The main branch has a close association with the Lung, and then the principal meridian emerges in the axilla, next to the axillary artery. From here it travels directly to the medial epicondyle of the elbow, and continues on, medially to the wrist. HT 7 is close to the pisiform as a marker. The last part of the channel runs through the palm to finish on the radial edge of the nail of the little finger.
Area covered	Chest, face, upper abdomen, medial aspect of the arm and forearm.
Areas affected by treatment	Emotions of all kinds (the Heart is the organ that houses all aspects of the Shen). Cardiac conditions – palpitations/chest pain. Throat and speech, including stammer and loss of voice. Circulation – cold hands/feet, Raynaud's disease.
Key points	HT 3, HT 4, HT 6, HT 7.

HT 1   Jiquan
Highest Spring

Myotome	None – superficial tissue
Dermatome	T1/T2

Location
At the centre of the axilla, medial to the axillary artery. Locate and treat with the arm lifted above the head.

To aid location, palpate the lateral border of the pectoralis major muscle.

Needling
0.5 to 1 cun perpendicular insertion.

Beware anatomy in this region. In many texts this is a forbidden point to needle.

Actions and indications
Although HT 1 *is a powerful point*, it is not very commonly employed in the modern-day acupuncture practice, because needling the axilla can be dangerous.

First, it treats *disorders of the axillary area* caused by *heat and fire in the Liver or Heart*. Symptoms include: axillary pain, swelling or lumps, inflammation of the sweat glands, lymphadenopathy, excessive sweating, skin diseases, intercostal neuralgia, and mastitis.

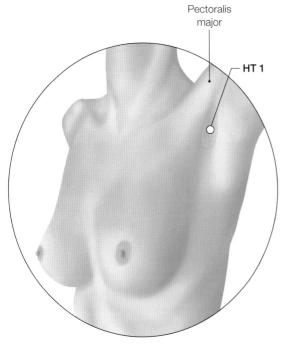

Pectoralis major

HT 1

Situated in the distinct trough of the channel pathway formed between the biceps brachii and triceps brachii muscles.

Situated along the course of the brachial artery and basilic vein.

To aid location, it is approximately one hand width proximal to HT 3. Palpate for the brachial artery pulse.

This is an extremely sensitive location due to the underlying vessels and nerves and in some traditional texts it is contraindicated to needling.

It is interesting to note that, depending on the exact site of stimulation at HT 2, the sensation can extend more toward the Pericardium channel (via the median nerve) or more toward the Heart channel (via the ulnar nerve). This is a clear demonstration of the interconnection of these two channels, which can be noticeably affected by this point. The name of this point implies a "clarifying" of the spirit, which is influenced by both these channels.

Second, HT 1 affects the *mobility of the shoulder and arm* and is used in the treatment of frozen shoulder, inability to raise the arm, paralysis of the upper limb and cold pain of the arm and elbow.

Third, it can be used for *diseases of the chest and Heart* due to heat and fire or Blood stasis, causing symptoms such as fullness and pain of the chest, hypochondrial pain, mental agitation, arrhythmia, and palpitations.

> **Main Areas**—Axilla. Shoulder. Chest. Heart.
> **Main Functions**—Clears heat. Regulates sweat. Regulates Heart Qi.

Needling
0.5 to 1 cun oblique angle or distal angle. Avoid the brachial artery.

Actions and indications
Not used freely as there are safer points to use for shoulder problems, but HT 2 can be used for difficulties in rasing the shoulder, e.g. frozen shoulder.

> **Main Areas**—Shoulder. Arm. Chest. Lungs.
> **Main Functions**—Regulates Qi. Alleviates pain.

HT 2   Qingling
Qing Spirit

Myotome	C5–C7
Dermatome	C8/T1

Location
3 cun proximal to the medial end of the transverse cubital crease. Locate with the elbow flexed.

HT 3   Shaohai
Lesser Sea

He-Sea point, Water point

Myotome	None – superficial tissue
Dermatome	C8/T1

175

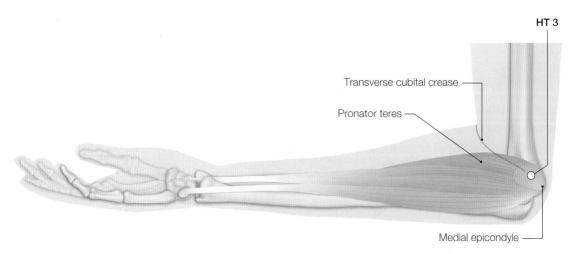

HT 3

Transverse cubital crease

Pronator teres

Medial epicondyle

Location

In the depression anterior to the medial epicondyle of the humerus, near the medial end of the transverse cubital crease. Locate and treat with the elbow flexed. Situated in the pronator teres muscle (superficially) and the brachialis muscle (deeper).

To aid location, it is approximately one finger-width diagonally anterior to the tip of the epicondyle.

Needling

0.3 to 1 cun perpendicular insertion.

Actions and indications

HT 3 is an important and widely used point to *clear both full and empty heat* and *transform phlegm while having a calming and soothing effect on the Heart and the mind.*

Indications include: insomnia, mental agitation, depression, poor memory, psychological disturbances, insanity, epilepsy, dizziness, chest pain, palpitations, lymphadenopathy, vomiting, headache, and fevers.

As a *local point*, HT 3 effectively treats pain and stiffness of the medial aspect of the elbow and forearm, tendinitis, golfer's elbow, atrophy of the medial forearm muscles (flexors), and weakness, trembling or numbness of the forearm.

> **Main Areas**—Elbow. Chest. Heart.
> **Main Functions**—Clears heat. Transforms phlegm. Soothes the Heart.

HT 4   Lingdao
Spirit Path

Jing-River point, Metal point

Myotome	C8/T1 at depth
Dermatome	C8

Location

On the radial side of the tendon of the flexor carpi ulnaris, 1.5 cun proximal to the transverse wrist crease (HT 7).

Situated in the depression between the flexor carpi ulnaris and the flexor digitorum superficialis. The pronator quadratus is situated in its deep position.

To aid location, if the tips of the four fingers are placed next to each other so that the index finger is located on HT 7, the middle finger will be on HT 6, the ring finger on HT 5, and the tip of the little finger will be on HT 4. Also, HT 4 is approximately level with LU 8.

Needling

0.3 to 0.5 cun perpendicular insertion.
0.5 to 1 cun oblique insertion distally down the channel to join with HT 5 or HT 6.

Actions and indications

HT 4 is not as commonly used as other Heart channel points; however, it does have similar

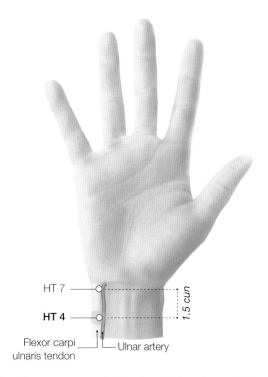

HT 7

HT 4

Flexor carpi
ulnaris tendon — Ulnar artery

1.5 cun

HT 5 Tongli

Inward Connection

Luo-Connecting point
Heavenly Star point

Myotome	None – superficial tissue
Dermatome	C8

Location
On the radial side of the tendon of the flexor carpi ulnaris, 1 cun proximal to the transverse wrist crease (HT 7).

Needling
0.3 to 0.5 cun perpendicular insertion.
0.5 to 1 cun oblique insertion proximally along the channel to join with HT 4.

Actions and indications
HT 5 is an important and widely used point to *regulate and tonify Heart Qi* and *calm the mind*. Indications include: palpitations or chest pain on exertion, spontaneous sweating, mental tiredness,

functions such as *calming the mind and regulating Heart Qi*. Having said that is one of the jing-river points which are used to indicate soft tissue/fascial tightness along the channel. Manual pressure here could be valuable in treating musculo-skeletal conditions of the arm and chest.

Treatment at HT 4 is primarily employed in *channel disorders* of the forearm, wrist and elbow. It is particularly indicated for hypertonicity of the ulnar wrist flexors, stiffness of the wrist or elbow and contraction of the fingers.

> **Main Areas**—Forearm. Wrist. Heart.
> **Main Functions**—Regulates Qi and Blood. Alleviates pain. Calms the mind.

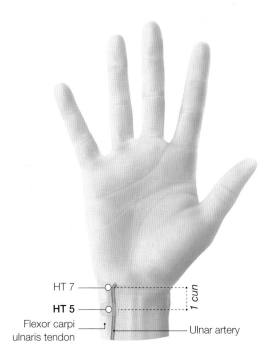

HT 7

HT 5

Flexor carpi
ulnaris tendon — Ulnar artery

1 cun

177

depression, dizziness, epilepsy, sadness, fright, shock, hysteria and even insanity.

HT 5 is also extensively used in the treatment of *disorders of the tongue and speech*, including: paralysis or stiffness of the tongue, pain of the throat, stuttering, aphasia, and other speech difficulties.

Another function of HT 5 is to *clear heat and benefit the urinary system* and lower jiao via the relationship of the Heart with the Small Intestine and Uterus. Symptoms include: dysuria, haematuria and excessive menstruation due to heat in the lower jiao.

> **Main Areas**—Heart. Tongue. Bladder. Wrist.
> **Main Functions**—Regulates and tonifies Heart Qi. Calms the mind. Benefits the tongue. Regulates speech.

HT 6   Yinxi
Yin Cleft

Xi-Cleft point

Myotome	None – superficial tissue
Dermatome	C8

Location
On the radial side of the tendon of the flexor carpi ulnaris, 0.5 cun proximal to the transverse wrist crease (HT 7).

Needling
0.3 to 0.5 cun perpendicular insertion.
0.5 to 1 cun oblique insertion distally down the channel to HT 7.

Alternative needling location
Insert the needle lateral to the tendon of the flexor carpi ulnaris, so that it passes under the tendon sheath.

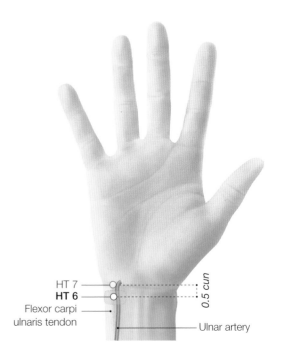

HT 7
HT 6
Flexor carpi ulnaris tendon
0.5 cun
Ulnar artery

Actions and indications
HT 6 is a *very important* and extensively used point because it effectively *clears heat and fire from the Heart and helps reduce excessive sweating and night sweating by securing the exterior*. It *cools Blood, nourishes Heart Yin and calms the mind*.

Indications include: excessive sweating, particularly night sweating, steaming bone syndrome, pain or fullness of the chest, angina pectoris, palpitations, tachycardia, arrhythmia, insomnia, mental restlessness, agitation, dizziness, epistaxis, haemoptysis, and sore throat.

HT 6, HT 4, HT 5 and HT 7 are all effective treatment sites for various *channel disorders and pain*. HT 6 is particularly indicated for acute stabbing pain along the channel pathway.

> **Main Areas**—Exterior. Heart. Mind. Wrist.
> **Main Functions**—Clears heat and fire. Calms the mind. Secures sweat.

HT 7   Shenmen
Shen Gate

神門

Shu-Stream point, Earth point
Yuan-Source point

Myotome	None – superficial tissue
Dermatome	C8

Location
In the transverse wrist flexion crease, in the small depression proximal to the pisiform bone on the radial side of the tendon of the flexor carpi ulnaris. Situated in the depression between the flexor carpi ulnaris and the flexor digitorum superficialis.

To aid location, HT 7 is level with the proximal border of the pisiform bone when the wrist is flexed. This usually falls on the distal wrist flexion crease. Also, it is approximately level with LU 9.

Needling
0.3 to 0.5 cun perpendicular insertion, directed in a slightly ulnar direction in order to avoid the ulnar artery.

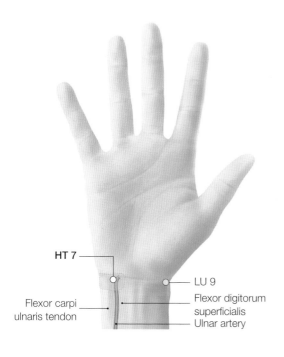

HT 7

Flexor carpi
ulnaris tendon

LU 9
Flexor digitorum
superficialis
Ulnar artery

0.3 to 0.5 cun oblique insertion distally under the pisiform bone, directed towards its ulnar side. This technique usually elicits the strongest deqi easier. Prick to bleed.

Actions and indications
HT 7 is one of the top *most commonly used and important points*. It is extensively employed to *calm the mind, reduce anxiety, clear heat and regulate the Heart*. It is particularly indicated for *deficiency conditions*, particularly if there is *depletion of Blood and Yin*.

Common indications include: palpitations, tachycardia, arrhythmia, chest pain, angina pectoris, dull complexion, and dizziness. Also, it is widely used for a variety of psychological disorders, including: insomnia, anxiety, worry, stress, depression, panic attacks, stage fright, hysteria, tendency to laugh too much, poor memory, and tiredness.

Additionally, it has been used for a diversity of symptoms and conditions, including: heat in the five hearts, burning of the palms, spitting blood, swollen painful throat, ulceration of the mouth and tongue, dyspnoea, loss of voice, epilepsy, speech impairment, drooling, redness of the face, enuresis, dysuria, and urinary tract infections.

HT 7 is also effective to treat *disorders of the wrist* such as pain, swelling and stiffness, ulnar flexor tendinitis, spasticity of the fingers, and atrophy of the forearm.

> **Main Areas**—Heart. Mind. Wrist.
> **Main Functions**—Calms the mind. Nourishes Heart Blood. Soothes the Heart. Clears heat.

HT 8　Shaofu
Lesser Mansion

Ying-Spring point, Fire point

Myotome	C8/T1
Dermatome	C7/C8

Location
On the palm, in the depression between the fourth and fifth metacarpal bones, on the distal transverse palmar crease (known as the heart line in palmistry).

To aid location, the tip of the little finger touches this point when a fist is made.

Needling
0.3 to 0.5 cun perpendicular insertion.

Actions and indications
HT 8 is a useful point to treat excess conditions caused by heat and fire in the Heart. Symptoms include: palpitations, tachycardia, sore throat, thirst, fever, ulceration of the tongue, itching, dysuria, heat in the palms, convulsions, insomnia, mental agitation, and even delirium.

In practice, however, it is not commonly used for these complaints. Its sphere of action lies mainly in the treatment of channel disorders such as inflammation and pain of the fingers and palm, hypertonicity of the little finger, and pain and stiffness of the forearm, arm and axilla.

> **Main Areas**—Hand. Heart. Mind.
> **Main Functions**—Clears Heart fire. Cools and calms the Heart. Benefits the palms.

HT 9　Shaochong
Lesser Surge

Jing-Well point, Wood point

Myotome	None – superficial tissue
Dermatome	C8

Location
On the radial side of the little finger, 0.1 cun proximal to the corner of the nail.

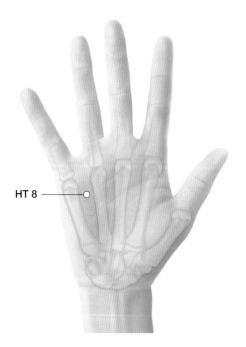

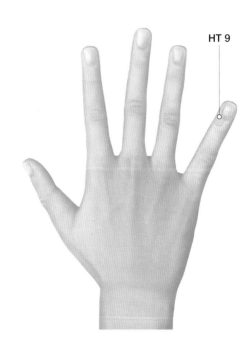

To aid location, it is at the intersection of the line following the radial border of the nail and the line following the base of the nail.

Needling
0.1 cun perpendicular insertion.
Prick to bleed.

Actions and indications
HT 9 is a *powerful point to open the orifices, clear the mind, resuscitate consciousness, regulate Heart Qi and clear heat.*

Indications include: arrhythmia, bradycardia, tachycardia, palpitations, angina pectoris, convulsions, pain and swelling of the throat, pain at the root of the tongue, fever, fainting, shock, coma, syncope, wind stroke, and mental tiredness.

Main Areas—Mind. Heart. Chest.
Main Functions—Resuscitates consciousness. Regulates Heart Qi.

13 Points of the Arm Tai Yang Small Intestine Channel

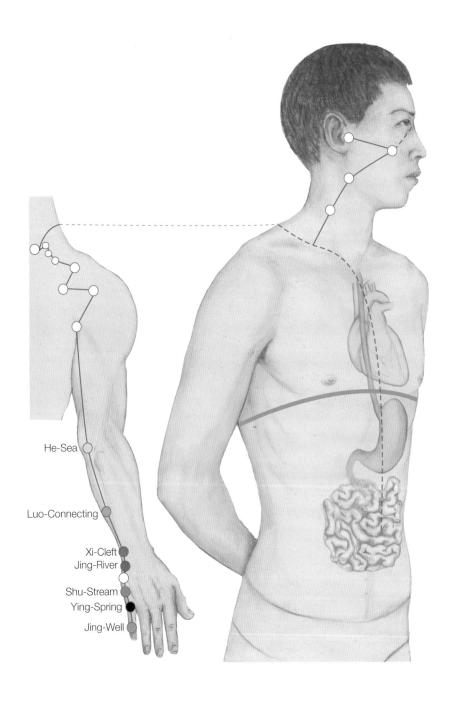

手太陽小腸經穴

He-Sea

Luo-Connecting

Xi-Cleft
Jing-River

Shu-Stream
Ying-Spring

Jing-Well

General	The Small Intestine channel starts on the little finger and runs across the medial border of the palm and hand, to cross the elbow at the ulnar groove near the medial epicondyle.
	Continuing up to the posterior aspect of the axilla, it then crosses the scapula in a zigzag fashion, eventually heading from the centre of the supraspinatus, across the trapezius and SCM, to behind the angle of the jaw. From here it crosses the cheek and is reflected back on itself, finishing in front of the tragus of the ear.
	The channel has 19 points. It is grouped with the Heart under the Fire element in five-element theory.
More specifically	The channel starts at the medial side of the nail of the little finger, opposite where the Heart channel has finished on the lateral aspect.
	It runs across the medial aspect of the palm, crossing the hypothenar muscles (SI 3 is situated within these), and crosses the wrist near the ulnar styloid. From here it ascends to the medial epicondyle of the humerus, with SI 8 being close to the ulnar groove. It then travels upwards along the triceps, and, crossing the posterior deltoid, it zigzags across the posterior deltoid, infraspinatus, supraspinatus and levator scapulae (see the diagram showing the course of the channel).
	SI 12, within the centre of the supraspinatus gives a branch that descends to connect with the Heart, its Yin partner. This affects the throat, diaphragm and Stomach in addition.
	The main branch continues from SI 12 upwards across the SCM to the site behind the angle of the mandible. Here, it spreads into the face, crossing the cheek to sit on the under border of the zygomatic arch, in line with the outer canthus of the eye (level with ST 3). It then moves posteriorly across the masseter, and the last point, SI 19, is situated in front of the tragus of the ear, on the skin in the depression just behind the condyloid process of the mandible. It sits between two other points – GB 2 below and TE 21 above.
Area covered	Little finger, hand, medial wrist, medial elbow, scapula and posterior neck. Cheek.
Areas affected with treatment	Digestive issues, particularly if associated with stress and emotional states. Injuries to the hand/wrist/elbow, Golfer's elbow and compartment syndrome affecting the hand, 'writer's cramp', carpal tunnel.
	Shoulder problems – frozen shoulder in particular, and subacromial impingement syndromes involving the supraspinatus and infraspinatus. Reverse scapula-humeral rhythm seen in shoulder problems.
	Musculo-skeletal issues with the neck, elevated shoulders, lack of rotation in the cervical spine. TMJ.
Key points	SI 3, SI 5, SI 8, SI 9, SI 10, SI 11, SI 12, SI 14, SI 18.

SI 1 Shaoze

Lesser Marsh

and restore consciousness in common with other jing-well points.

Another important traditional use for this point is to *clear the chest, benefit the breasts and promote lactation.*

Jing-Well point, Metal point

Myotome	None – superficial tissue
Dermatome	C8

Location

On the ulnar side of the little finger, about 0.1 cun proximal to the base of the nail, at the intersection of two lines following the ulnar border and the base of the nail.

Needling

0.1 to 0.2 cun perpendicular insertion (7 or 13mm needle).

Actions and indications

SI 1 is not very commonly used, although it has been traditionally employed to *release the exterior, clear wind and heat and calm the mind*

Main Areas—Breast. Mind.
Main Functions—Promotes lactation. Restores consciousness. Releases the exterior.

SI 2 Qiangu

Front Valley

Ying-Spring point, Water point

Myotome	None – superficial tissue
Dermatome	C8

Location

On the ulnar side of the base of the little finger, in the depression formed just distal to the base of the fifth metatarsal bone.

To aid location, form a loose fist.

Needling

0.2 to 0.5 cun perpendicular or oblique insertion.

Actions and indications

Although SI 2 is traditionally indicated to clear wind and heat from the sense organs, it is not commonly used for these purposes.

Although it is primarily used as a local point to treat pain and stiffness of the little finger or MCP joint, SI 2 has a beneficial effect on the entire channel and has been traditionally indicated for pain and stiffness of the neck, shoulder, arm and wrist.

Main Areas—Shoulder. Arm. Chest. Lungs.
Main Functions—Regulates Qi. Alleviates pain.

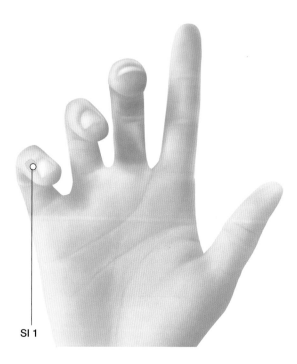

SI 1

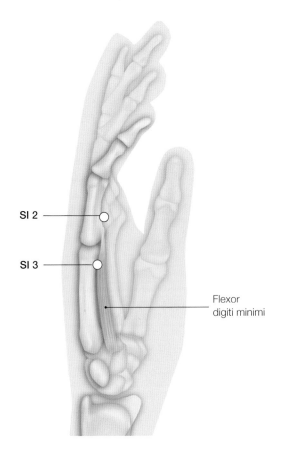

SI 2

SI 3

Flexor
digiti minimi

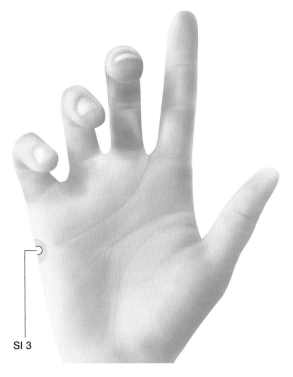

SI 3

SI 3 Houxi
Back Stream

後谿

Shu-Stream point, Wood point
Opening point of the Governor Vessel

Myotome	C8/T1
Dermatome	C8

Location
When a loose fist is formed, this point is found
at the ulnar end of the distal transverse palmar
crease, in the depression between the muscle and
the bone, just proximal to the head of the fifth
metacarpal bone.

To aid location, SI 3 is in the visible depression
formed slightly proximal and dorsal to the skin fold
formed at the end of the transverse palmar crease
when a loose fist is formed.

Needling
Needle with the palm in a relaxed position so that
the fingers are slightly flexed.
0.3 to 0.7 cun perpendicular insertion into the space
between the bone and the hypothenar muscles.

Actions and indications
SI 3 is a very *important and widely used point* for
a variety of disorders. Its primary functions are to
regulate the Yang Qi, whether it is excessive or
deficient, and to *benefit the Governor Vessel*.

It is effective to *descend excessive Yang, clear heat,
calm the mind and benefit the neck, spine and sense
organs*. However, SI 3 can also be used to tonify
and warm the Yang Qi. Furthermore, it *releases the
exterior and dispels wind, cold and heat*.

Indications include: pain and stiffness of the spine,
particularly the neck, upper back and shoulders,
headache, especially occipital, migraine, dizziness
and vertigo, chills and fever, tinnitus, inflammation
of the eyes, spasms, convulsions and epilepsy,
hypertension, palpitations and tachycardia, and
mental restlessness and insomnia.

As a *local point*, SI 3 can treat pain and stiffness of the wrist and fingers.

It has a very strong but effective deqi sensation and clients should be aware of this because they may try to pull away.

> **Main Areas**—Hand. Neck. Spine. Sense organs. Mind. Brain. Nervous system. Heart.
> **Main Functions**—Descends Yang. Clears heat. Opens the Governor Vessel. Benefits the spine.

SI 4   Wangu   腕骨
Wrist Bone

Yuan-Source point

Myotome	None – superficial tissue
Dermatome	C8

Location
On the ulnar border of the hand, in the depression between the base of the fifth metacarpal bone and the process of the triquetrum bone. In its deep position, it is located between the triquetrum and hamate bones.

To aid location, make a loose fist.

Needling
Needle with the palm in a relaxed position so that the fingers are slightly flexed.
0.3 to 1 cun perpendicular insertion. The needle should be directed into the joint space between the process of the triquetrum and the hamate bones.

Actions and indications
SI 4 is an excellent point for *pain and stiffness of the fingers, wrist and forearm*, although it is not often employed for its traditional indications that include such diverse conditions as: jaundice, cholecystitis, gastritis, diabetes, emaciation, tinnitus, toothache, sore throat, thirst, and febrile diseases.

> **Main Areas**—Wrist. Hand.
> **Main Function**—Alleviates swelling and pain.

SI 5   Yanggu   陽谷
Yang Valley

Jing-River point, Fire point

Myotome	None – superficial tissue
Dermatome	C8

Location
On the ulnar border of the wrist, in the depression of the wrist joint space between the ulna and the

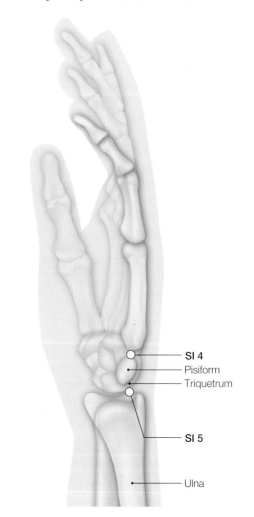

SI 4
Pisiform
Triquetrum

SI 5

Ulna

triquetrum bone, slightly anterior to the styloid process of the ulna.

To aid location, it is on the transverse wrist crease formed when the wrist is flexed in an ulnar direction.

Needling
0.3 to 1 cun perpendicular insertion. The needle should be directed into the joint space between the ulna and the triquetrum bone.

Actions and indications
Similarly to *SI 4*, SI 5 is particularly effective for *problems of the wrist* such as stiffness, pain and arthritis. However, it also *clears heat and calms the mind* and can be used in psychosomatic disturbances. As one of the jing-river points, it is used to treat soft tissue/ fascial tightness along the channel. Manual pressure here could be valuable in treating musculo-skeletal conditions of the arm, shoulder and face/ TMJ.

> **Main Areas**—Wrist. Hand.
> **Main Function**—Alleviates swelling and pain.

SI 6 Yanglao 養老
Support the Aged

Xi-Cleft point

Myotome	None – superficial tissue
Dermatome	C8

Location
On the posterior aspect of the ulnar head in the bony cleft between the tendons of the extensor digiti minimi and the extensor carpi ulnaris.

To aid location, place your index finger on the head of the ulna and slowly turn the palm so that it faces towards the chest. The narrow cleft between the tendons of the extensor digiti minimi and extensor carpi ulnaris becomes palpable on the ulnar head. Extending the little finger and wrist defines these tendons.

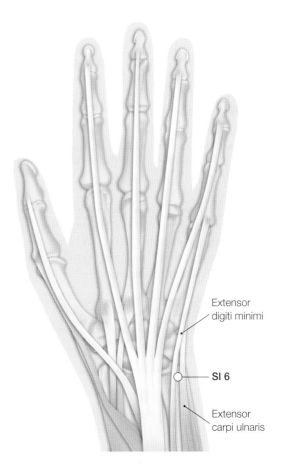

Extensor digiti minimi

SI 6

Extensor carpi ulnaris

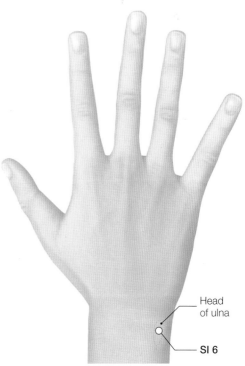

Head of ulna

SI 6

Needling

0.3 to 0.5 cun perpendicular insertion into the small space between the ulna and the tendon of the extensor digitorum longus.

Actions and indications

SI 6 is a particularly effective point to *stop pain anywhere along the Small Intestine channel*, and is especially useful for pain of the wrist, elbow and shoulder.

It has also been traditionally used to *increase vitality in the elderly* and alleviate symptoms such as lumbar pain, failing vision and deafness. Additionally, it has been employed to treat hernia pain, appendicitis and hemiplegia.

> **Main Areas**—Arm. Wrist. Shoulder.
> **Main Functions**—Regulates Qi and Blood. Alleviates pain.

SI 7   Zhizheng
Branching Point

Luo-Connecting point

Myotome	C8/T1
Dermatome	C8

Location

5 cun proximal to SI 5 in a depression medial to the border of flexor carpi ulnaris and anterior to the ulnar shaft.

Needling

0.5 to 1 cun perpendicular insertion.
0.5 to 1.5 cun oblique insertion proximally or distally.

Beware: Needling deeply can injure the underlying ulnar artery.

Actions and indications

Although SI 7 is the Luo point, it is not as commonly used as other points of the Small Intestine channel. It can, however, be very effective to release the exterior in TaiYang syndromes and to treat pain and stiffness along the course of the channel.

SI 7 is also traditionally indicated to calm the Shen and treat anxiety.

> **Main Areas**—Forearm. Hand. Head.
> **Main Functions**—Releases the exterior. Clears heat. Calms the Shen. Regulates Qi and Blood. Alleviates pain.

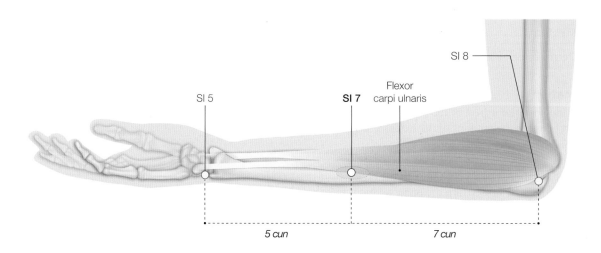

SI 8

Flexor carpi ulnaris

SI 5   SI 7

5 cun   7 cun

SI 8 Xiaohai

Small Sea

小海

Main Areas—Elbow. Forearm. Ulnar nerve.
Main Functions—Regulates Qi and Blood.
Alleviates pain.

He-Sea point, Earth point

Myotome	None – superficial tissue
Dermatome	C8

Location

In the shallow depression of the flat area between the olecranon process of the ulna and the medial epicondyle of the humerus. *Situated along the course of the ulnar nerve.* Locate with the elbow flexed.

To aid location, palpate firmly with the fingertip for the noticeable cord-like ulnar nerve.

Needling

0.3 to 0.5 cun perpendicular insertion.
0.5 to 1 cun oblique distal insertion.

Do not puncture the ulnar nerve – this lies extremely close to this point.

Actions and indications

SI 8 is an effective point for *disorders of the ulnar nerve, elbow, forearm and shoulder*, including pain, weakness and atrophy.

SI 9 Jianzhen

True Shoulder

肩貞

Myotome	C5/C6
Dermatome	C5

Location

On the posterior aspect of the shoulder, in a depression below the posterior border of the deltoid muscle, approximately 1 cun above the superior end of the posterior axillary crease. Situated below the infraglenoid tubercle, in the teres major muscle.

To aid location, find the end of the posterior axillary crease with the arm in adduction.

Needling

0.5 to 1.5 cun perpendicular insertion.

Actions and indications

SI 9 to SI 12 are all very *useful points for many disorders of the shoulder and arm*. They are primarily used to treat: impaired mobility, difficulty in abducting and lifting the arm, frozen shoulder, and atrophy, paralysis, pain and inflammatory conditions of the shoulder and arm. Pain and

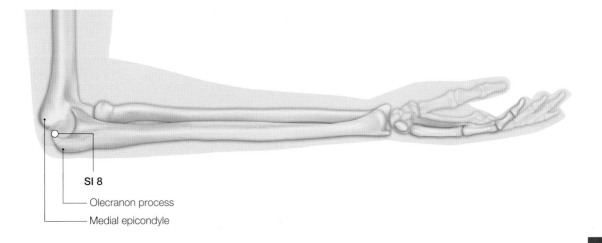

SI 8
Olecranon process
Medial epicondyle

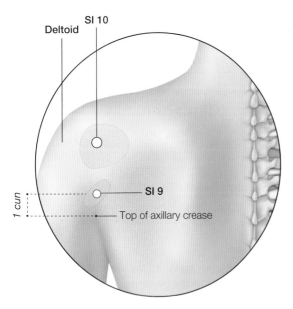

stiffness should be reduced after treatment at these points. Particularly useful for impaired lateral rotation of the shoulder joint.

Main Areas—Shoulder. Scapula. Arm.
Main Functions—Regulates Qi and Blood. Alleviates pain.

SI 10   Naoshu   臑俞
Upper Arm Point

Intersection of the Yang Wei Mai and Yang Qiao Mai on the Small Intestine channel

Myotome	C5/C6
Dermatome	C4/C5

Location
Directly above SI 9, in the depression directly below the scapular spine. Situated in the posterior portion of the deltoid muscle, and in its deep position, situated in the infraspinatus.

To aid location, a visible depression appears when the arm is raised above the head (abducted).

Needling
0.5 to 1.5 cun perpendicular insertion, angled slightly downward.

Actions and indications
Similar to SI 9. Additionally, SI 10 has an effect on the *axillary lymph glands* and helps *reduce swelling.*

Main Areas—Shoulder. Scapula. Arm.
Main Functions—Regulates Qi and Blood. Alleviates pain.

SI 11   Tianzong   天宗
Upper Esteemed Point

Myotome	C5/C6
Dermatome	T2

Location
At the centre of the scapula, midway between its medial and lateral borders, one third of the distance along the line joining the midpoint of the lower border of the scapular spine to the inferior angle of scapula. In a dip felt one third down from the centre of the spine of scapula, in the infraspinatus muscle.

To aid location, create an equilateral triangle between SI 9, SI 10 and SI 11.

Needling
0.5 to 1.5 cun perpendicular or oblique insertion in various directions.

Beware of too deep perpendicular needling due to potential foramen within the centre of the spine of scapula.

Actions and indications
SI 11 is probably the most widely used point of the region, having *a very powerful relaxing effect on the entire shoulder*. It has been extensively employed to treat most shoulder problems.

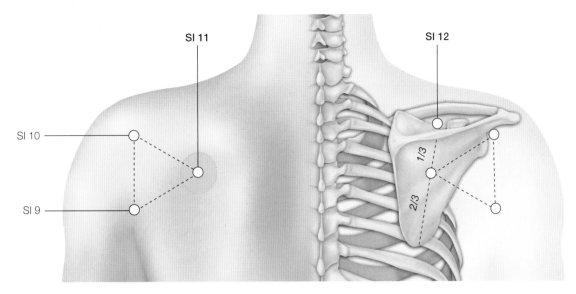

SI 11 also has a *calming effect on the digestive system*, particularly the stomach, liver and gallbladder, and treats symptoms such as indigestion, acid reflux, abdominal pain, irritable bowel, diarrhoea, dysphagia and hypochondrial pain.

Additionally, it can be used for complaints of the breasts such as pain, lumpiness and insufficient lactation. It has also been traditionally used to treat breathing difficulties and coughs.

> **Main Areas**—Shoulder. Scapula. Arm. Chest.
> **Main Functions**—Regulates Qi and Blood.
> Alleviates pain. Relaxes the chest.

SI 12 Bingfeng
Grasping the Wind

Intersection of the Gallbladder, Triple Energizer and Large Intestine on the Small Intestine channel

Myotome	C5/C6
Dermatome	C4

Location
At the centre of the suprascapular fossa directly above SI 11. Situated superficially in the trapezius, and deeper, in the supraspinatus muscle.

To aid location, a visible depression is formed at SI 12 when the arm is abducted.

Needling
0.5 to 1 cun oblique insertion, medially along the supraspinal fossa towards SI 13.
0.3 to 1 cun perpendicular insertion into the belly of the supraspinatus muscle, in a slightly posterior direction.

Do not needle deeply in an anterior direction, because of danger of puncturing the apex of the lung.

Actions and indications
Similar to SI 9, SI 10, SI 11, SI 13 and SI 14. Considering its name, this point is primarily used for muscular issues that have resulted in tight, dry muscles. Because of its connection with the GB, TE and LI channels its sphere of influence around the shoulder, neck and face is considerable.

> **Main Areas**—Scapula. Supraspinatus.
> **Main Functions**—Regulates Qi and Blood.
> Alleviates pain.

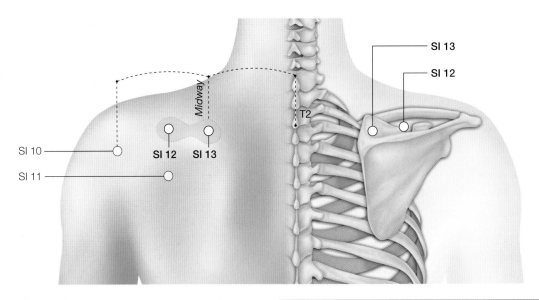

SI 13   Quyuan
Crooked Wall

曲垣

Main Areas—Scapula. Supraspinatus.
Main Functions—Regulates Qi and Blood.
Alleviates pain.

Myotome	C5/C6
Dermatome	C4

Location
At the medial end of the suprascapular fossa.
Situated superficially in the trapezius, and deeper,
in the supraspinatus muscle.

To aid location, it is approximately midway between
SI 10 and the spinous process of T2.

Needling
0.5 to 1 cun perpendicular insertion. Also oblique
lateral insertion. Important to stay away from being
too medial and missing the medial border of the
scapula and thus becoming unsafe heading towards
the ribs and lungs.

Treatment and applications
Similar to SI 12 and SI 14. Choose between these
points, depending on which is more reactive during
pressure palpation. SI 13 is also a known trigger
point position within medial supraspinatus, in which
case needling will follow trigger point theory.

SI 14   Jianwaishu
Outer Shoulder Point

肩外俞

Myotome	C4/C5 and T1/T2
Dermatome	C4

Location
3 cun lateral to the lower border of the spinous
process of the first thoracic vertebra, on the line of
the medial border of the scapula. Situated in the
trapezius and serratus posterior superior. In its deep
position lies the iliocostalis muscle and the levator
scapulae insertion.

To aid location, it is in line with the outer Bladder
channel points. Also, it is level with GV 13.

Needling
0.3 to 0.5 cun perpendicular insertion.
0.5 to 1 cun oblique medial insertion.

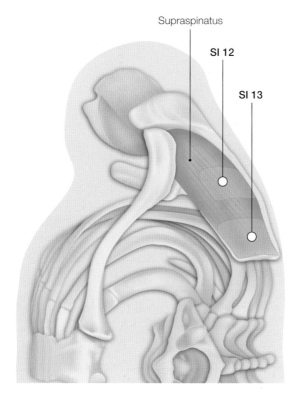

Supraspinatus

SI 12

SI 13

Do not needle deeply at a perpendicular angle, because this holds a considerable risk of puncturing the lung.

Actions and indications

SI 13 and SI 14 have similar actions to the other surrounding Small Intestine points. They effectively improve the flow of Qi and Blood and stop pain in the shoulder and arm, upper back and neck.

SI 14 can also be used as a levator scapulae muscle trigger point.

> **Main Areas**—Shoulder. Neck. Levator scapulae muscle.
> **Main Functions**—Regulates Qi and Blood. Alleviates pain.

SI 15　Jianzhongshu 肩中俞
Middle Shoulder Point

Myotome	C3–C5
Dermatome	C3/C4

Location
2 cun lateral to the lower border of C7, approximately at the end of the transverse process of T1. Situated in the trapezius and levator scapulae muscles.

To aid location, it is level with GV 14.

Needling
0.3 to 0.5 cun perpendicular insertion.
0.5 to 1 cun oblique medial insertion.

Do not needle deeply, because this holds a considerable risk of puncturing the lung.

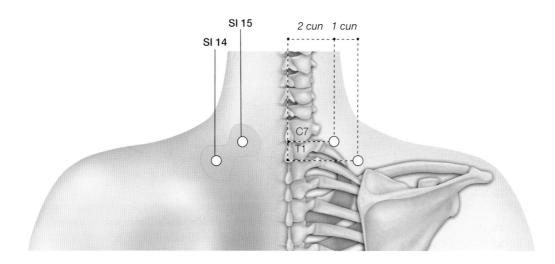

SI 15

SI 14

2 cun　1 cun

C7

T1

Actions and indications

SI 15 is primarily used to treat *disorders of the neck, shoulder, upper limb and lungs.*

Symptoms include: stiffness of the shoulders and neck, asthma, cough, chills and fever, and absence of sweating in exterior diseases (see also SI 14).

> **Main Areas**—Neck. Shoulder. Chest.
> **Main Functions**—Regulates Qi and Blood.
> Alleviates pain. Relaxes the chest.

SI 16   Tianchuang
Upper Window

 天窗

Window of the Sky point

Myotome	Accessory nerve, C1–C5
Dermatome	C3

Location

On the lateral aspect of the neck, at the posterior border of the SCM muscle, directly lateral to LI 18.

To aid location, define the SCM muscle by asking the person to turn their head away from the side to be palpated while applying resistance to the chin.

Needling

0.5 to 1 cun maximum perpendicular insertion.

Treatment and applications

Similar to LI 17 and LI 18. However, because SI 16 is situated exactly on the superficial cervical plexus nerve block point, it is even more sensitive than LI 17.

> **Main Areas**—Throat. Neck. Ears. Shoulder.
> **Main Functions**—Regulates Qi and Blood.
> Alleviates pain. Relieves swelling.

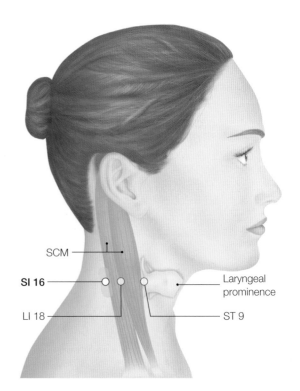

SI 17   Tianrong
Upper Magnitude

天容

Window of the Sky point

Myotome	C1/C2
Dermatome	C3

Location

In the depression immediately posterior to the angle of the mandible and anterior to the border of the SCM. More deeply it is situated at the inferior margin of the posterior belly of the digastric muscle, and deeper still, anterior to the external carotid artery.

To aid location, define the SCM muscle by asking the person to turn their head away from the side to be palpated while applying resistance

Needling

0.5 to 1 cun perpendicular insertion towards the root of the tongue, directed anterior to the carotid artery.

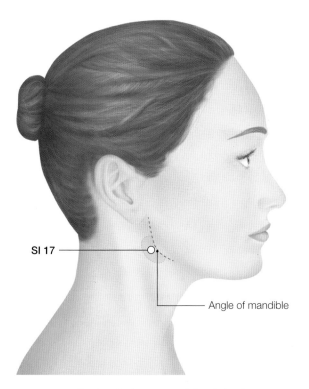

SI 17

Angle of mandible

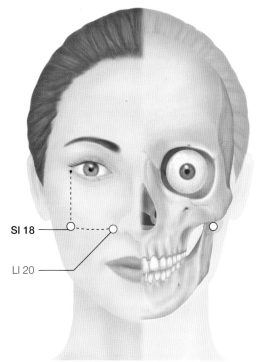

SI 18

LI 20

Do not needle deeply, because of the risk of puncturing the numerous vessels located at this site.

Actions and indications

SI 17 is a *very effective point for disorders of the ear, cheek, throat and tongue* and is particularly indicated for pain, swelling and nodules in these areas.

Main Areas—Throat. Ears.
Main Functions—Regulates Qi and Blood. Alleviates pain. Relieves swelling.

SI 18   Quanliao   顴髎
Cheek Bone Hole

Intersection of the Triple Energizer and Gallbladder on the Small Intestine channel

Myotome	Trigeminal nerve
Dermatome	Facial nerve

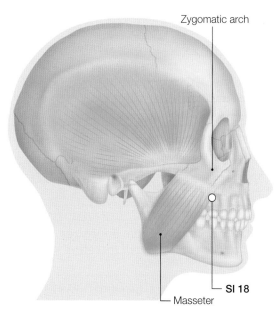

Zygomatic arch

SI 18

Masseter

Location

In the depression at the lower border of the zygomatic arch, directly below the outer canthus of the eye. Situated at the anterior border of the masseter muscle.

To aid location, SI 18 is approximately level with LI 20 and ST 3.

Needling
0.2 to 0.6 cun perpendicular insertion. Transverse or subcutaneous insertion in various directions: medially towards the nose, laterally along the curve of the zygomatic arch towards ST 7, and inferiorly or posteriorly towards ST 5 or ST 6.

Be aware of complex facial anatomy in this region.

Actions and indications
SI 18 is *effective for problems of the cheeks, eyes and teeth,* including: facial paralysis, trigeminal neuralgia, spasm of the cheek muscles, and inflammatory conditions such as sinusitis, otitis, parotitis and swelling of the cheeks.

SI 18 clears heat and can be used for *aesthetic problems* of the skin such as redness, thread veins and acne. Applying manual techniques at this location, TENS or electro-acupuncture can help *tonify the zygomatic muscles, giving a face-lifting effect.*

> **Main Areas**—Cheeks. Face.
> **Main Functions**—Clears heat. Dissipates cold. Tonifies the cheeks.

SI 19   Tinggong   聽宮
Palace of Hearing

Intersection of the Triple Energizer and Gallbladder on the Small Intestine channel

Myotome	None – superficial tissue
Dermatome	Facial nerve

Location
Anterior to the tip of the tragus, in the depression posterior to the condyloid process of the mandible, in line with GB 2 and TE 21.

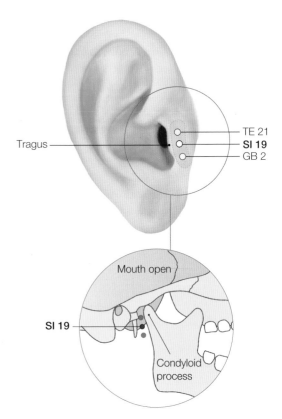

To aid location, when the patient opens their mouth, the condyloid process of the mandible slides forwards to reveal the depression.

This is a sensitive point and care should be taken in all forms of treatment.

Needling
0.3 to 1 cun perpendicular needling, directed slightly posteriorly. Insert the needle with the patient's mouth open. After insertion, the patient can close the mouth.

Actions and indications
In common with GB 2 and TE 21, SI 19 is very effective for many problems of the ears, including acute inflammation, tinnitus and deafness. See also GB 2.

Treatment at SI 19, GB 2 and TE 21 can occasionally bring about a tinnitus-like buzzing in the ears or the sound of moving water. This is due to an increase in blood circulation or other reaction in the inner ear as a result of the treatment. It could, however, mean that the needle is touching the artery, or that excessive heat from moxibustion has been applied.

It is also effective for other disorders of the local area, including: stiffness or injury of the jaw, TMJ syndrome, temporal headache, toothache, facial pain and trigeminal neuralgia.

SI 19 is also traditionally considered to *calm the mind.*

> **Main Areas**—Ears. Temple. Jaw.
> **Main Functions**—Improves hearing and benefits the ears. Regulates Qi and Blood. Alleviates pain. Clears heat.

足
太
陽
膀
經
穴

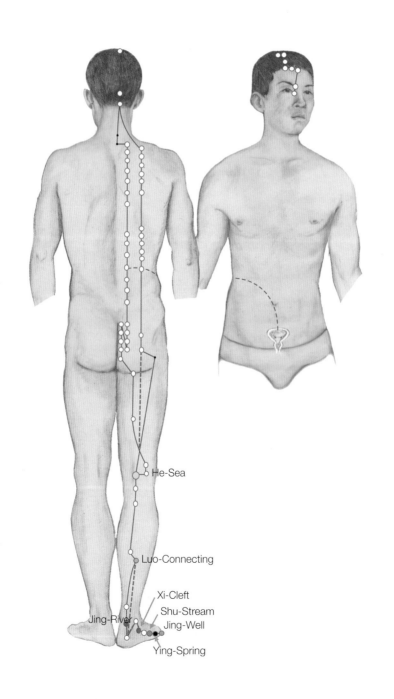

He-Sea

Luo-Connecting

Xi-Cleft

Shu-Stream

Jing-Well

Jing-River

Ying-Spring

General	The Bladder channel is the longest channel in the series of the twelve main pathways. Starting at the medial corner of the eye socket, it travels up and over the head, close to the midline, over the occiput and down the spine in two lines. These sit over the trapezius, erector spinae, longissimus and latissimus dorsi.
	The channel reaches the sacrum and doubles back on itself to sit over the sacral foramina. From here it branches off down the back of the leg, passing over the ischial tuberosity, down the hamstrings, and veers laterally to sit over the lateral hamstrings in the lower third of the thigh. Moving back into the midline, the channel then continues in the leg down through the gastrocnemius and over the Achilles, again moving slightly more laterally and finishing over the lateral aspect of the foot, all the way to the edge of the little toe.
	AT BL 40, behind the knee, the numbering system confusingly jumps back up to the spine and the outer Bladder line, which sits 3 cun from the midline and extends from T2 (BL 41) down to the piriformis at BL 54.
	The channel has 67 points. It is grouped with the Kidney under the Water element in five-element theory.
More specifically	Starting in the inner canthus of the eye, BL 1 is a powerful but very delicate point. The channel ascends to the medial edge of the eyebrow, and then on upwards into the hairline. Points along the scalp are often tender in headaches and situated above/within the occipitofrontalis. A connection with GV 20 occurs at the vertex.
	The channel continues over the occiput to BL 9 at the external occipital protuberance. A powerful point for treatment for the head and headaches, BL 10 sits immediately lateral to the upper fibres of the trapezius.
	Continuing in a straight line into the cervical spine, the channel divides at the level of approximately C4 into two lines. The inner Bladder line continues all the way down the spine at a distance of 1.5 cun from the midline. Anatomically, the sympathetic ganglia are located at this same distance from the midline, obviously deeper and more anteriorly, but the inner Bladder line has a special part to play in conditions affecting the autonomic nervous system. Points along the spine are supplied by the posterior rami of these nerves, explaining the far-reaching visceral and emotional effect that these Bladder points can have.
	A set of the inner Bladder points (BL 11 through BL 28) have been named the back-shu (or transporting) points, and these have specific effects on targeted organs and 'whole health'. These points are also situated above the costotransverse joints in the thoracic spine.
	The outer Bladder line sits more over the angles of the ribs in the thoracic region, at 3 cun from the midline, and continues on this line down into the buttock. Some of these points have a strong effect on the Shen and all things spiritual – especially if linked with chronic illness.
	BL 54 in the buttock is the most accurate point for targeting the piriformis, and there is a branch from the Bladder channel connecting with GB 30 in the buttock. This region often has pain from the lumbar area refer to it, and these points can be very useful in both a Chinese medical model and a Western anatomical sense.

	The two lines merge again at the knee (BL 40), with the path having followed the sciatic nerve and the gaps and furrows within the hamstrings, veering laterally. After descending through the gastrocnemius, the channel passes behind the lateral malleolus and finishes along the lateral border of the foot, to reach BL 67 on the lateral aspect of the nail of the little toe.
Area covered	Forehead. Occiput. Cervical, thoracic, lumbar, sacral spine. Buttock, hamstrings and calf. Sciatic nerve.
Areas affected with treatment	Whole body/well-being/emotional health. Specifically, calf, knee, hamstrings, buttock and low back, spinal problems, head and neck. Eyesight.
Key points	BL 10, BL 11–28, BL 36, BL 39, BL 40, BL 41–54, BL 57, BL 60, BL 67.

BL 1   Jingming
Bright Eyes

睛明

Intersection of the Small Intestine, Stomach, Gallbladder, Triple Energizer, Governor Vessel, Yin Qiao Mai and Yang Qiao Mai on the Bladder channel

Myotome	None – non-muscular tissue
Dermatome	Facial nerve

Location
Approximately 0.1 cun medial and superior to the inner canthus of the eye. Locate and treat with the eyes closed. Superior to the medial palpebral ligament. In its deep position, situated in the medial rectus muscle and the superior oblique muscle.

To aid location, the best needling site is usually at the centre of the visible depression just above the inner canthus.

Needling
0.3 to 1 cun perpendicular insertion.

BL 1

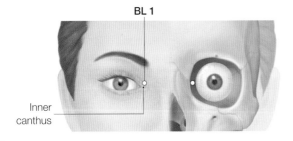
Inner canthus

Support the medial side of the eyeball with the index finger and push it laterally holding it gently but firmly. Insert the needle slowly with the other hand. Do not manipulate the needle. Use the thinnest needle possible.

Needling this location is potentially dangerous and requires special skill and experience. Great care should be taken, as wrongly angled insertion can damage the eye.

The patient should keep the eyes as relaxed and still as possible during needle retention and avoid unnecessary blinking. It is best that the eyes remain closed for the duration of the treatment, until after the needle is removed, to avoid the skin being pulled. Apply pressure with a cotton pad for up to 1 minute after removing the needle.

BL 1 can bruise easily. If any slight swelling is observed, remove the needle immediately and apply pressure and a cold compress. If bruising occurs, apply the cold compress for 2–5 minutes. The bruising should disappear within a week and will not affect the eyesight.

Beware of considerable delicate anatomy in this region.

Actions and indications
BL 1 is a *very important point*, used in a wide variety of eye disorders. Its primary functions are to *clear and brighten the eyes, dispel wind and heat, moisten and cool the eyes, nourish Yin and improve vision.*

Symptoms include: tired, dry, inflamed, sensitive eyes, itching or inflammation of the inner canthus, excessive lacrimation, chronic or acute eye pain, disorders of the optic nerve, poor or diminishing vision, blurred vision, colour blindness, night blindness and diseases of the eye such as conjunctivitis, keratitis, irregular refraction and iritis.

It is also a *major beauty point* and *helps improve the appearance of the surrounding skin*. It effectively treats dark circles, visible capillaries, bags and swollen eyelids.

> **Main Area**—Eyes.
> **Main Functions**—Clears and brightens the eyes. Improves vision. Dispels wind and clears heat. Alleviates pain. Nourishes Yin. Improves appearance.

BL 2   Zanzhu
Gathered Bamboo

攢竹

Myotome	Facial nerve
Dermatome	Trigeminal nerve

Location
Near the medial end of the eyebrow, in a small depression superior to BL 1. More deeply, it is situated in the corrugator supercilii muscle.

To aid location, feel for the tender spot by palpating laterally from the medial end of the eyebrow.

Needling
0.2 to 0.3 cun perpendicular or oblique insertion.

BL 2

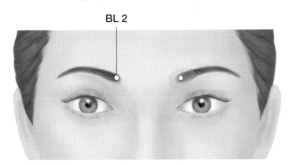

0.3 to 0.5 cun transverse insertion medially towards the base of the nose (nasion) or Yintang.
0.5 to 1 cun lateral transverse insertion towards Yuyao.

Actions and indications
BL 2 is a *major point for disorders of the eyes and forehead* because it *dispels wind, clears heat, regulates Qi and Blood* and *alleviates pain*.

It has been extensively employed in such cases as: frontal headache, migraine, sinusitis, facial paralysis, chronic or acute pain and other disorders of the eyes.

> **Main Areas**—Eyes. Forehead.
> **Main Functions**—Regulates Qi and Blood. Alleviates pain. Dispels wind. Clears heat.

BL 3   Meichong
Eyebrow Ascension

眉衝

Myotome	None – superficial tissue
Dermatome	Trigeminal nerve

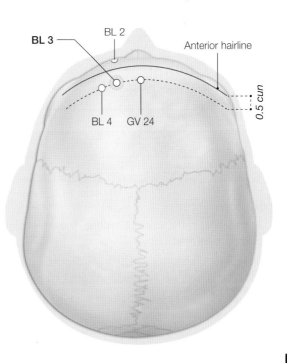

Location

Directly superior to BL 2, 0.5 cun within the anterior hairline.

To aid location, it is level with GV 24 and BL 4.

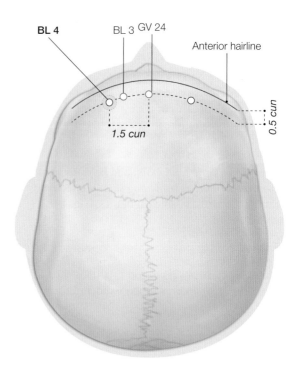

Needling

0.3 to 1 cun transverse insertion, either posteriorly along the course of the channel or in other directions depending on the area to be treated.

Pick up the cutaneous tissue of the scalp and insert the needle under the galea aponeurotica parallel to the bone. If the scalp is very tight, this may be difficult, making perpendicular insertion 0.1 to 0.2 cun the only alternative.

Actions and indications

Although BL 3 is primarily used as a *local point* to *dispel wind, clear the head and relieve stasis and pain*, it also has more internal functions, including *clearing heat and calming the mind.*

Indications include: headache, sinusitis, epilepsy, dizziness, disorders of the eyes, and facial paralysis.

> **Main Area**—Head.
> **Main Functions**—Dispels wind. Clears heat. Alleviates pain.

BL 4 Quchai
Deviating Curve

曲差

Myotome	None – superficial tissue
Dermatome	Trigeminal nerve

Location

1.5 cun lateral to the anterior midline, 0.5 cun within the anterior hairline.

To aid location, it is one third of the distance between GV 24 and ST 8.

Needling

0.3 to 1 cun transverse insertion, either posteriorly along the course of the channel or in other directions depending on the area to be treated.

Pick up the cutaneous tissue of the scalp and insert the needle under the galea aponeurotica parallel to the bone. If the scalp is very tight, this may be difficult, making perpendicular insertion 0.1 to 0.2 cun the only alternative.

Actions and indications

BL 4 is primarily used as a *local point, to dispel wind, clear heat and alleviate pain.* It is particularly indicated for *disorders of the nose.*

Indications include: headache, fever, sinusitis, rhinitis, nasal congestion, epistaxis, epilepsy, eye disorders, and facial paralysis.

> **Main Areas**—Nose. Head.
> **Main Functions**—Dispels wind. Clears heat. Alleviates pain.

BL 5   Wuchu   五處
Fifth Position

Myotome	None – superficial tissue
Dermatome	Trigeminal nerve, C2

Location
1.5 cun lateral to the anterior midline, 1 cun within the anterior hairline.

To aid location, it is 1.5 cun lateral to GV 23, or 0.5 cun posterior to BL 4.

Needling
0.3 to 1 cun transverse insertion, either posteriorly along the course of the channel or in other directions depending on the area to be treated.

Pick up the cutaneous tissue of the scalp and insert the needle under the galea aponeurotica parallel to the bone. If the scalp is very tight, this may be difficult, making perpendicular insertion 0.1 to 0.2 cun the only alternative.

Actions and indications
Although BL 5 is not a very commonly used point, it can help *clear the head, eyes* and *nose and dispel wind, descend rising Yang and clear heat.*

Indications include: headache, heavy feeling in the head, dizziness, epilepsy, poor or diminishing eyesight, painful eyes, and nasal congestion.

> **Main Areas**—Head. Eyes. Nose.
> **Main Functions**—Dispels wind. Clears heat. Descends Yang.

BL 6   Chengguang   承光
Receiving Light

Myotome	None – superficial tissue
Dermatome	C2

Location
2.5 cun within the anterior hairline, 1.5 cun lateral to the midline.

To aid location, it is 1.5 cun posterior to BL 5.

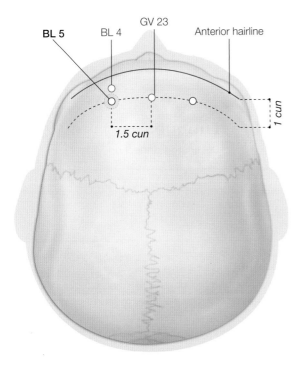

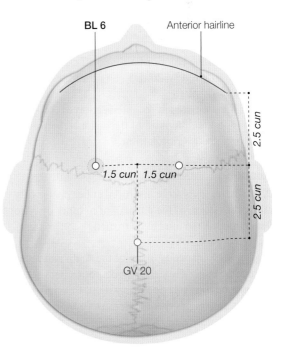

Needling

0.3 to 1 cun transverse insertion, either posteriorly along the course of the channel or in other directions depending on the area to be treated.

Pick up the cutaneous tissue of the scalp and insert the needle under the galea aponeurotica parallel to the bone. If the scalp is very tight, this may be difficult, making perpendicular insertion 0.1 to 0.2 cun the only alternative.

Actions and indications

In common with BL 4 and BL 5, BL 6 helps to dissipate *wind and clear heat from the head* and *benefits the eyes and nose*. Use pressure palpation to decide which of these points are more reactive.

> **Main Areas**—Head. Eyes. Nose.
> **Main Functions**—Dispels wind. Clears heat.

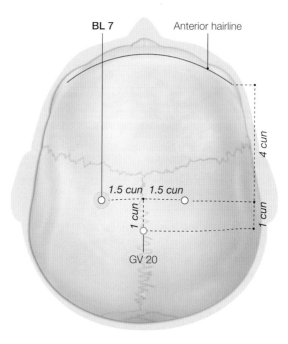

BL 7   Tongtian
Reaching Upward
通天

Myotome	None – superficial tissue
Dermatome	C2

Location

4 cun within the anterior hairline, 1.5 cun lateral and 1 cun anterior to GV 20, 1.5 cun posterior to BL 6.

To aid location, it is at the intersection of the anterior and middle third of the distance between the anterior and posterior hairlines.

Needling

0.3 to 1 cun transverse insertion, either posteriorly along the course of the channel or in other directions depending on the area to be treated.

Pick up the cutaneous tissue of the scalp and insert the needle under the galea aponeurotica parallel to the bone. If the scalp is very tight, this may be difficult, making perpendicular insertion 0.1 to 0.2 cun the only alternative.

Actions and indications

BL 7 is useful to treat *disorders of the head and nose*. It helps to *dispel wind* and *clear phlegm and heat*.

Indications include: headache, dizziness, facial paralysis, loss of sense of smell, nasal congestion, soreness of the nose, and epistaxis. For the latter symptoms, it is often combined with GV 23.

> **Main Areas**—Head. Eyes. Nose.
> **Main Functions**—Dispels wind. Clears heat.

BL 8   Luoque
Declining Connection
絡卻

Myotome	None – superficial tissue
Dermatome	C2

Location

5.5 cun within the anterior hairline, 1.5 cun lateral to the midline, 1.5 cun posterior to BL 7.

To aid location, BL 8 is 1.5 cun lateral and 0.5 cun posterior to GV 20.

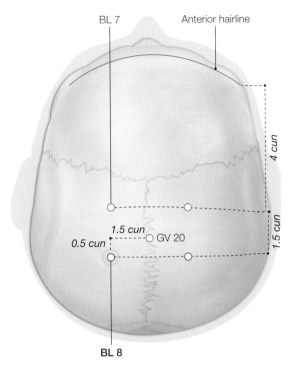

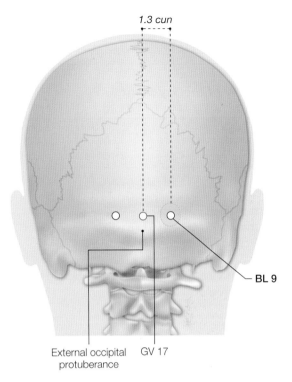

Needling

0.3 to 1 cun transverse insertion, either posteriorly along the course of the channel or in other directions depending on the area to be treated.

Pick up the cutaneous tissue of the scalp and insert the needle under the galea aponeurotica parallel to the bone. If the scalp is very tight, this may be difficult, making perpendicular insertion 0.1 to 0.2 cun the only alternative.

Actions and indications

Useful to treat *disorders of the head and nose. Brightens the eyes.*

Main Areas—Head. Nose. Eyes.
Main Functions—Dispels wind. Clears heat.

BL 9   Yuzhen   玉枕
Jade Pillow

Myotome	None – superficial tissue
Dermatome	C2

Location

In a shallow depression just above the superior nuchal line, 1.3 cun lateral to GV 17, approximately 2.5 cun within the posterior hairline.

To aid location, GV 17 is in the depression superior to the external occipital protuberance.

Needling

0.3 to 0.5 cun transverse inferior insertion. For needling method, see BL 3.

Do not puncture the occipital artery and vein, or the greater occipital nerve.

Actions and indications

BL 9 can be effective to alleviate pain, dispel wind and clear the sense organs (especially the eyes), in common with GV 17. Often this is a sore and tense spot in tension headaches.

Main Areas—Head. Eyes. Sense organs.
Main Functions—Dispels wind. Clears the eyes.

BL 10 Tianzhu
Upper Pillar

天柱

Window of the Sky point

Myotome	Accessory nerve, C1/C2
Dermatome	C3

Location
On the lateral part of the descending portion of the trapezius muscle, 0.5 cun within the posterior hairline, approximately 1.3 cun lateral to GV 15.

To aid location, GV 15 is directly superior to the spinous process of C2.

Needling
0.5 to 1 cun perpendicular insertion.

Do not needle deeply or in an upward direction.

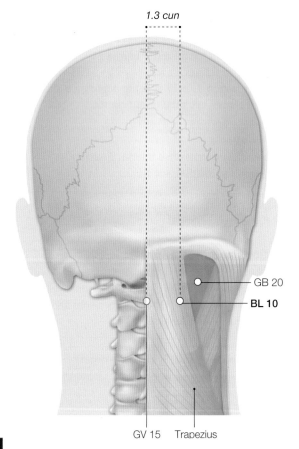

1.3 cun

GB 20
BL 10
GV 15   Trapezius

Actions and indications
BL 10 is a *very important point to treat the neck, upper back, head and entire Tai Yang area*. It is primarily used to *dispel wind and cold, regulate Qi and Blood circulation*, and *alleviate pain*.

Indications include: occipital headache, stiffness of the neck, pain of the body, sore throat, chills and fever, nasal congestion, pain and inflammation of the eyes, excessive lacrimation, blurred vision, epilepsy, and dizziness.

BL 10 is also very effective to *calm the mind* and *relax the body* by *increasing parasympathetic activity*, in common with other adjacent points such as GB 20. This is due to the cranial output of the PSNS.

> **Main Areas**—Neck. Head. Tai Yang area. Entire body.
> **Main Functions**—Dispels wind and cold. Regulates Qi and Blood. Calms the mind.

BL 11 Dazhu
Great Vertebra

大杼

Influential point of Bone
Intersection of the Small Intestine, Triple Energizer, Governor Vessel and Gallbladder on the Bladder channel
Sea of Blood point

Myotome	C3–C7 and dorsal rami of segmental thoracic vertebrae
Dermatome	C5/C6

Location
1.5 cun lateral to the lower border of the spinous process of T1.

Needling
0.4 to 1 cun oblique medial insertion.
0.5 cun oblique inferior insertion.

Do not needle deeply or at a different angle.
This poses considerable risk of puncturing the lung.
This goes for ALL back-shu points up to BL 23.

Actions and indications

BL 11 is useful in the treatment of *disorders of the bones and spine* and has been used to assist the *healing of bone* after fracture and to treat *bone diseases* due to *weakness of Jing and Blood*, including osteoporosis and kyphosis of the spine.

BL 11 also *effectively releases the exterior, dispels wind and cold, regulates Lung Qi* and *alleviates cough*, in common with BL 12 and BL 13.

Indications include: chills and fever, aversion to cold, absence of sweating, headache, pain of the upper back and shoulders, stiffness and pain of the neck, sore throat, dyspnoea, and cough.

BL 11 is mentioned as one of the *Eight Points to Clear Heat from the Chest* (together with BL 12, LU 1 and ST 12) and is therefore considered an *important point to clear heat from the upper jiao*.

> **Main Areas**—Bones. Chest. Lungs. Neck.
> **Main Functions**—Releases the exterior.
> Regulates Lung Qi and alleviates cough.
> Nourishes Blood. Benefits the bones.

BL 12   Fengmen
Wind Gate

Intersection of the Governor Vessel on the Bladder channel

Myotome	C3–C7 and dorsal rami of segmental thoracic vertebrae
Dermatome	C5/T1

Location

1.5 cun lateral to the lower border of the spinous process of T2.

Needling

0.4 to 1 cun oblique medial insertion.
0.5 cun oblique inferior insertion.

Actions and indications

In common with BL 13, BL 12 is widely used in *exterior disorders to clear the Tai Yang area*, particularly at the *initial stage of wind cold invasion*.

Additionally, BL 12 is mentioned as one of the *Eight Points to Clear Heat From the Chest* (together with BL 11, LU 1 and ST 12) and is considered important to *clear heat from the upper jiao*.

Indications include: chills and fever, aversion to cold, absence of sweating, headache, dizziness, heaviness of the eyes, sneezing, runny or blocked nose, epistaxis, susceptibility to catching colds, sore throat, high fever, retching, haemoptysis, dyspnoea, cough, and pain or stiffness of the neck, shoulders and upper back.

> **Main Areas**—Lungs. Chest. Exterior. Upper back.
> **Main Functions**—Dispels wind and cold.
> Regulates Lung Qi. Clears heat.

The Back-Shu Points (Inner Bladder Line)

Location

All the points on the inner Bladder line are located at the highest part of the erector spinae muscle group (longissimus muscle), 1.5 cun lateral to the posterior midline and level with the lower border of their relevant spinous process.

To aid location, these points are usually at the highest point of the prominence of the paraspinal muscles, in a depression where the muscle fibres divide on pressure.

For the *thoracic points*, the 1.5 cun distance is measured midway between the posterior midline and the vertebral (medial) border of the scapula. It is possible to palpate small dips in the tissue in this region.

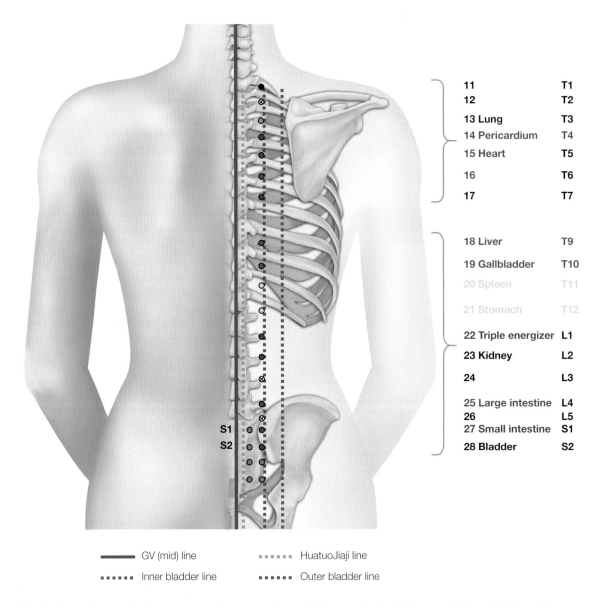

11	T1
12	T2
13 Lung	T3
14 Pericardium	T4
15 Heart	T5
16	T6
17	T7

18 Liver	T9
19 Gallbladder	T10
20 Spleen	T11
21 Stomach	T12
22 Triple energizer	L1
23 Kidney	L2
24	L3
25 Large intestine	L4
26	L5
27 Small intestine	S1
28 Bladder	S2

——— GV (mid) line ⋅⋅⋅⋅⋅ HuatuoJiaji line

▪▪▪▪▪ Inner bladder line ▪▪▪▪▪ Outer bladder line

The back varies greatly from person to person, and cases of kyphosis, scoliosis and other variations of the spine must be taken into account.

Needling

In general, the *thoracic points* are needled obliquely 0.4 to 1 cun (or slightly more in some cases) in a medial direction. However, the points on the outer Bladder line should be needled slightly more superficially than those on the inner line.

Another common way to needle these points is at an oblique angle, to a depth of 0.5 cun in an inferior direction.

Points on the back between T1 and L2 should not be needled deeply at a perpendicular angle, or in a lateral oblique direction. This poses a considerable risk of puncturing the lungs and other organs.

The *lumbar points below L2* are needled perpendicularly to a depth of up to 1.5 cun, depending on individual build.

The *sacral points*, however, can be needled deeper, up to 3 cun.

BL 13 Feishu
Lung Shu

Back-Shu point of the Lung

Myotome	C4–C7 and dorsal rami of segmental thoracic vertebrae
Dermatome	T3

Location
1.5 cun lateral to the lower border of the spinous process of T3. Situated in the trapezius, rhomboid and, more deeply, the longissimus muscles.

Needling
0.4 to 1 cun oblique medial insertion.
0.5 cun oblique inferior insertion.

Actions and indications
BL 13 is widely employed for both *interior and exterior Lung disorders*. It effectively *dispels wind and releases the exterior, transforms phlegm* and *descends rebellious Lung Qi*. It also *tonifies Lung Qi, cools and moistens the Lungs* and *nourishes Yin*.

Indications include: chronic or acute cough, productive or dry cough, chronic or acute respiratory diseases, asthma, fever, thirst, aversion to cold, chronic breathing difficulty, dyspnoea, shortness of breath, chest pain, chronic tiredness, spontaneous sweating, night sweating, low-grade fever, steaming bone syndrome, haemoptysis, rhinitis, nasal discharge, nasal congestion, occipital headache, and pain at the back of the head and neck.

As a *local point*, it has been successfully employed to treat kyphosis and pain of the upper back.

BL 13 helps release stuck emotional states, particularly grief and sadness.

BL 14 Jueyinshu
Absolute Yin Shu

Back-Shu point of the Pericardium

Myotome	C4–C7 and dorsal rami of segmental thoracic vertebrae
Dermatome	T4

Location
1.5 cun lateral to the lower border of the spinous process of T4. Situated in the trapezius, rhomboid and, more deeply, the longissimus muscles.

Needling
0.4 to 1 cun oblique medial insertion.
0.5 cun oblique inferior insertion.

Actions and indications
BL 14 is an important point to *regulate Heart* and *Liver Qi* and unbind the chest.

Indications include: palpitations, mental agitation, dyspnoea, coughing, retching, vomiting, and thoracic oppression, pain and fullness.

As a *local point*, BL 14 can also be used for pain and stiffness of the upper back.

BL 15   Xinshu
Heart Shu

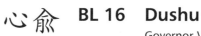

BL 16   Dushu
Governor Vessel Shu

Back-Shu point of the Heart

Myotome	C4–C7 and dorsal rami of segmental thoracic vertebrae
Dermatome	T5

Location
1.5 cun lateral to the lower border of the spinous process of T5. Situated in the trapezius, rhomboid major and, more deeply, the longissimus muscles.

Needling
0.4 to 1 cun oblique medial insertion.
0.5 cun oblique inferior insertion.

Actions and indications
BL 15 is widely used to *nourish, cool* and *soothe the Heart,* and *calm the mind.* It is also important to *regulate chest Qi* and *dispel stasis.*

Indications include: palpitations, arrhythmia, dyspnoea, circulation disorders, angina pectoris, and tightness, oppression or pain of the chest.

In addition, BL 15 treats a *wide range of psychosomatic disturbances,* including: poor memory, amnesia, depression, insomnia, mental restlessness, anxiety, grief, dream-disturbed sleep, nightmares, aphasia, speech disorders, panic attacks, phobias, and even insanity.

It has also been used for an assortment of other symptoms, including: coughing, haemoptysis, epistaxis, nasal congestion, pain of the eyes, retching and vomiting, epilepsy, wind stroke, hemiplegia, fever, and heat in the palms and soles.

As a *local point,* BL 15 can also be used for pain and stiffness of the upper back.

> **Main Areas**—Chest. Heart.
> **Main Functions**—Regulates Qi and Blood in the chest. Tonifies Heart Qi. Calms the mind.

Governor Vessel Shu point

Myotome	Dorsal rami of segmental thoracic vertebrae. Due to latissimus dorsi supply, also C6–C8
Dermatome	T6

Location
1.5 cun lateral to the lower border of the spinous process of T6.

Needling
0.4 to 1 cun oblique medial insertion.
0.5 cun oblique inferior insertion.

Actions and indications
Although BL 16 is not as commonly used as the other back-shu points, it can be useful to *regulate Qi, dispel stasis* and *alleviate pain from the chest, abdomen and spine.*

It has a special place in terms of anatomy, because the spinal cord is at its thickest at this level, and so mobility within this region and the spinal canal is very important. Lack of movement here, can lead to lack of movement of all four limbs, and also lack of movement of emotions, due to the strong interconnection of the sympathetic chain and the viscera at this level. The viscera and enteric nervous system are inherently connected to our emotional state, so this could almost be called the Emotional Shu point.

Other indications include: abdominal pain and distension, thoracic pain, alopecia, and skin disorders such as dryness, scaling and itching of the skin.

> **Main Areas**—Chest. Abdomen. Spine. Skin.
> **Main Functions**—Regulates Qi and Blood in the chest and abdomen. Dispels stasis and pain.

BL 17   Geshu
Diaphragm Shu

 膈俞

Diaphragm (Blood) Shu point
Influential point of Blood

Myotome	Dorsal rami of segmental thoracic vertebrae. Due to latissimus dorsi supply, also C6–C8
Dermatome	T7

Location
1.5 cun lateral to the lower border of the spinous process of T7.

Needling
0.4 to 1 cun oblique medial insertion.
0.5 cun oblique inferior insertion.

Actions and indications
BL 17 is a *very important point and widely used for many disorders of the Blood*. Specifically, it is used both to *nourish* and *invigorate Blood* and dispel stasis, as well as to *cool Blood* and *arrest bleeding*.

BL 17 and BL 19 are also known as the *Four Flowers* and are indicated for fevers and to arrest bleeding. Also they are used for Blood stasis, which in western medical terms would be considered cramp and spasm within the spinal muscles.

Indications include: fever with or without sweating, tidal fever, night sweating, thirst, anaemia, dry eyes, headache, dizziness, asthma, dyspnoea, coughing, amenorrhoea, dysmenorrhoea, dry skin conditions, rashes, mental restlessness, depression, insomnia, and tightness, oppression and pain of the chest. It is also indicated for pain of the whole body, including the skin and muscles.

BL 17 also effectively *benefits the diaphragm, harmonises the Stomach and descends rebellious Qi.* Indications include: abdominal pain and distension, spasm of the diaphragm, hiccup, difficulty swallowing, heartburn, retching, nausea, and vomiting.

BL 17 is also very effective to treat *pain and stiffness of the spine and mid-upper back.*

> **Main Areas**—Diaphragm. Chest. Abdomen. Entire body.
> **Main Functions**—Nourishes Blood. Invigorates Blood and dispels stasis. Clears Blood heat. Relaxes the diaphragm. Benefits the skin.

BL 18   Ganshu
Liver Shu

 肝俞

Back-Shu point of the Liver

Myotome	Dorsal rami of segmental thoracic vertebrae. Due to latissimus dorsi supply, also C6–C8
Dermatome	T9

Location
1.5 cun lateral to the lower border of the spinous process of T9.

Needling
0.4 to 1 cun oblique medial insertion.
0.5 cun oblique inferior insertion.

Actions and indications
BL 18 is very *important to regulate Liver Qi, invigorate Blood and nourish Yin and Blood.* Additionally, it *clears heat and fire from the Liver and sedates interior wind.*

Indications include: tightness or pain of the chest and abdomen, shortness of breath, palpitations, hypertension, epilepsy, dizziness, hypochondrial pain and distension, jaundice, bitter taste in the mouth, nausea and vomiting, coughing or spitting blood, liver and gallbladder disease, painful palpable masses in the abdomen, enlargement of the liver or spleen, pain of the axilla, breast pain, irritability, insomnia, mental restlessness, mood swings, premenstrual syndrome, infertility, dysmenorrhoea, oligomenorrhoea, and amenorrhoea.

BL 18 is also an important point to benefit the eyes and relax the sinews and muscles.

Indications include: diminishing vision, glaucoma, excessive lacrimation, chronic inflammation, pain or dryness of the eyes, stiffness, tightness or cramping of the muscles, arthritis, and pains in the spine and joints.

As a *local point*, BL18 can be used to treat pain and stiffness of the back.

> **Main Areas**—Liver. Hypochondrium. Abdomen. Eyes.
> **Main Functions**—Regulates Liver Qi. Dispels stasis. Nourishes Blood. Clears heat and dampness. Benefits the eyes.

BL 19   Danshu   膽俞
Gallbladder Shu

Back-Shu point of the Gallbladder

Myotome	Dorsal rami of segmental thoracic vertebrae. Due to latissimus dorsi supply, also C6–C8
Dermatome	T10

Location
1.5 cun lateral to the lower border of the spinous process of T10.

Needling
0.4 to 1 cun oblique medial insertion.
0.5 cun oblique inferior insertion.

Actions and indications
BL 19 is a useful point to *clear dampness and heat from the Liver and Gallbladder* and to *regulate Liver and Gallbladder Qi*. It is useful in disorders of the gallbladder and liver, including jaundice, cholecystitis and hepatitis.

Additionally, it can treat disorders of the ShaoYang with symptoms such as alternating chills and fever,

sore throat, headache, hypochondrial pain and distension, bitter taste in the mouth, nausea, and vomiting.

BL 19 can be used to tonify the Gallbladder channel in psycho-emotional disorders such as mental restlessness, anxiety, fright, panic attacks, timidity and indecisiveness.

BL 17 and BL 19 are also known as the *Four Flowers* and are indicated for fevers and to arrest bleeding. Also they are used for Blood stasis, which in western medical terms would be considered cramp and spasm within the spinal muscles.

As a *local point*, BL 19 can be used to treat pain and stiffness of the back.

> **Main Areas**—Gallbladder. Liver. Hypochondrium. Abdomen.
> **Main Functions**—Regulates Gallbladder and Liver Qi. Dispels stasis. Alleviates pain. Clears dampness and heat. Dispels shaoYang pathogens.

BL 20   Pishu   脾俞
Spleen Shu

Back-Shu point of the Spleen

Myotome	Dorsal rami of segmental thoracic vertebrae. Due to latissimus dorsi supply, also C6–C8
Dermatome	T11

Location
1.5 cun lateral to the lower border of the spinous process of T11.

Needling
0.4 to 1 cun oblique medial insertion.
0.5 cun oblique inferior insertion.

Actions and indications

BL 20 is important to *tonify and lift Spleen Qi, boost the middle jiao, nourish Blood* and *resolve dampness*. It has been extensively employed for most symptoms of *Spleen deficiency*, including *Qi, Yang and Blood deficiency*.

Indications include: tiredness and weakness of the limbs and body, sweating, flaccidity of the muscles, tendency to gain weight, water retention, swelling, oedema, abdominal distension, loose stools, chronic diarrhoea, undigested food in the stools, poor appetite, indigestion, infertility, oligomenorrhoea, and amenorrhoea.

Furthermore, it can treat *urinary and digestive disorders caused by dampness accumulation*. Indications include: diarrhoea, vomiting, jaundice, productive cough, dysuria, cystitis, urethritis, and leucorrhoea.

As a *local point*, BL 20 can be useful for pain and stiffness of the lower thoracic region.

> **Main Areas**—Spleen. Stomach. Intestines. Digestive system. Muscles. Entire body. Lower thoracic area.
> **Main Functions**—Boosts Spleen and Stomach Qi. Boosts transformation and movement. Clears dampness.

BL 21   Weishu
Stomach Shu

Back-Shu point of the Stomach

Myotome	Dorsal rami of segmental thoracic vertebrae. Due to latissimus dorsi supply, also C6–C8
Dermatome	T10

Location

1.5 cun lateral to the lower border of the spinous process of T12.

To aid location, the spinous process of T12 is usually visibly smaller than that of L1. Also, to locate T12, it is best to count up from L5.

Needling

0.4 to 1 cun oblique medial insertion.
0.5 cun oblique inferior insertion.

Actions and indications

BL 21 is *important to regulate the Stomach, harmonise the middle jiao* and *descend rebellious Qi*. Furthermore, it *boosts Stomach Qi and aids in Blood production*. Indications include: heartburn, belching, nausea, vomiting, jaundice, poor appetite, loose stools, diarrhoea, and epigastric or abdominal heaviness, distension, and pain.

> **Main Areas**—Digestive system. Stomach.
> **Main Functions**—Regulates Stomach Qi. Benefits the digestion. Descends rebellious Qi.

BL 22   Sanjiaoshu
Triple Energizer Shu

Back-Shu point of the Triple Energizer

Myotome	Dorsal rami of segmental thoracic vertebrae. Due to latissimus dorsi supply, also C6–C8
Dermatome	T12/L1

Location

1.5 cun lateral to the lower border of the spinous process of L1.

Needling

0.4 to 1 cun oblique medial insertion.
0.5 cun oblique inferior insertion.

Actions and indications

BL 22 is important to *resolve dampness, open the water passages and promote urination*. Additionally, it *harmonises the middle jiao* and *boosts Spleen Qi*. It has been extensively employed to treat: water retention, urinary disorders, and swelling and oedema of the abdomen, limbs or entire body.

> **Main Area**—Urinary system.
> **Main Functions**—Resolves dampness. Opens the water passages. Harmonises the Triple Energizer.

BL 23   Shenshu
Kidney Shu

Back-Shu point of the Kidneys

Myotome	Dorsal rami of segmental thoracic vertebrae. Due to latissimus dorsi supply, also C6–C8
Dermatome	T10

Location
1.5 cun lateral to the lower border of the spinous process of L2. Situated in the latissimus dorsi, erector spinae and, in its deep position, the quadratus lumborum muscle.

To aid location, BL 23 is approximately level with the thinnest part of the waist – the 'anatomical waist'.

Needling
0.5 to 1.5 cun perpendicular insertion.
0.5 to 1.5 cun oblique medial insertion.

Actions and indications
BL 23 is *extremely important to tonify both the Yin and Yang aspects of the Kidneys.*

Common indications include: chronic tiredness, weakness and exhaustion, spontaneous sweating, night sweating, palpitations, chronic weak breathing and coughing, diminishing vision and hearing, chronic diarrhoea, lower abdominal pain and distension, oedema, and all chronic disorders in general.

BL 23 is a *very important point to regulate the water passages* and *benefit the lower jiao, genitourinary system and uterus.*

Indications include: frequent urination, chronic urinary tract infections, dysuria, haematuria, renal colic, infertility, amenorrhoea, dysmenorrhoea, oligomenorrhoea, leucorrhoea, diminishing libido, impotence, spermatorrhoea, premature ejaculation, and prostatitis.

BL 23 is also a major point for many disorders of the spine, lumbar area, lower limbs and bones.

Indications include: chronic lumbar pain and weakness, disorders of the lumbar spine, spasm of the lumbar muscles, difficulty walking, chronic weakness or paralysis of the lower limbs, cold in the lower back, knees and legs, sciatica, pain in the bones and steaming bone syndrome.

Moxibustion is particularly effective to tonify and warm the *Kidney Yang and mobilise the Qi in the lower jiao.*

> **Main Areas**—Kidneys. Lumbar area. Abdomen. Genitourinary system. Entire body.
> **Main Functions**—Boosts the Kidneys. Tonifies Yang and warms the lower jiao. Nourishes Yin and cools empty heat. Resolves dampness. Benefits urination. Alleviates pain.

BL 24   Qihaishu
Sea of Qi Shu

Sea of Qi Shu point

Myotome	Dorsal rami of segmental thoracic vertebrae. Due to latissimus dorsi supply, also C6–C8
Dermatome	L2/L3

Location
1.5 cun lateral to the lower border of the spinous process of L3.

Needling

0.5 to 1.5 cun perpendicular insertion.
0.5 to 1.5 cun oblique medial insertion.

Actions and indications

Although BL 24 can be used to *strengthen the Kidneys* in common with BL 23, it is not as frequently employed for internal disorders as the other back-shu points. It is, however, effective to treat regional pain and to strengthen the lumbar area, abdomen and lower limbs.

> **Main Area**—Lumbar area.
> **Main Functions**—Regulates Qi and Blood. Alleviates pain.

BL 25   Dachangshu
Large Intestine Shu

Back-Shu point of the Large Intestine

Myotome	Dorsal rami of segmental thoracic vertebrae. Due to latissimus dorsi supply, also C6–C8
Dermatome	L2/L3

Location

1.5 cun lateral to the lower border of the spinous process of L4.

Needling

0.5 to 1.5 cun perpendicular insertion.
0.5 to 1.5 cun oblique medial insertion.

Actions and indications

BL 25 is very important for many *disorders of the Large Intestine*. Indications include: chronic constipation or diarrhoea, undigested food in the stools, abdominal rumbling, and abdominal distension and pain.

Furthermore, it *strengthens the lumbar region and lower limbs* and *alleviates pain and sciatica*.

At an emotional level, it has been quoted *as being effective in letting go of emotional waste*, due to the Large Intestine holding things in and not letting go of physical waste as well as emotional waste.

> **Main Areas**—Intestines. Lumbar area.
> **Main Functions**—Alleviates constipation and diarrhoea. Regulates Qi and alleviates pain.

BL 26   Guanyuanshu
Original Qi Gate Shu

Original Qi Gate Shu point

Myotome	Dorsal rami of segmental thoracic vertebrae. Due to latissimus dorsi supply, also C6–C8
Dermatome	L2/L3

Location

1.5 cun lateral to the lower border of the spinous process of L5.

Needling

0.5 to 1.5 cun perpendicular insertion.
0.5 to 1.5 cun oblique medial insertion.

Actions and indications

BL 26 is effective *to regulate the lower jiao and urinary system, treat pain and stiffness of the lumbosacral joint and strengthen the lumbar region and lower limbs*.

> **Main Areas**—Lumbosacral joint. Genitourinary system.
> **Main Functions**—Benefits the urinary system. Clears dampness and heat. Regulates Qi and alleviates pain.

BL 27 Xiaochangshu 小腸俞
Small Intestine Shu

Back-Shu point of the Small Intestine

Myotome	Dorsal rami of segmental thoracic vertebrae
Dermatome	S1

Location
1.5 cun lateral to the posterior midline, level with the first sacral foramen. Situated over the sacroiliac joint.

To aid location, it is just medial to the superior border of the PSIS, over the sacroiliac joint.

Needling
0.5 to 1.5 cun perpendicular insertion, slightly laterally between the PSIS and the sacrum, towards the sacroiliac joint.

Actions and indications
BL 27 is important for *disorders of the urinary system and intestines*. It *clears dampness and heat, harmonises the intestines and Bladder and aids the Small Intestine function of 'separating the pure from the impure'.*

Indications include: dysuria, haematuria, dark or turbid urine, frequent or urgent urination, diarrhoea, and lower abdominal pain.

As a *local point*, it can be useful in the treatment of lower backache, sciatica and *disorders of the sacroiliac joint.*

> **Main Areas**—Small Intestine. Sacroiliac joint. Urinary system.
> **Main Functions**—Benefits the urinary system. Clears dampness and heat. Regulates Qi and alleviates pain.

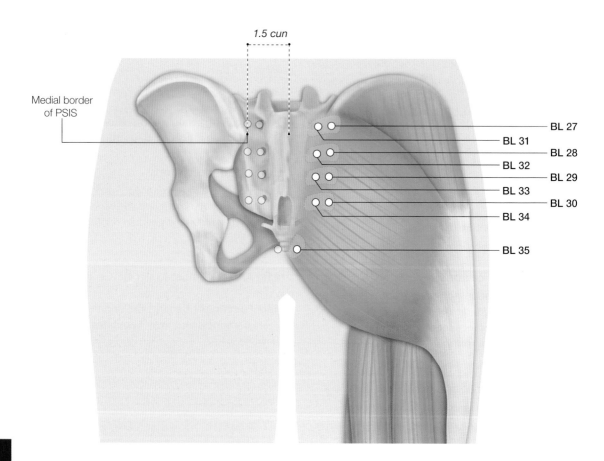

1.5 cun

Medial border of PSIS

BL 27
BL 31
BL 28
BL 32
BL 29
BL 33
BL 30
BL 34
BL 35

BL 28 Pangguangshu 膀胱俞
Bladder Shu

Back-Shu point of the Bladder

Myotome	Dorsal rami of segmental sacral vertebrae
Dermatome	S2

Location
At the level of the second sacral foramen (BL 32), 1.5 cun lateral to the posterior midline.

To aid location, it is just medial to the lower border of the PSIS, over the sacroiliac joint.

Needling
0.5 to 1.5 cun perpendicular insertion.

Actions and indications
BL 28 is *important to clear dampness and heat from the lower jiao and regulate the Bladder*.

Indications include: urinary tract infections, dysuria, haematuria, turbid urine, frequent or urgent urination, enuresis, diarrhoea, leucorrhoea, spermatorrhoea, impotence, and pain or inflammation of the genitals.

Furthermore, it *dispels stasis, alleviates pain and benefits the sacroiliac joint, lumbar region and legs*.

> **Main Areas**—Bladder. Sacroiliac joint. Urinary system.
> **Main Functions**—Regulates the Bladder. Benefits the urinary system. Clears dampness and heat. Alleviates pain.

BL 29 Zhonglushu 中膂俞
Middle Spine Shu

Backbone Shu point

Myotome	Dorsal rami of segmental sacral vertebrae
Dermatome	S3

Location
At the level of the third sacral foramen, 1.5 cun lateral to the posterior midline.

To aid location, BL 29 is usually slightly more medial to BL 28 because the line of the sacral foramina converges slightly towards the midline as it descends.

Needling
0.5 to 1.5 cun perpendicular insertion.

Actions and indications
BL 29 is primarily used as a *local point to dispel stasis from the channel and alleviate pain*. It can, however, also help *dissipate cold from the lower jiao* and treat such disorders as weakness and cold of the lower back and legs, diarrhoea, hernia and lower abdominal pain.

> **Main Area**—Sacrum.
> **Main Functions**—Regulates Qi and Blood. Alleviates pain.

BL 30 Baihuanshu 白環俞
White Ring Shu

Perineum (White Ring) Shu point

Myotome	Dorsal rami of segmental sacral vertebrae
Dermatome	S3/S4

Location

At the level of the fourth sacral foramen, 1.5 cun lateral to the posterior midline.

To aid location, BL 30 is usually slightly more medial to BL 28 and BL 29 because the line of the sacral foramina converges slightly towards the midline as it descends.

Needling

0.5 to 1 cun perpendicular insertion.

Actions and indications

BL 30 is an important point for *disorders of the anal and genital region.*

Indications include: leucorrhoea, impotence, premature ejaculation, haemorrhoids, diarrhoea, irregular menstruation, and amenorrhoea.

Benefits the lumbar and sacral regions and can help dispel cold and stasis and alleviate pain.

> **Main Areas**—Sacrum. Anus. Genitals.
> **Main Functions**—Regulates Qi and Blood. Alleviates pain. Benefits the anus.

BL 31   Shangliao
Upper Bone Hole

Intersection of the Gallbladder on the Bladder channel

Myotome	Dorsal rami of segmental sacral vertebrae
Dermatome	S1

Location

Over the first sacral foramen, level with BL 27.

To aid location, it is approximately midway between the PSIS and the posterior midline.

Needling

0.5 to 1 cun perpendicular insertion.
1 to 2.5 cun perpendicular insertion, directed slightly medially and inferiorly into the sacral foramen.

Actions and indications

BL 31 is an important point for *disorders of the sacral, anal and genital area.*

Indications include: lumbar or sacral pain, irregular menstruation, leucorrhoea, vaginal prolapse, dysmenorrhoea, impotence, and difficult urination or defecation.

BL 31 is one of the *eight sacral foramina points, known as 'The Eight Bone Holes'* (Baliao). These points are particularly useful when treated simultaneously; see also BL 32 and Ex B 2.

> **Main Areas**—Sacrum. Genitals.
> **Main Functions**—Regulates Qi and Blood. Alleviates pain.

BL 32   Ciliao
Second Bone Hole

Additional (Uterus) Back-Shu point

Myotome	Dorsal rami of segmental sacral vertebrae
Dermatome	S2

Location

Over the second sacral foramen, level with BL 28, inferior and slightly medial to BL 31.

To aid location, BL 32 is approximately midway between the PSIS and the posterior midline.

BL 32 is one of the eight sacral foramina points, known as 'The Eight Bone Holes' (Baliao). These points are particularly useful when treated simultaneously; see also BL 31 and Ex B 2.

Needling

0.5 to 1 cun perpendicular insertion.
1 to 2.5 cun perpendicular insertion, directed slightly medially and inferiorly into the sacral foramen.

Actions and indications

BL 32 is an important point for *disorders of the sacrum, anal and genital region* and is particularly indicated for *disorders of the uterus and menstruation.*

Indications include: lumbar or sacral pain, sciatica, numbness and weakness of the lower limbs, irregular menstruation, amenorrhoea, infertility, leucorrhoea, vaginal prolapse, dysmenorrhoea, lower abdominal pain, impotence, and difficult urination or defecation.

BL 32 can be used *during labour for pain relief* as well as to induce contractions and help the *cervix dilate.* Additionally, it is very useful in the treatment of dysmenorrhoea.

The eight sacral foramina points, bilateral BL 31, BL 32, BL 33, and BL 34, when treated simultaneously offer a very powerful pain-relieving treatment during labour. A combination of moxibustion, massage and needling over the eight sacral foramina points is most effective to treat pain during labour and help the cervix dilate.

> **Main Areas**—Sacrum. Uterus. Genitals.
> **Main Functions**—Regulates Qi and Blood.
> Alleviates pain. Induces labour.

BL 33   Zhongliao
Middle Bone Hole

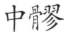

Myotome	Dorsal rami of segmental sacral vertebrae
Dermatome	S3

Location

Over the third sacral foramen, level with BL 29, inferior and slightly medial to BL 32.

Needling

0.5 to 1 cun perpendicular insertion.
1 to 2.5 cun perpendicular insertion, directed slightly medially and inferiorly into the sacral foramen.

Actions and indications

BL 33 is one of the eight sacral foramina points, known as 'The Eight Bone Holes' (Baliao). These points are particularly useful when treated simultaneously; see also BL 32 and Ex B 2.

> **Main Areas**—Sacrum. Uterus. Genitals.
> **Main Functions**—Regulates Qi and Blood.
> Alleviates pain. Induces labour.

BL 34   Xialiao
Lower Bone Hole

Intersection of the Gallbladder on the Bladder channel

Myotome	Dorsal rami of segmental sacral vertebrae
Dermatome	S4

Location

Over the fourth sacral foramen, level with BL 30, inferior and slightly medial to BL 33.

Needling

0.5 to 1 cun perpendicular insertion.
1 to 2.5 cun perpendicular insertion, directed slightly medially and inferiorly into the sacral foramen.

Actions and indications

BL 34 is one of the eight sacral foramina points, known as 'The Eight Bone Holes' (Baliao). These points are particularly useful when treated simultaneously; see also BL 32 and Ex B 2.

> **Main Areas**—Sacrum. Uterus. Genitals.
> **Main Functions**—Regulates Qi and Blood.
> Alleviates pain. Induces labour.

BL 35 Huiyang 會陽
Meeting of Yang

Myotome	Dorsal rami of segmental sacral vertebrae
Dermatome	S5

Location
0.5 cun lateral to the posterior midline, level with the tip of the coccyx.

Needling
0.5 to 1 cun perpendicular insertion.

Actions and indications
BL 35 is an *important point for regional disorders*, particularly associated with the *coccyx, anus and genitals*. Its primary functions are to *clear damp heat, regulate Qi in the lower jiao and benefit the anus*.

Indications include: haemorrhoids painful defecation, diarrhoea, coccygeal and sacral pain, impotence, genital pain or itching, and dysmenorrhoea.

> **Main Areas**—Coccyx. Anus. Genitals.
> **Main Functions**—Regulates Qi and Blood. Alleviates pain and swelling.

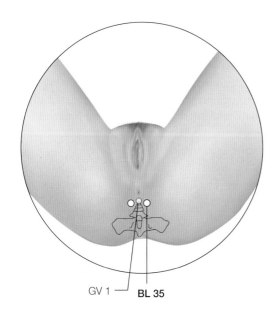

GV 1 — BL 35

BL 36 Chengfu 承扶
Hold and Support

Myotome	L5/S1/S2
Dermatome	S2

Location
At the centre of the transverse gluteal crease, in a sizeable depression, just below the inferior border of the gluteus maximus muscle, between the biceps femoris and semitendinosus muscles.

Needling
0.5 to 1.5 cun perpendicular insertion.

Actions and indications
BL 36 in *an important point for disorders of the lower limbs, buttocks and lumbar region* and is widely used to treat sciatica, pain, weakness and atrophy of the lower limbs. Also worth considering in hamstring injuries.

Furthermore, it treats such cases as haemorrhoids, constipation, genital pain, and dysuria.

> **Main Areas**—Buttock. Thigh. Lower limb. Sciatic nerve.
> **Main Functions**—Regulates Qi and Blood. Alleviates pain.

BL 37 Yinmen 殷門
Hamstring Gate

Myotome	L5/S1/S2
Dermatome	S2

Location
6 cun distal to the transverse gluteal crease, on the line connecting BL 36 with BL 40, in the depression between the biceps femoris and semitendinosus muscles.

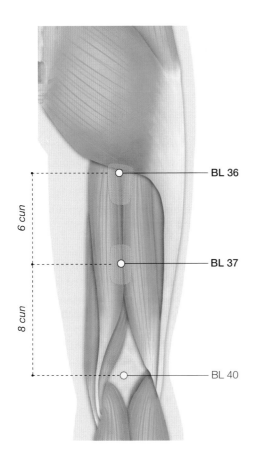

BL 36

BL 37

BL 40

6 cun

8 cun

To aid location, BL 37 is approximately two hand-widths distal to BL 36, or 1 cun proximal to the middle of the line joining BL 40 to BL 36.

Needling
0.5 to 1.5 cun perpendicular insertion.

Actions and indications
BL 37 is an *effective point for disorders of the lower limbs* and is widely used to treat sciatica and pain, weakness or atrophy of the lower limbs.

> **Main Areas**—Thigh. Lower limb.
> **Main Functions**—Regulates Qi and Blood. Alleviates pain and sciatica.

BL 38 Fuxi
Superficial Cleft

Myotome	L5/S1/S2
Dermatome	L2/L3

Location
1 cun above BL 39, on the medial side of the biceps femoris.

To aid location, the patient's knee should be slightly flexed.

Needling
0.5 to 1.5 cun perpendicular insertion.

Actions and indications
Clears Heat and aids constipation. Also local injuries involving hamstrings and back pain with sciatica.

> **Main Area**—Knee.
> **Main Function**—Regulates Qi and Blood.

BL 39 Weiyang
Lateral End of the Crease

Lower He-Sea point of the Triple Energizer

Myotome	None – superficial tissue
Dermatome	L5

Location
Lateral end of the popliteal crease, on the medial side of the biceps femoris tendon (lateral to BL 40). Locate with the knee flexed. If the client is prone, and the knee is flexed beyond 30 degrees, a dip appears medial to the biceps femoris tendon. (N.B., on the medial aspect, the corresponding dip next to the medial semimembranosus hamstring, is KI 10.)

Needling
0.5 to 1 cun perpendicular insertion.

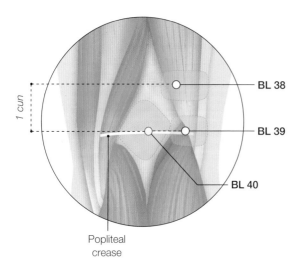

Popliteal
crease

Actions and indications

BL 39 is used to *harmonise the Triple Energizer,
open the water passages and regulate urination.*

Indications include: dysuria, urinary retention,
incontinence, water retention, swelling, and oedema.

BL 39 *regulates Qi and Blood* and treats *lower
back pain, sciatica* and *disorders of the knee.* It
is said to be more useful for sciatic symptoms,
which feel as if a *tight rope is down the back of
the thigh.*

> **Main Areas**—Knee. Lower limbs. Urinary system.
> **Main Functions**—Regulates urination and opens
> the water passages. Regulates Qi and alleviates
> pain.

BL 40   Weizhong

Middle of the Crease

He-Sea point, Earth point
Command point of the back
Heavenly Star point

Myotome	None – superficial tissue
Dermatome	L5–S2

Location

At the midpoint of the popliteal crease, midway
between the tendons of the biceps femoris and
semitendinosus muscles. Locate with the knee
flexed.

To aid location, it is at the site where the pulse of the
popliteal artery can be palpated, and usually where
it is most sensitive on pressure palpation.

Do not apply any form of treatment to BL 40 if the
possibility of thrombosis has not been ruled out.

Needling

0.5 to 1.5 cun perpendicular insertion.
Prick to bleed. Bleeding BL 40 is used for skin
diseases characterised by red skin rashes.
Plum blossom needling is also applicable.

Do not needle deeply and be aware of popliteal
anatomy.

Actions and indications

BL 40 is one of the *most important points to treat
lower back problems of both acute and chronic
nature.* BL 40 also helps *strengthen the spine and
Kidneys.* Indications include: most types of lumbar
pain, sciatica, weakness of the lower limbs, and
disorders of the knees.

BL 40 is an important point to *clear interior heat
and cool the Blood.*

Indications include: fevers, epistaxis, headache,
sore throat, epilepsy, loss of consciousness, night
sweating, rashes and other skin disorders, itching,
eczema, psoriasis, abdominal pain, diarrhoea, and
vomiting. It is also mentioned as one of *Seven
Points for Draining Heat from the Extremities*
alongside LI 15, LU 2 and GV 2.

BL 40 is also important in the treatment of *disorders
of the urinary system.*

Indications include: frequent, painful or turbid
urination, haematuria, incontinence, water retention,
oedema, and lower abdominal pain.

> **Main Areas**—Lower back. Knee. Lower limbs. Urinary system. Skin.
> **Main Functions**—Regulates Qi and Blood. Alleviates pain. Clears heat. Alleviates itching.

The Outer Bladder Line

Location

The points on the *outer Bladder line* are situated on the iliocostalis muscle, 3 cun lateral to the posterior midline, measured between the vertebral (medial) border of the scapula and the midline. All the thoracic outer Bladder points should be located in the intercostal spaces and level with the lower border of the spinous process of their relevant segment. The 3 cun distance is usually slightly smaller in the lumbar region as the Bladder channel converges slightly here. The 3 cun can be measured by doubling the distance from the medial border of the PSIS to the posterior midline.

The back varies greatly from person to person, and cases of kyphosis, scoliosis and other variations of the spine must be taken into account.

Needling

In general, the *thoracic points* are needled obliquely 0.4 to 1 cun (or slightly more in some cases) in a medial direction. However, the points on the outer Bladder line should be needled slightly more superficially than those on the inner line.

Another common way to needle these points is at an oblique angle, to a depth of 0.5 cun in an inferior direction.

Points on the back between T1 and L2 should not be needled deeply at a perpendicular angle, or in a lateral oblique direction. This poses a considerable risk of puncturing the lungs and other organs.

The *lumbar points below L2* are needled perpendicularly to a depth of up to 1.5 cun, depending on individual build.

The *sacral points*, however, can be needled deeper, up to 3 cun.

BL 41 Fufen
Outer Branch

Intersection of the Small Intestine on the Bladder channel

Myotome	T1–T4
Dermatome	T2

Location

3 cun lateral to the lower border of the spinous process of T2, in the depression just medial to the vertebral border of the scapula. Situated in the trapezius, rhomboid minor and serratus posterior superior muscles, and, in its deep position, the iliocostalis muscle.

To aid location, it is level with BL 12. The 3 cun line corresponds to a line just medial to the vertebral border of the scapula when the shoulder is relaxed.

Needling

0.4 to 1 cun transverse oblique medial insertion (towards BL 12).
0.5 cun oblique inferior insertion.

Actions and indications

Similar to SI 14 and BL 12. Extremely useful for neck and upper thoracic musculo-skeletal problems.

> **Main Areas**—Shoulder. Upper back. Lungs.
> **Main Function**—Regulates Qi and Blood.

BL 42 Pohu
Door of the Corporeal Soul

Myotome	T1–T4
Dermatome	T3

Location

3 cun lateral to the lower border of the spinous process of T3, in the depression just medial to the

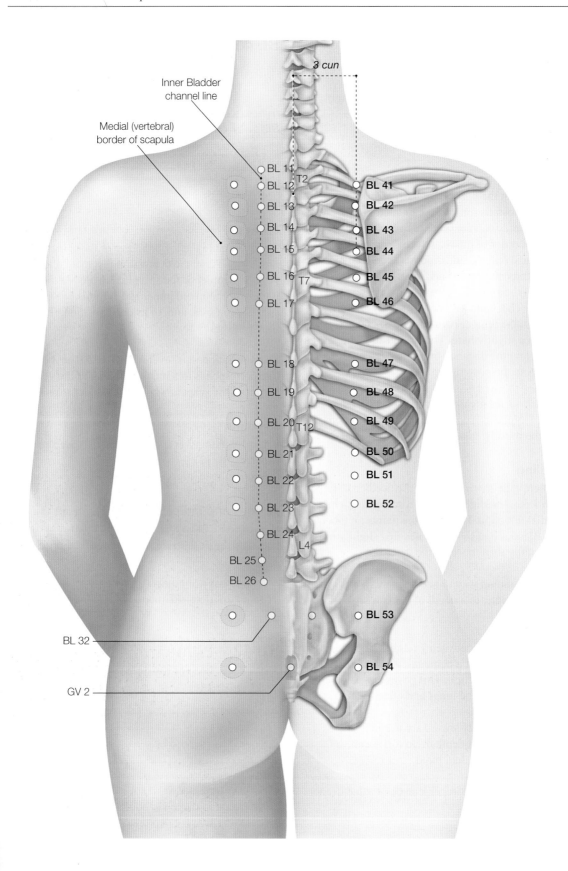

3 cun

Inner Bladder
channel line

Medial (vertebral)
border of scapula

BL 11
BL 12 T2
BL 13
BL 14
BL 15
BL 16 T7
BL 17
BL 18
BL 19
BL 20 T12
BL 21
BL 22
BL 23
BL 24
BL 25
BL 26 L4

BL 32

GV 2

BL 41
BL 42
BL 43
BL 44
BL 45
BL 46
BL 47
BL 48
BL 49
BL 50
BL 51
BL 52
BL 53
BL 54

vertebral border of the scapula. Situated in the trapezius, rhomboid major and serratus posterior superior muscles, and, in its deep position, the iliocostalis muscle.

To aid location, it is level with BL 13. The 3 cun line corresponds to a line just medial to the vertebral border of the scapula when the shoulder is relaxed.

Needling

0.4 to 1 cun transverse oblique medial insertion (towards BL 13).
0.5 cun oblique inferior insertion.

Actions and indications

BL 42 can be *considered as the back-shu point for the Corporeal Soul* and is mainly used to treat *psychological disturbances* caused by *disharmony of the Corporeal Soul*, Lungs and Metal element in general.

BL 42 has similar actions and indications to BL 13. As a *local point*, it can help treat pain of the shoulder, neck and upper back. Useful for the deep seated tightness that can form in the rhomboids in particular.

> **Main Areas**—Chest. Upper back. Lungs. Mind.
> **Main Functions**—Regulates Lung Qi. Balances the Corporeal Soul. Alleviates pain.

BL 43 Gaohuangshu 膏肓俞
Vital Region Shu

Myotome	T1–T4
Dermatome	T4

Location

3 cun lateral to the lower border of the spinous process of T4, in the depression just medial to the vertebral border of the scapula. Situated in the trapezius, rhomboid major and serratus posterior superior muscles, and, in its deep position, the iliocostalis muscle.

To aid location, it is level with BL 14. The 3 cun line corresponds to a line just medial to the vertebral border of the scapula when the shoulder is relaxed.

Needling

0.4 to 1 cun transverse oblique medial insertion (towards BL 14).
0.5 cun oblique inferior insertion.

Actions and indications

BL 43 is an *important point traditionally indicated for any chronic, serious diseases, particularly those affecting the chest, lungs and heart*. It is considered to *strengthen the Lungs, Heart, Kidneys, Spleen and Stomach and is indicated to resolve phlegm, nourish Yin, clear empty heat and tonify yuan Qi (original Qi)*. Furthermore, it is *effective to calm the mind*, by virtue of its relationship to the Heart.

Indications include: chronic cough, dry cough, productive cough, haemoptysis, dyspnoea, shortness of breath, emaciation, exhaustion, and low-grade fever.

As a *local point*, it can help treat pain of the shoulder, neck and upper back.

> **Main Areas**—Chest. Lungs. Heart. Upper back.
> **Main Functions**—Regulates chest Qi. Strengthens the Lungs and Heart. Alleviates pain.

BL 44 Shentang 神堂
Spirit Hall

Myotome	T1–T4 and dorsal rami of adjacent thoracic segments
Dermatome	T5

Location

3 cun lateral to the lower border of the spinous process of T5, in the depression just medial to the vertebral border of the scapula. Situated in the trapezius and rhomboid major muscles, and, in its deep position, the iliocostalis muscle.

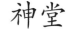

To aid location, it is level with BL 15. The 3 cun line corresponds to a line just medial to the vertebral border of the scapula when the shoulder is relaxed.

Needling
0.4 to 1 cun transverse oblique medial insertion (towards BL 15).
0.5 cun oblique inferior insertion.

Actions and indications
BL 44 can be *considered as the back-shu point for the mind or Shen* and is used mainly to treat *psychological disorders* relating to disharmony of the Heart and all aspects and levels of consciousness, especially on an *emotional and psycho-spiritual level.*

Symptoms include: anxiety, restlessness, insomnia, dream-disturbed sleep, nightmares, depression, convulsions, and even insanity.

BL 44 helps *regulate Qi and Blood in the chest* and is indicated in the treatment of dyspnoea, coughing, asthma, thoracic pain, cardiac pain, and pain of the upper back and ribs.

> **Main Areas**—Chest. Heart. Upper back.
> **Main Functions**—Regulates chest Qi. Benefits the Heart. Balances the mind. Alleviates pain.

BL 45 Yixi
That Hurts!

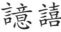

Myotome	Dorsal rami of adjacent thoracic segments
Dermatome	T6

Location
3 cun lateral to the lower border of the spinous process of T6, level with BL 16.

To aid location, apply pressure palpation to the area just medial to the vertebral border of the scapula and locate BL 45 at the most painful spot

(hence the point's name). BL 45 is sometimes slightly further lateral to the previous Bladder channel points.

Needling
0.4 to 1 cun transverse oblique medial insertion towards BL 16.
0.5 cun inferior oblique insertion.

Actions and indications
BL 45 is a useful point to *regulate Qi and Blood, dispel stasis and alleviate pain.* Furthermore, it *expels wind, clears heat and descends Lung Qi.*

Indications include: pain and stiffness of the back and shoulder, rib pain, intercostal neuralgia, chest pain, acute and chronic cough, and dyspnoea.

> **Main Areas**—Chest. Back.
> **Main Functions**—Regulates Qi and Blood. Alleviates pain.

BL 46 Geguan
Diaphragm Gate

Myotome	Dorsal rami of adjacent thoracic segments
Dermatome	T7

Location
3 cun lateral to the lower border of the spinous process of T7.

To aid location, it is level with BL 17 and slightly further lateral to the previous Bladder channel points.

Needling
0.4 to 1 cun transverse oblique medial insertion (towards BL 17).
0.5 cun oblique inferior insertion.

Actions and indications
Similar to BL 17 and other adjacent points.

> **Main Areas**—Diaphragm. Back.
> **Main Functions**—Regulates Qi and Blood.
> Alleviates pain.

BL 47   Hunmen
Gate of the Ethereal Soul

Myotome	Dorsal rami of adjacent thoracic segments, and through its association with latissimus dorsi, C6–C8
Dermatome	T8/T9

Location
3 cun lateral to the lower border of the spinous process of T9. Situated in the latissimus dorsi and iliocostalis muscles.

To aid location, it is level with BL 18.

Needling
0.4 to 1 cun transverse oblique medial insertion (towards BL 18).
0.5 cun oblique inferior insertion.

Actions and indications
BL 47 can be considered as the *back-shu point for the Ethereal Soul (Hun)* and is used mainly to treat *psychological disorders* relating to disharmony of the ethereal soul and Liver.

Symptoms include: irritability, anxiety, dream-disturbed sleep, insomnia, depression, timidity, boredom, and lack of inspiration, initiative or goals in life.

BL 47 helps *regulate Liver Qi and harmonise the middle jiao*. Indications include: enlargement of the liver or spleen, hepatitis, diarrhoea, and hypochondrial, epigastric or thoracic pain.

As a *local point*, it can help treat regional pain and stiffness of the back and ribs. Worthy of note is that many thoracic points in this region can help with upper thoracic and cervical problems due to the low attachment of many of the cervical muscles.

> **Main Areas**—Hypochondrium. Abdomen. Liver.
> **Main Functions**—Regulates Qi and Blood. Balances the Ethereal Soul.

BL 48   Yanggang
Linking to the Gallbladder

Myotome	Dorsal rami of adjacent thoracic segments, and through its association with latissimus dorsi, C6–C8
Dermatome	T9/T10

Location
3 cun lateral to the lower border of the spinous process of T10. Situated in the latissimus dorsi and serratus posterior inferior muscles, and, more deeply, the iliocostalis muscle.

To aid location, it is level with BL 19.

Needling
0.4 to 1 cun transverse oblique medial insertion (towards BL 19).
0.5 cun oblique inferior insertion.

Actions and indications
BL 48 can be useful to *harmonise the Gallbladder and Spleen, regulate Qi* and *clear dampness and heat* from the middle jiao.

Indications include: diarrhoea, gastroenteritis, cholecystitis, and jaundice.

As a local point, it can help treat regional pain and stiffness of the back and ribs.

> **Main Areas**—Gallbladder. Spleen. Digestive system.
> **Main Functions**—Clears heat and dampness. Regulates Qi in the middle jiao.

BL 49 Yishe
Abode of Thought

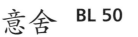

BL 50 Weicang
Stomach Granary

Myotome	Dorsal rami of adjacent thoracic segments, and through its association with latissimus dorsi, C6–C8
Dermatome	T10/T11

Myotome	Dorsal rami of adjacent thoracic segments, and through its association with latissimus dorsi, C6–C8
Dermatome	T12/L1

Location
3 cun lateral to the lower border of the spinous process of T11. Situated in the latissimus dorsi and serratus posterior inferior muscles, and, more deeply, the iliocostalis muscle.

To aid location, it is level with BL 20.

Location
3 cun lateral to the lower border of the spinous process of T12. Situated in the latissimus dorsi and serratus posterior inferior muscles, and, more deeply, the iliocostalis muscle.

To aid location, it is level with BL 21.

Needling
0.4 to 1 cun transverse oblique medial insertion (towards BL 20).
0.5 cun oblique inferior insertion.

Needling
0.4 to 1 cun transverse oblique medial insertion (towards BL 21).
0.5 cun oblique inferior insertion.

Actions and indications
BL 49 can be considered as the *back-shu point for Thought (Yi)* and is primarily employed in the treatment of *psychological disorders* caused by *disharmony of the Spleen* and the Earth element in general, particularly in relation to mental processing.

Indications include: excessive thinking and worry, poor concentration, diminishing memory, and depression.

Furthermore, BL 49 *harmonises the Spleen and Stomach* and helps *clear dampness and heat.* Indications include: abdominal or hypochondrial distension, nausea, vomiting, jaundice, loose stools, diarrhoea, abdominal rumbling, and indigestion.

As a *local point*, it can help treat regional pain and stiffness of the back.

Actions and indications
BL 50 is a useful point to *harmonise the Stomach and middle jiao and benefit the digestion.*

Indications are similar to those of BL 21.

> **Main Area**—Stomach.
> **Main Functions**—Tonifies Stomach Qi. Descends rebellious Qi.

BL 51 Huangmen
Vitals Gate

Myotome	Dorsal rami of adjacent thoracic segments, and through its association with latissimus dorsi, C6–C8
Dermatome	T12/L1

> **Main Areas**—Spleen. Mind.
> **Main Functions**—Boosts the Spleen. Improves concentration and thinking.

Location

3 cun lateral to the lower border of the spinous process of the first lumbar vertebra. Situated in the latissimus dorsi, serratus posterior inferior and iliocostalis muscles, and, in its deep position, the quadratus lumborum muscle.

To aid location, it is level with BL 22. The 3 cun can be measured by doubling the distance from the medial border of the PSIS to the posterior midline.

Needling

0.4 to 1 cun transverse oblique medial insertion (towards BL 22).
0.5 cun oblique inferior insertion.

Actions and indications

Similar to BL 22 and other adjacent points.

> **Main Areas**—Abdomen. Epigastrium.
> **Main Functions**—Regulates Qi in the chest and abdomen.

BL 52　Zhishi
Willpower Room

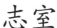 志室

Myotome	Dorsal rami of adjacent thoracic segments, and through its association with latissimus dorsi, C6–C8
Dermatome	L1/L2

Location

3 cun lateral to the lower border of the spinous process of L2. Situated in the latissimus dorsi, internal abdominal oblique and iliocostalis muscles, and, in its deep position, the quadratus lumborum muscle.

To aid location, it is in a soft depression approximately level with the thinnest part of the waist, the 'anatomical waist', in line with BL 23.

Needling

0.5 to 1.5 cun perpendicular insertion.
1 to 2 cun oblique medial insertion towards BL 23.

Do not needle deeply or in a superior direction, particularly on the right side. This poses considerable risk of injuring the kidney.

Actions and indications

BL 52 can be considered as the *back-shu point for the Willpower (Zhi)* and is used to treat *Kidney deficiency and psychological disorders* relating to disharmony of the Kidneys and the willpower.

BL 52 helps *regulate urination and strengthen the lumbar area*. Indications are similar to BL 23.

It is often close to quadratus lumborum and can be a very useful addition in treating lumbar pain.

> **Main Areas**—Kidneys. Lumbar area. Lower jiao.
> **Main Functions**—Boosts the Kidneys. Increases vitality. Strengthens the willpower.

BL 53　Baohuang
Bladder's Vitals

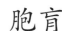 胞肓

Myotome	L4/L5, S1/S2
Dermatome	S1/S2

Location

3 cun lateral to the lower border of the spinous process of S2, level with BL 28 and BL 32. Situated in the gluteus maximus and medius muscles. To aid location, feel for the most tender spot by palpating laterally from the lower border of the PSIS.

Needling

1 to 2 cun perpendicular insertion.

Actions and indications

Extremely useful point for problems with the low back and sacroiliac joints.

> **Main Areas**—Sacrum. Buttock. Genitourinary system.
> **Main Functions**—Regulates Qi and Blood in the lower jiao. Alleviates pain.

BL 54   Zhibian
Lowermost in Order

秩邊

Myotome	L4/L5, S1/S2
Dermatome	S3

Location
On the highest point of the buttock, level with the sacral hiatus, 3 cun lateral to the posterior midline. Situated in the gluteus maximus and medius muscles, and, more deeply, the piriformis muscle.

To aid location, it is level with GV 2.

Needling
1 to 2.5 cun perpendicular insertion. The needle will enter the medial bulk of piriformis muscle belly during deep insertion. The sciatic nerve should pass beneath piriformis but in some cases there

is an anomaly and the nerve can either sit on top of piriformis, or pass through its bulk. Slow and responsive needling can avoid any stimulation to the nerve itself, so be aware and ask for constant feedback from your client.

Actions and indications
BL 54 is a *very effective point for the treatment of pain of the lower back, sacrum and buttocks*, sciatica and *disorders of the lower limbs. Regulates Qi in the lower jiao* and benefits the *anus and genitourinary system.*

> **Main Areas**—Sacrum. Buttock. Lower limbs. Anus.
> **Main Functions**—Regulates Qi and Blood in the lower jiao. Alleviates pain.

BL 55   Heyang
Yang Confluence

合陽

Myotome	S1/S2
Dermatome	L4–S1

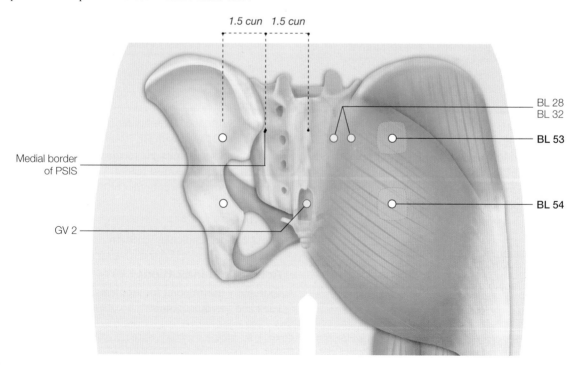

Location

2 cun distal to BL40, on the line connecting BL 40 and BL 57, in the depression between the two heads of the gastrocnemius muscle.

To aid location, BL 55 is one quarter of the distance between BL 40 and BL 57.

Needling

0.5 to 1 cun perpendicular insertion.

Actions and indications

BL 55 is indicated for *disorders of the gynaecological system*, especially abnormal uterine bleeding, leucorrhoea and intense genital pain.

BL 55 is effective to *regulate Qi and Blood and alleviate pain* of the channel and can be used in similar cases to BL 56.

An extremely useful point for lower limb injuries involving the calf and Achilles tendon.

Main Areas—Calf. Knee. Genitals.
Main Functions—Regulates Qi and Blood in the lower jiao. Alleviates regional pain.

BL 56   Chengjin
Sinew Support

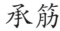

Myotome	S1/S2
Dermatome	L4–S1

Location

At the centre of the belly of the gastrocnemius muscle, 5 cun distal to BL 40, midway between BL 55 and BL 57.

Needling

0.5 to 1 cun perpendicular insertion.

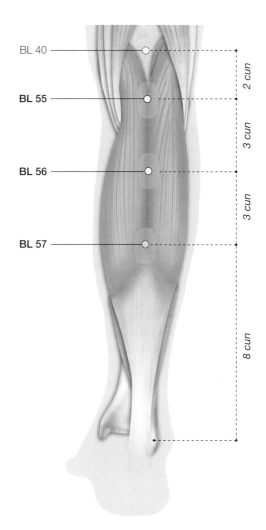

BL 40

BL 55

BL 56

BL 57

2 cun

3 cun

3 cun

8 cun

Actions and indications

BL 56 is a very *effective local point* to treat pain, cramping, stiffness or weakness of the calf. It is also useful in the treatment of sciatica, atrophy or paralysis of the lower limbs and lumbar pain.

In common with BL 57, it is also indicated for *constipation, haemorrhoids and other disorders of the anus*.

Main Areas—Anus. Calf and leg.
Main Functions—Regulates Qi and Blood. Alleviates pain. Treats haemorrhoids.

BL 57 Chengshan
Mountain Support

承山

BL 58 Feiyang
Taking Flight

飛揚

Heavenly Star point

Myotome	S1/S2
Dermatome	L4–S1

Luo-Connecting point

Myotome	S1/S2
Dermatome	S1

Location

At the centre of the calf, in the depression below the two bellies of the gastrocnemius muscle, approximately 8 cun inferior to BL 40, or midway between BL 40 and the insertion of the Achilles tendon on the heel.

To aid location, contract the gastrocnemius by asking the patient to press the ball of their foot against the resistance of your hand; then run your finger up the midline, from the Achilles tendon until it naturally slips into the depression.

Location

7 cun proximal to BL 60, on the posterior border of the fibula, at the lateral margin of the gastrocnemius muscle. Approximately 1 cun distal and lateral to BL 57.

To aid location, BL 58 is 1 cun distal to the midpoint of the line joining BL 60 with the lateral end of the popliteal crease.

Needling

0.5 to 1 cun perpendicular insertion.

Needling

0.5 to 1 cun perpendicular insertion.

Actions and indications

BL 57 is an *important point for disorders of the channel pathway* and has been extensively used to treat: sciatica, lumbar pain, and atrophy, paralysis, pain, cramping, stiffness or weakness of the calf and leg. Also for Achilles tendinitis.

In addition, BL 57 is *important in the treatment of disorders of the anal and genital region* and is especially indicated for: haemorrhoids, constipation, rectal prolapse, pain of the perineum or anus, and dysmenorrhoea.

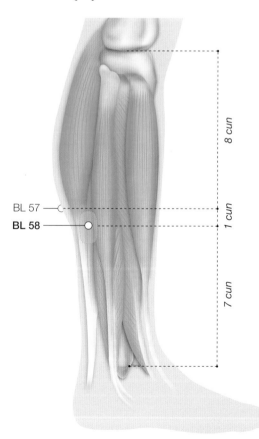

> **Main Areas**—Anus. Calf and leg.
> **Main Functions**—Regulates Qi and Blood.
> Alleviates pain. Treats haemorrhoids.

Actions and indications

BL 58 is a useful point to *clear the Tai Yang and dispel wind, dampness and heat* as well as to *regulate Qi and Blood and alleviate pain.*

Main indications include: sciatica, lumbar pain, pain or cramping of the calf and weakness, stiffness or swelling of the legs. It has also been successfully used to treat such cases as: haemorrhoids, chills and fever, headache, dizziness, epilepsy, nasal congestion, and epistaxis.

> **Main Areas**—Lower limbs. Anus. Tai Yang area. Lower back.
> **Main Functions**—Dispels wind, dampness and heat. Clears the Tai Yang. Regulates Qi and Blood. Alleviates pain.

BL 59   Fuyang
Tarsus Yang

Xi-Cleft point of the Yang Qiao Mai

Myotome	S1/S2
Dermatome	S1

Location

3 cun (one hand-width) directly proximal to BL 60, between the Achilles tendon and the posterior border of the fibula.

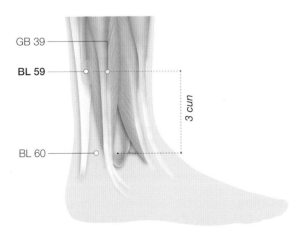

GB 39
BL 59
BL 60
3 cun

Needling

0.5 to 1 cun perpendicular insertion.

Actions and indications

BL 59 is a useful point to *dispel wind and dampness and clear the Tai Yang.*

Indications include: headache, dizziness, nasal congestion, lower backache, and pain, atrophy, numbness or swelling of the calf or ankle.

> **Main Areas**—Calf. Head.
> **Main Functions**—Dispels wind and dampness. Clears the Tai Yang. Alleviates pain.

BL 60   Kunlun
Kunlun (Mountains)

Jing-River point, Fire point
Heavenly Star point

Myotome	None – superficial tissue
Dermatome	S1

Location

At the centre of the large depression formed between the lateral malleolus and the Achilles tendon, level with the prominence of the lateral malleolus when the foot is at right angles to the leg. Situated in the triangle-shaped depression posterior to the tendon sheath of the fibularis longus and brevis and anterior to the Achilles tendon.

To aid location, BL 60 is opposite and slightly inferior to KI 3. Grasp the Achilles tendon between the finger and the thumb to locate both points.

Note: The deep position of BL 60 and KI 3 is approximately at the same anatomical point and both needling and acupressure treatment can access it. Additionally, the two points can be joined.

Needling

0.3 to 5 cun perpendicular insertion.

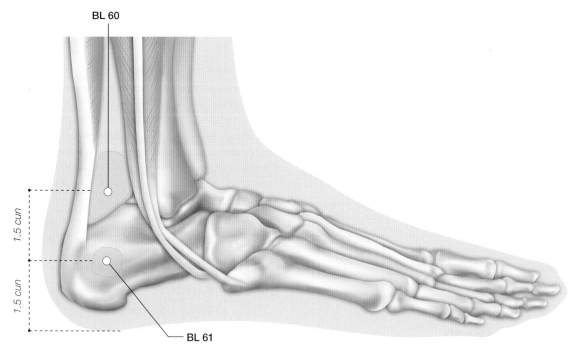

0.5 to 1 cun perpendicular insertion to join with KI 3.

If needling to join with KI 3, ensure that the vessels on the medial side are not punctured, particularly the tibial nerve and the posterior tibial artery and veins.

Actions and indications

BL 60 is a *very dynamic point* and is *very important in the treatment of any blockage along the course of the Bladder channel*, particularly if there is pain. It is widely used to *clear the Tai Yang, treat interior and exterior wind, descend rising Yang and clear heat, particularly from the head and upper body.* BL 60 is also used to *strengthen the lumbar region and tonify the Kidneys.*

Indications include: headache, stiffness of the neck, heat sensation in the head, inflammation of the eyes, epistaxis, dizziness, hemiplegia, convulsions, chills and fever, acute and chronic lumbar pain, sciatica, and pain of the lateral aspect of the leg and heel.

Additionally, BL 60 has a *powerful effect on the uterus, relieving Blood stasis, alleviating pain and promoting labour.*

Traditionally, BL 60 has also been used to treat a variety of other symptoms and conditions,

including: infantile epilepsy, malaria, diarrhoea, infertility, toothache, fullness of the chest, dyspnoea, and cough.

> **Main Areas**—Tai Yang area. Lower limb. Ankle. Lumbus. Spine. Neck. Head. Uterus.
> **Main Functions**—Clears the Tai Yang and expels exterior pathogens. Descends rising Yang, subdues wind and clears heat. Regulates Qi and Blood and dispels stasis from the lower jiao. Promotes labour. Alleviates pain.

BL 61   Pucan
Subservient Visitor

Intersection of the Yang Qiao Mai on the Bladder channel

Myotome	None – superficial tissue
Dermatome	S1

Location

On the lateral aspect of the foot, directly inferior to BL 60, in a depression on the calcaneus, at the junction of the skin of the plantar and dorsal aspects of the foot.

Needling
0.3 to 0.5 cun perpendicular insertion.
Oblique/sub-cutaneous insertion towards the toes.

Actions and indications
BL 61 is primarily used as a *local point* for regional pain, stiffness or swelling.

> **Main Areas**—Ankle. Heel.
> **Main Function**—Alleviates pain.

BL 62   Shenmai
Extending Vessel

Opening point of the Yang Qiao Mai
Fifth Ghost point

Myotome	None – superficial tissue
Dermatome	S1

Location
Directly inferior to the lateral malleolus, in the small space between the tendons of the fibularis longus and brevis muscles. Approximately 0.5 cun inferior to the inferior border of the lateral malleolus.

Alternative locations
If the site between the tendons is very tight, treat BL 62 in the posterior to the tendon of the fibularis longus. Alternatively, locate slightly more superiorly in the joint space between the talus and the calcaneus.

Needling
0.3 to 0.4 cun perpendicular insertion between the two tendons. If the tendons are very tight, apply manual pressure to loosen them before needling. 0.3 to 0.5 cun oblique inferior insertion posterior to the tendons.

Actions and indications
BL 62 is important to *regulate the flow of Yang Qi, descend rising Yang, clear heat and calm the mind. Clears the Tai Yang area and dissipates exterior wind, cold and heat.*

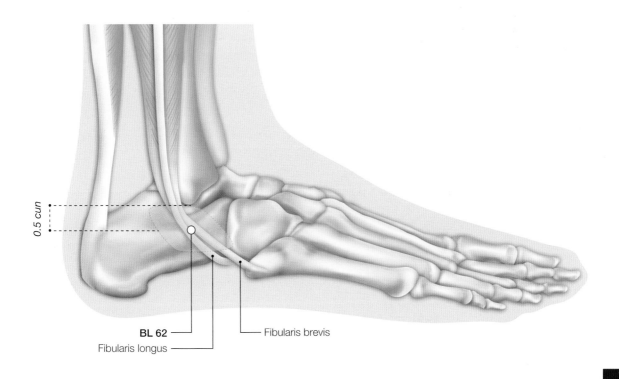

0.5 cun

BL 62
Fibularis longus
Fibularis brevis

Indications include: headache, stiffness of the neck, redness of the face, dizziness, tinnitus, facial paralysis, wind stroke, hemiplegia, convulsions, epilepsy, fever, chills, epistaxis, inflammation and pain of the eyes, palpitations, depression, fright, irritability, and insomnia.

Furthermore, BL 62 *regulates the flow of Qi and Blood in the channel pathway and alleviates pain.* Indications include: sciatica, lumbar pain, stiffness and pain of the neck, and stiffness or swelling of the ankle.

Other indications include dysmenorrhoea, swelling of the axilla and fullness of the chest.

> **Main Areas**—Head. Spine. Lower limb. Ankle.
> **Main Functions**—Descends rising Yang and clears heat. Subdues interior wind. Clears the head. Calms the mind. Alleviates pain.

BL 63　Jinmen

Golden Gate

Xi-Cleft point
Intersection of the Yang Wei Mai
on the Bladder channel

Myotome	None – superficial tissue
Dermatome	S1

Location
On the lateral aspect of the foot, inferior and anterior to BL 62, in the depression of the cuboid bone, posterior and superior to the tuberosity of the fifth metatarsal.

Alternative location
BL 63 can be alternatively treated further down, posterior to the tuberosity of the fifth metatarsal bone, between the fibularis brevis tendon and the abductor digiti minimi muscle. Use pressure palpation to determine which location is most reactive.

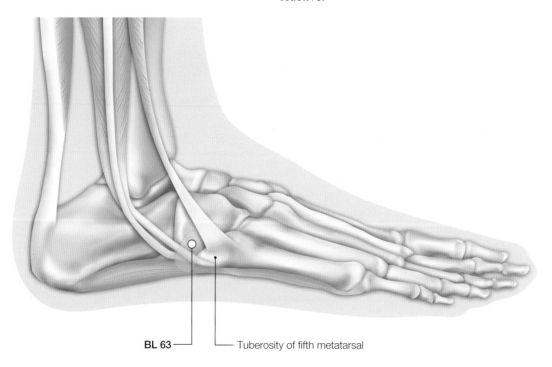

BL 63 ——　└—— Tuberosity of fifth metatarsal

Needling

0.3 to 0.5 cun perpendicular insertion.
Oblique/sub-cutaneous insertion towards the toes.

Actions and indications

In common with the other xi-cleft points, BL 63 helps *moderate acute conditions and relieve pain*. It is particularly effective for acute pain and cramping along the course of the Bladder channel, especially lumbar pain and sciatica.

> **Main Areas**—Bladder channel. Spine and lumbar region. Lower limbs.
> **Main Functions**—Regulates Qi and Blood. Alleviates pain.

BL 64　Jinggu
Metatarsal Tuberosity

Yuan-Source point

Myotome	None – superficial tissue
Dermatome	S1

Location

On the lateral aspect of the foot, in the depression anterior and inferior to the tuberosity of the fifth metatarsal bone, at the junction of the skin of the plantar and dorsal aspects of the foot.

Alternative locations

Some sources place this point directly lateral to the tuberosity of the fifth metatarsal bone, whereas others place it posterior and inferior to it.

To aid location, apply pressure palpation to the area directly inferior to the tuberosity in order to determine the reactive site that causes a sensation to extend outwards from the point.

Needling

0.3 to 0.5 cun perpendicular insertion.
Oblique/sub-cutaneous insertion towards the toes.

Actions and indications

BL 64 is primarily indicated to *dispel wind and clear heat*, especially from the *head and eyes*. It is also used to *calm the mind*.

Indications include: headache, stiffness of the neck, chills and fever, heat sensation in the head,

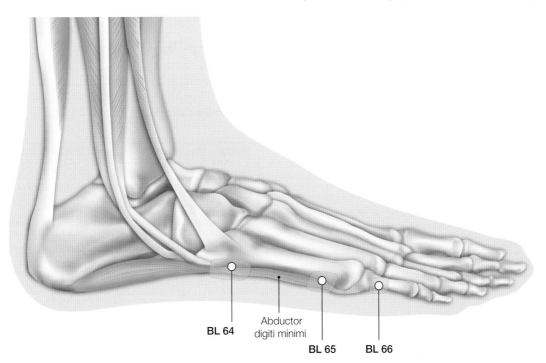

BL 64
Abductor digiti minimi
BL 65
BL 66

epistaxis, pain and inflammation of the eyes, dizziness, fright, epilepsy, palpitations, lower backache, and stiffness or pain along the course of the channel pathway.

> **Main Areas**—Head. Eyes. Bladder channel.
> **Main Functions**—Dispels wind and clears heat. Calms the mind. Alleviates pain.

BL 65   Shugu
Metatarsal Head

Shu-Stream point, Wood point

Myotome	None – superficial tissue
Dermatome	S1

Location
On the lateral aspect of the foot, in the depression proximal and slightly inferior to the head of the fifth metatarsal bone, at the junction of the skin of the plantar and dorsal surface.

Needling
0.2 to 0.5 cun perpendicular insertion.
Oblique/sub-cutaneous insertion towards the toes.

Actions and indications
Used to treat excess conditions of the head and upper back through its channel connection. As a Wood point, it is useful in treating muscular problems, as the Wood element is associated with all things muscular. Headache within the occipital region.

> **Main Areas**—Foot. Metatarsal. Head.
> **Main Functions**—Dispels wind and clears heat. Alleviates pain.

BL 66   Zutonggu
Foot Valley Passage

Ying-Spring point, Water point

Myotome	None – superficial tissue
Dermatome	S1

Location
On the lateral aspect of the foot, distal and inferior to the fifth MTP joint, at the junction of the skin of the plantar and dorsal aspects of the foot.

Needling
0.2 to 0.3 cun perpendicular insertion.

Actions and indications
Clears disorders of the *head (occipital region in particular) upper thoracic spine, cervical spine and eyes.*

> **Main Areas**—MTP joint. Toe. Head.
> **Main Functions**—Dispels wind and clears heat. Alleviates pain.

BL 67   Zhiyin
Reaching Yin

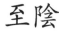

Jing-Well point, Metal point

Myotome	None – superficial tissue
Dermatome	S1

Location
0.1 cun proximal to the lateral corner of the base of the nail, at the intersection of two lines following the lateral border of the nail and the base of the nail.

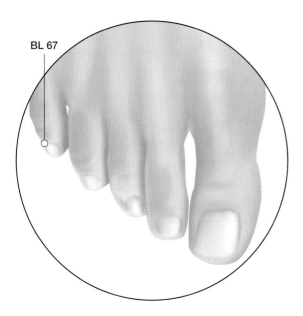

BL 67

Contraindicated during pregnancy.

Needling

0.1 cun perpendicular insertion.

Actions and indications

BL 67 has a *powerful effect on the uterus* by *activating the Yang Qi of the Bladder and Kidney*. It is therefore contraindicated during pregnancy, except in the case of *breech presentation*, in which event the application of moxibustion is employed to turn the foetus during the seventh and eighth month. It is also used to *induce labour and expedite delivery* of the baby and placenta.

Furthermore, BL 67 *dispels wind, clears heat and benefits the head and eyes*.

Indications include: chills and fever, headache, stiff neck, inflammation of the eyes, nasal congestion, and epistaxis.

> **Main Areas**—Uterus. Head.
> **Main Functions**—Corrects position of the foetus. Dispels exterior pathogens and clears the Tai Yang.

Points of the Leg Shao Yin Kidney Channel

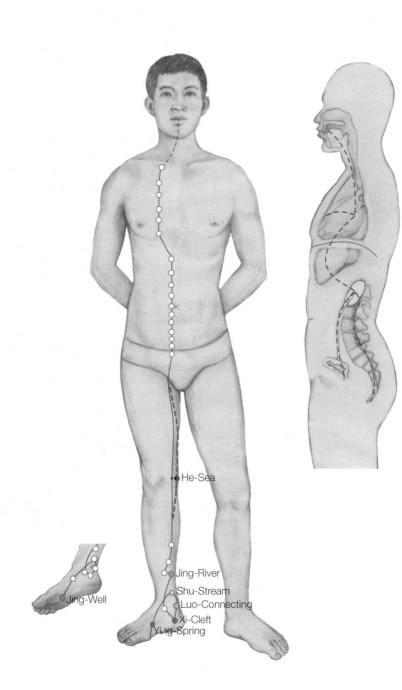

He-Sea

Jing-River

Shu-Stream
Luo-Connecting

Jing-Well

Xi-Cleft
Ying-Spring

足少陰腎經穴

General	The Kidney channel starts on the sole of the foot – KI 1 being the only acupuncture point on this surface. It moves up across the instep, and, circling the medial malleolus, then travels up the medial aspect of the leg, veering backwards to sit at KI 10 between the two medial hamstrings at the posterior aspect of the knee. Continuing in a line up through the gracilis and moving forwards again, the channel emerges at the perineum at GV 1. Its internal pathway works upwards through the spine, but its accessible channel travels up only half a cun from the midline, all the way up the front of the body, over the abdominals. Moving laterally at the breast, it finishes just below the clavicle in a dip at its medial end. The channel has 27 points. It is grouped with the Bladder under the Water element in five-element theory.
More specifically	There are many connecting channels that intersect with the Kidney, and rightly give it a place of extreme importance in the channel network. As an organ, it forms the Shao Yin division along with the Heart – the two most fundamental organs of life. The KI 1 point is akin to the solar plexus point in reflexology, and lies at the junction of the top and middle thirds of a line drawn on the sole of the foot from the heel to the toes. The channel wraps around the medial arch of the foot, and from KI 3 travels back down a small way, creating an elaborate circle around the medial malleolus. The channel gets going again 2 cun above the malleolus, at KI 7 and KI 8, and then travels upwards and slightly posteriorly, via SP 6, to meet at KI 10, in a dip in between the two medial hamstrings. Crossing the adductor muscles and following the path of the gracilis, it moves up the thigh, from back to front, and crosses the perineum. It has a connection with GV 1 at this point. From here it sends internal connections as it moves upwards through the body to the Bladder channel and both the Conception and Governor Vessels at CV 3, CV 4 and CV 7. (The Bladder is the Kidney's Yang paired organ.) Aspects of this channel reach as far as the tongue, the back of the head at BL 10 and around the Heart, emphasising the strong medical connection between Heart function and Kidney function. Other aspects are said to be more structurally internal, as the tendino-muscular channel runs up the *front* of the spine, leading to upright posture and hence providing an open working environment for all the other internal organs.
Area covered	Foot, medial knee and groin, pelvic floor, spine (especially lumbar), chest.
Areas affected with treatment	Chest – breathing/asthma, lumbar spine weakness, pelvic floor and all urogenital conditions, knee and hamstrings, instep of foot/plantar fascia.
Key points	KI 1, KI 3, KI 7, KI 8, KI 10, KI 16.

KI 1   Yongquan
Bubbling Spring

涌泉

Jing-Well point, Wood point

Myotome	S2/S3
Dermatome	L5

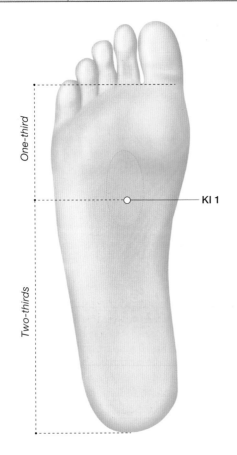

One-third

Two-thirds

KI 1

Location
On the sole of the foot, in the visible depression formed when the foot is plantar flexed, between the second and third metatarsal bones, approximately one third of the distance from the base of the second toe to the heel. Situated in the second lumbrical muscle, between the tendons of the flexor digitorum

brevis and longus muscles attaching to the second and third toes.

To aid location, use pressure palpation to determine the exact site that is most reactive.

Needling
0.5 to 1 cun perpendicular insertion.

KI 1 can be very painful when needled. You may need to use slightly thicker needles if the plantar skin is hard. In general, needling is rarely applied here exactly because it can be so painful.

Actions and indications
KI 1 is an important point to *clear heat and fire, descend excessive Yang* and *subdue wind*. It is mostly indicated for excess conditions, particularly when the upper body is affected. Furthermore, it has a powerful *relaxing and calming effect* on the body and mind.

Indications include: headache on the vertex or whole head, dizziness, vertigo, insomnia, mental agitation, poor memory, mental confusion, night sweats, sore or swollen throat, blurred vision, aversion to cold, cyanosis, hypertension, loss of consciousness, shock, wind stroke, epilepsy, epistaxis, constipation, difficult urination, lower abdominal pain, infertility, impotence, lumbar pain, sciatica, weakness or paralysis of the lower limbs, heat in the soles of the feet, and pain of the sole of the foot and toes.

If a client seems to be getting panicky and showing signs of an extreme stress response, firm pressure on KI 1 can help 'bring them down' and settle them.

> **Main Areas**—Head. Mind. Entire body. Sole of the foot.
> **Main Functions**—Clears fire. Sedates interior wind. Calms the mind. Resuscitates.

KI 2   Rangu
Blazing Valley

Ying-Spring point, Fire point

Myotome	None – superficial tissue
Dermatome	L5

Location
On the medial side of the foot, in the depression inferior and slightly anterior to the navicular tuberosity, along the line joining KI 1 to KI 3.

To aid location, the navicular tuberosity is the most prominent bony landmark on the medial side of the foot.

Needling
0.5 to 1 cun perpendicular insertion.

Actions and indications
KI 2 is primarily used to *clear empty fire and heat* due to *Kidney Yin deficiency*. It treats symptoms such as insomnia, restlessness, night sweating, fever, emaciation, pain of the bones and spine which is worse at night, thirst, sore or swollen throat, coughing blood, dry unproductive cough, and loss of voice.

Additionally, KI 2 *regulates menstruation and benefits the uterus*. Indications include: uterine prolapse, genital itching, leucorrhoea, infertility, irregular menstruation, and excessive menstrual bleeding.

It is also used for other *disorders of the lower jiao*, including: dysuria, haematuria, turbid urination, urethritis, cystitis, prostatitis, impotence, and premature ejaculation.

KI 2 can be used to *tonify Kidney Yang and warm the lower jiao*, particularly if treated with moxibustion.

> **Main Areas**—Kidneys. Spine. Entire body.
> **Main Functions**—Clears empty fire. Nourishes Kidney Yin. Benefits the genitourinary system.

KI 3   Taixi
Great Stream

Shu-Stream point, Earth point
Yuan-Source point

Myotome	None – superficial tissue
Dermatome	S1

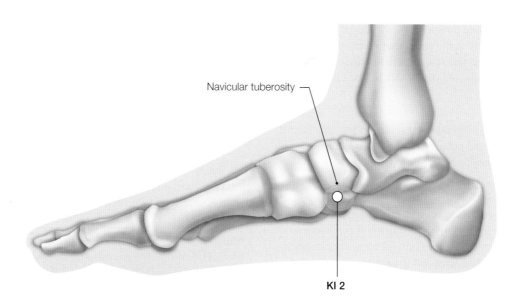

Navicular tuberosity

KI 2

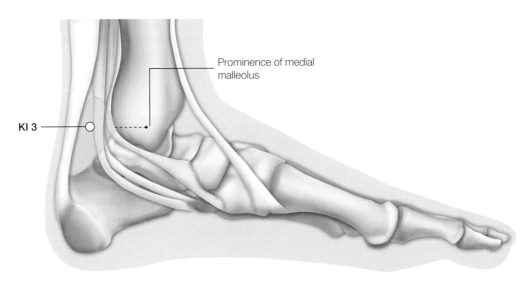

Prominence of medial malleolus

KI 3

Location

In the depression midway between the posterior border of the medial malleolus and the anterior border of the Achilles tendon, level with the prominence of the medial malleolus when the foot is at right angles to the leg.

To aid location, KI 3 is opposite and slightly superior to BL 60. Grasp the Achilles tendon between the finger and the thumb to locate both these points. Furthermore, it is usually most reactive at the visible centre of the depression, therefore locating it visually may be more helpful (this does not apply in cases of swelling or deformity of the ankle).

Note: The deep position of KI 3 and BL 60 is approximately at the same anatomical point and both needling and acupressure treatment can access it. Additionally, the two points can be joined.

Needling

0.3 to 1 cun perpendicular insertion towards BL 60. Palpate for the pulse of the posterior tibial artery and insert the needle posterior to it.

Actions and indications

KI 3 one of the top most commonly used points with a wide range of applications. It is a major tonifying point for the Kidneys because it *augments the Kidney Yin, Yang* and jing and is of particular importance in the treatment of disorders of the lower jiao, Kidneys, Bladder, reproductive system and spine. It is used in the treatment of *many chronic diseases* because it *tonifies the Original Qi (yuan Qi)* that stems from the Kidney Yin and Yang.

Indications include: exhaustion, diminished hearing and sight, tinnitus, dizziness, hypertension, heat in the five hearts (hands, feet and chest), fever, night sweating, insomnia, dream-disturbed sleep, emaciation, thirst, sore throat, infertility, impotence, premature ejaculation, spermatorrhoea, amenorrhoea, irregular menstruation, menopausal syndromes, frequent and abundant urination, dribbling urination, dysuria, dark urine, enuresis, constipation, swelling of the legs, oedema, abdominal pain, chronic lower backache, and coldness and weakness of the lower back, abdomen, knees and legs.

It is a commonly used point for *Achilles tendon issues and ankle sprains* with swelling.

KI 3 has a *beneficial influence on the Lungs and breathing* and can help the Kidneys in the function of *grasping Qi from the Lungs*.

Indications include: chronic cough, haemoptysis, epistaxis, chest pain, shallow breathing, and asthma due to Kidney and Lung disharmony.

Main Areas—Kidneys. Spine. Entire body.
Main Functions—Augments Kidney Yin and Yang. Tonifies yuan Qi. Benefits the genitourinary system. Increases fertility.

KI 4   Dazhong

Large Bell

 大鐘

Luo-Connecting point

Myotome	None – superficial tissue
Dermatome	S1

Location

In a small depression approximately 0.5 cun inferior and posterior to KI 3, at the anterior border of the Achilles tendon.

To aid location, find the midpoint of the line joining KI 3 to KI 5 and, from here, move posteriorly to the point just anterior to the Achilles tendon.

Needling

0.3 to 0.5 cun perpendicular or oblique anterior insertion.

Actions and indications

KI 4 has been extensively employed to *strengthen the Kidneys* both in the physical and in the psycho-emotional sense. It is traditionally indicated to increase the *willpower and dispel* fear and has been used to treat such cases as: propensity to fright, chronic phobias, psychological insecurity, lack of confidence, introverted behaviour, lack of willpower, sleepiness, anxiety, irritability, fright palpitations, insomnia, and other psychological disturbances.

KI 4 is important to *harmonise the Kidney and Lung* and helps draw down excess causing various respiratory disorders. Symptoms include: shallow breathing, asthma, cough, haemoptysis, and dryness and soreness of the mouth and throat.

Symptoms relating to *disharmony of the Kidney luo-connecting channel* include: lumbar pain, weakness of the lower limbs, pain of the ankle or heel, oppression of the chest, palpitations, cardiac pain, vomiting, abdominal distension and fullness, dysuria, and urinary retention.

KI 4 also treats other symptoms of *Kidney weakness*, including: exhaustion, chronic constipation, impotence, infertility, and irregular menstruation.

> **Main Areas**—Mind. Kidneys. Lungs.
> **Main Functions**—Reinforces the Kidneys. Strengthens willpower. Harmonises the Kidney and Lung.

KI 5   Shuiquan

Water Spring

 水泉

Xi-Cleft point

Myotome	None – superficial tissue
Dermatome	L4

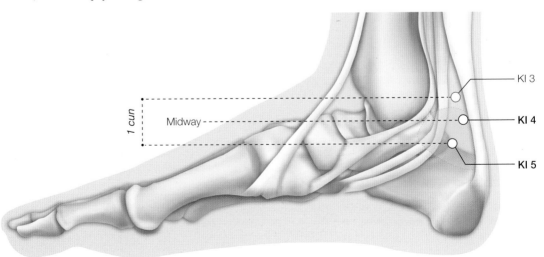

Location

1 cun inferior to KI 3, in the depression anterior and superior to the insertion of the Achilles tendon at the calcaneal tuberosity. Locate with the foot at a right angle to the leg.

Needling

0.3 to 0.5 cun perpendicular or oblique anterior insertion.

Actions and indications

KI 5 is important to regulate the *flow of Qi and Blood in the lower jiao and harmonise the Conception Vessel and Chong Mai*. It is used to *nourish Blood* as well as to *dispel Blood stasis*.

Indications include: abdominal pain, dysmenorrhoea, amenorrhoea, irregular menstruation, infertility, uterine prolapse, frequent urination, dysuria, and dribbling.

KI 5 has been traditionally used to treat *disorders of the eyes*, including nearsightedness and diminishing or unclear vision.

> **Main Areas**—Lower jiao. Gynaecological and urinary system. Eyes.
> **Main Functions**—Dispels Blood stasis. Nourishes Blood. Regulates the Conception Vessel and Chong Mai.

KI 6 Zhaohai
Shining Sea
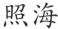

Opening point of the Yin Qiao Mai

Myotome	None – superficial tissue
Dermatome	L4

Location

In the depression approximately 1 cun below the prominence of the medial malleolus, between the tendons of the tibialis posterior and flexor digitorum longus muscles.

To aid location, define the tendons by plantar flexing and inverting the foot.

Alternative location

If the tendons are very stiff and tight, treat KI 6 in the depression directly below the sustentaculum tali.

Needling

0.3 to 0.5 cun perpendicular insertion in a slightly superior direction. The needle should go between the two tendons. However, if this location is very tight, it will be painful and so needling should be applied below the sustentaculum tali.

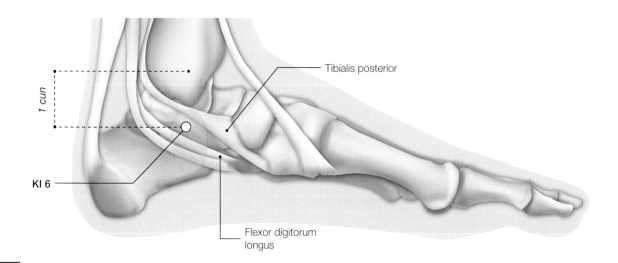

1 cun

Tibialis posterior

KI 6

Flexor digitorum longus

Actions and indications

KI 6 is one of the most important points to *nourish and moisten Yin, cool the body and clear empty heat.*

Indications include: night sweating, heat in the five hearts, low-grade fever, hot flushes, menopausal syndromes, impotence, headache, dizziness, palpitations, epilepsy, exhaustion, chronic thirst and dry mouth, chronic sore or swollen throat, pharyngitis, dryness and pain of the eyes, photophobia, diminishing vision, tinnitus, soreness of the lower back and pain in the bones.

KI 6 is also a significant point for the treatment of *gynaecological complaints* such as infertility, irregular menstruation, amenorrhoea, excessive menstrual bleeding, post partum abdominal pain, excessive lochia, leucorrhoea, uterine prolapse, and genital itching and dryness.

KI 6 helps to *calm the mind* in cases of anxiety, restlessness and insomnia.

Main Areas—Head. Eyes. Ears. Throat. Mind. Lower jiao. Uterus. Entire body.
Main Functions—Nourishes Yin. Cools empty heat. Regulates the Yin Qiao Mai.

KI 7   Fuliu
Continuing Flow
復溜

Jing-River point, Metal point

Myotome	None – superficial tissue but close to soleus, S1/S2
Dermatome	L4

Location

2 cun proximal to KI 3, in the depression anterior to the border of the Achilles tendon and inferior to the soleus muscle.

Needling

0.5 to 1 cun perpendicular insertion.

Actions and indications

KI 7 is a *very important point to tonify Kidney Yang* and *promote the body's water metabolism* thus *regulating sweat, urination and movement of interstitial fluids.* It has been extensively used to treat: oedema, frequent urination, dribbling urination, anuria, lower backache and spontaneous, excessive or lack of sweating.

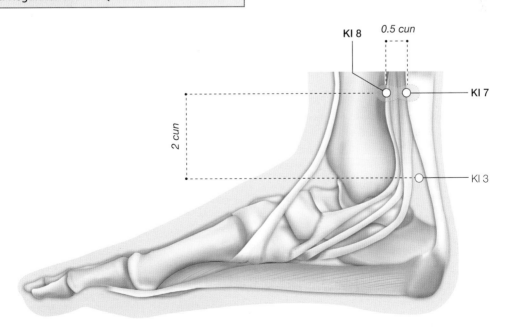

In terms of back pain, KI 7 can have a dramatic *effect on the tension within iliopsoas* if this is tight and adding to hip and back issues.

KI 7 is important to *clear damp heat* and has been employed to treat such cases as: night sweating, tidal fever, urinary tract infections, leucorrhoea, abdominal distension, diarrhoea, haemorrhoids and pus and blood in the stools.

Additionally, KI 7 treats other symptoms of *Kidney deficiency*, including: exhaustion, depression, lack of motivation, and other psychological disorders.

> **Main Areas**—Water passages. Lower jiao.
> **Main Functions**—Regulates sweat and urination. Reduces swelling. Tonifies Kidney Yang.

KI 8   Jiaoxin
Intersecting with Spleen

Xi-Cleft point of the Yin Qiao Mai
Intersection of the Yin Qiao Mai and Kidney channel

Myotome	None – superficial tissue but close to flexor digitorum longus L4/L5, S1/S2
Dermatome	L4

Location
0.5 cun anterior to KI 7, posterior to the medial border of the tibia, 2 cun proximal to KI 3.

Needling
0.5 to 1 cun perpendicular insertion.

Actions and indications
KI 8 is a *useful point to harmonise the Conception Vessel and Chong Mai* and *regulate menstruation*. Furthermore, it *clears dampness and heat and benefits the lower jiao*.

Indications include: irregular or excessive menstrual bleeding, dysmenorrhoea, amenorrhoea, uterine

prolapse, genital itching, urinary tract infections, urinary retention, diarrhoea, and lumbar pain.

> **Main Areas**—Genitourinary system.
> **Main Functions**—Regulates menstruation. Clears dampness and heat.

KI 9   Zhubin
Strong Knees

Xi-Cleft point of the Yin Wei Mai

Myotome	S1/S2
Dermatome	L4

Location
On the medial aspect of the calf, along the line joining KI 3 to KI 10, approximately 5 cun proximal

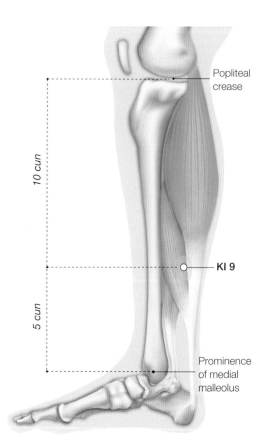

to KI 3, in the depression below the belly of the gastrocnemius muscle, just anterior to the border of the Achilles tendon.

To aid location, it is approximately one third of the distance along the line joining the prominence of the medial malleolus and the popliteal crease (or KI 3 to KI 10).

Also, it is approximately 1 cun posterior to LR 5.

Needling
0.5 to 1.5 cun perpendicular insertion.

Actions and indications
KI 9 is primarily indicated to *calm the mind, clear the Heart* and *transform phlegm*, at the same time as tonifying the Kidney Yin and jing. Its use is therefore recommended in the treatment of psycho-emotional disorders, including insomnia, epilepsy, anger, fright, and even insanity.

KI 9 has been used in the treatment of other related disorders, including: vomiting, oppression of the chest, palpitations, goitre, urinary tract infections, hernia, and abdominal pain and swelling.

As a *local point*, it can be helpful in cases of pain and spasm of the calf muscles.

> **Main Areas**—Heart. Mind. Lower jiao.
> **Main Functions**—Clears and calms the Heart and mind. Regulates Qi.

KI 10 Yingu
Yin Valley

陰谷

He-Sea point, Water point

Myotome	L5, S1/S2
Dermatome	L3

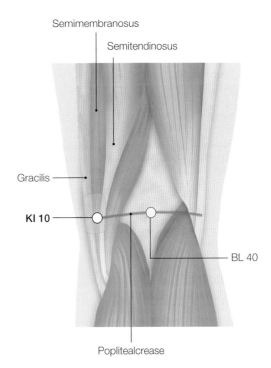

Semimembranosus
Semitendinosus
Gracilis
KI 10
BL 40
Poplitealcrease

Location
At the medial end of the popliteal crease, between the tendons of the semitendinosus and gracilis, level with BL 39 and BL 40. In its deep position, situated in the semimembranosus muscle. Locate with the knee flexed.

To aid location, the semitendinosus and gracilis are the two most prominent tendons at the medial posterior aspect of the knee. Define them by asking the patient to flex the knee against resistance.

KI 10 and BL 39 are best treated with the patient prone and with their knee flexed to at least 50–60 degrees, and supported on a pillow. This way, the dips that house K 10 and BL 39 become easily accessed and even visible.

Needling
0.5 to 1.5 cun perpendicular insertion.

Actions and indications
KI 10 is an *important point to transform dampness, clear heat, nourish Yin and benefit the lower jiao.*

It has been extensively employed to treat such symptoms as: dysuria, haematuria, frequent urination, impotence, chronic leucorrhoea, abnormal uterine bleeding, and pain of the lower back and knees.

> **Main Areas**—Lower jiao. Genitourinary system.
> **Main Functions**—Nourishes Yin and cools lower jiao heat. Transforms dampness.

KI 11   Henggu
Pubic Bone

Intersection of the Chong Mai on the Kidney channel

Myotome	None – superficial tissue
Dermatome	T12/L1

Location
On the superior border of the pubic symphysis, 0.5 cun lateral to the anterior midline level with CV 2.

To aid location, the 0.5 cun can be approximated by using a finger's breadth. However, it is 5 cun below the level of the umbilicus.

Alternative location
A number of sources place the points KI 11 to KI 17, slightly further laterally at a distance of 1 cun from the anterior midline.

Needling
0.5 to 1 cun perpendicular insertion.

Do not needle deeply, particularly if the patient is very thin. This poses the risk of puncturing a full bladder.

Actions and indications
KI 11 has similar functions to CV 2 and is primarily used to *treat disorders of the genitourinary system,* including: infertility, genital pain, dysuria, urinary retention, incontinence, prostatitis, and impotence.

> **Main Areas**—Bladder. Genitals. Lower jiao.
> **Main Functions**—Benefits the lower jiao. Improves sexual function and fertility.

KI 12   Dahe
Big Plentifulness

Intersection of the Chong Mai on the Kidney channel

Myotome	T7–T12
Dermatome	T12

Location
1 cun superior to KI 11. Level with CV 3.

Needling
0.5 to 1 cun perpendicular insertion.

Actions and indications
Genital pain and *penile disorders*. Uterine prolapse and pelvic floor insufficiency.

> **Main Areas**—Bladder. Genitals. Uterus. Lower jiao.
> **Main Functions**—Benefits the lower jiao.

KI 13   Qixue
Kidney Qi Cave

Intersection of the Chong Mai on the Kidney channel

Myotome	T7–T12
Dermatome	T11

Location
2 cun superior to KI 11. Level with CV 4.

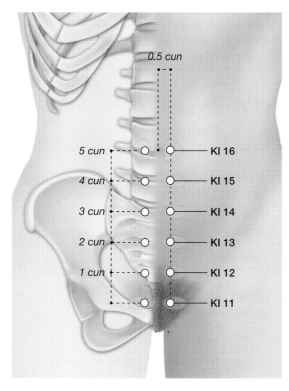

0.5 cun

5 cun — KI 16

4 cun — KI 15

3 cun — KI 14

2 cun — KI 13

1 cun — KI 12

KI 11

Needling

0.5 to 1 cun perpendicular insertion. Beware a full bladder. Ask client to empty bladder before treating in this region.

Actions and indications

Gynaecological symptoms, irregular menstruation, infertility. In particular it is a key point in the *treatment of running piglet Qi*, which is extreme panic and visceral feelings of collapse. Sensations rush upward from the lower jiao to the chest and throat.

> **Main Areas**—Uterus. Lower jiao. Emotional panic and anxiety.
> **Main Functions**—Benefits the lower jiao. Consolidates Qi in the lower jiao.

KI 14 Siman

Fourth for Fullness

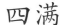

Intersection of the Chong Mai on the Kidney channel

Myotome	T7–T12
Dermatome	T11

Location

2 cun inferior to KI 16. Level with CV 5.

Needling

0.5 to 1 cun perpendicular insertion.

Actions and indications

Gynaecological symptoms, irregular menstruation, painful menstruation, a point for *running piglet Qi,* which is extreme panic and visceral feelings of collapse. Sensations rush upward from the lower jiao to the chest and throat.

Also, other issues with the *digestive tract involving distension and bloating* in the lower jiao.

> **Main Areas**—Large intestine, Lower jiao.
> **Main Functions**—Benefits the lower jiao. Reduces bloating and pain. Centers running piglet Qi.

KI 15 Zhongzhu

Pouring into the Middle

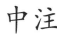

Intersection of the Chong Mai on the Kidney channel

Myotome	T7–T12
Dermatome	T11

Location

1 cun inferior to KI 16. Level with CV 7.

Needling

1 cun perpendicular insertion.

Actions and indications

Useful point for intestinal problems such as *constipation, diarrhoea, irregular menstruation.* Another centering area for *running piglet Qi.*

> **Main Areas**—Intestines. Lower jiao.
> **Main Functions**—Benefits the lower jiao. Improves digestive tract function. Calms running piglet Qi.

KI 16 Huangshu
Vital Tissues Shu

Intersection of the Chong Mai on the Kidney channel

Myotome	T7–T12
Dermatome	T10

Location

At the centre of the abdomen, 0.5 cun lateral to the centre of the umbilicus (CV 8). To aid location, it is usually just at the edge of the umbilicus.

Alternative location

A number of sources place the points KI 11 to KI 17, slightly further laterally, 1 cun from the anterior midline.

Needling

0.5 to 1.5 cun perpendicular insertion.

Actions and indications

In common with CV 8, ST 25 and SP 15, KI 16 *warms and regulates Qi in the abdomen and intestines and helps alleviate pain.* Symptoms include: constipation, dry stools, diarrhoea, vomiting, and abdominal pain, distension or swelling.

> **Main Areas**—Umbilicus. Abdomen. Intestines.
> **Main Functions**—Warms the abdomen. Regulates intestinal Qi. Alleviates pain.

KI 17 Shangqu
Metal Bend

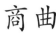

Intersection of the Chong Mai on the Kidney channel

Myotome	T7–T12
Dermatome	T8/T9

Location

2 cun superior to KI 16. Level with CV 10.

Needling

1 cun perpendicular insertion.

Actions and indications

Vomiting, constipation, diarrhoea. Loss of appetite and pain in the intestines.

> **Main Areas**—Abdomen. Epigastrium.
> **Main Functions**—Regulates Qi. Benefits the abdomen. Alleviates pain.

KI 18 Shiguan
Stone Gate

Intersection of the Chong Mai on the Kidney channel

Myotome	T7–T2
Dermatome	T7/8

Location

3 cun above the umbilicus, 0.5 cun lateral to the anterior midline.

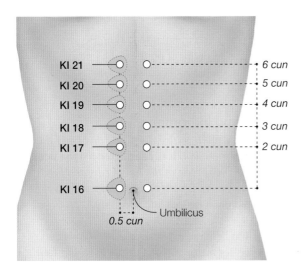

To aid location, it is level with CV 11 and ST 22.

Alternative location
A number of sources place the points KI 18 to KI 21 further laterally, at a distance of 1.5 cun from the anterior midline.

Needling
1 cun perpendicular insertion. Beware deep needling.

Actions and indications
Although KI 18 is not a very commonly used point, it can be used to *harmonise the Stomach* and treat symptoms such as nausea and vomiting, indigestion, epigastric or abdominal pain, and acid reflux.

Traditionally it is especially indicated for hard abdominal masses that may feel like 'stone'. This could be interpreted as extreme constipation.

Main Areas—Epigastrium. Stomach.
Main Functions—Harmonises the Stomach.
Descends rebellious Qi. Alleviates pain.

KI 19   Yindu
Yin Metropolis

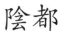

Intersection of the Chong Mai on the Kidney channel

Myotome	T7–T12
Dermatome	T7

Location
4 cun above the umbilicus, 0.5 cun lateral to the anterior midline.

To aid location, it is level with CV 12 and ST 21.

Alternative location
A number of sources place the points KI 18 to KI 21 further laterally, at a distance of 1.5 cun from the anterior midline.

Needling
0.5 to 1 cun perpendicular insertion

Actions and indications
Settles the Stomach in the case of nausea, distension and discomfort within the epigastrium. Aids constipation. Also helps clear upward pressure onto the diaphragm resulting in difficulty in breathing.

Main Areas—Epigastrium. Stomach.
Main Functions—Harmonises the Stomach.
Descends rebellious Qi. Alleviates pain.

KI 20   Futonggu
Abdominal Food

Passage
腹通谷

Intersection of the Chong Mai on the Kidney channel

Myotome	T7–T12
Dermatome	T6/T7

Location

5 cun above the umbilicus, 0.5 cun lateral to the anterior midline.

To aid location, it is level with CV 13 and ST 20.

Alternative location

A number of sources place the points KI 18 to KI 21 further laterally, at a distance of 1.5 cun from the anterior midline.

Needling

1 to 1.5 cun perpendicular insertion.

Actions and indications

Another point to help *clear constipation and undigested food* in the stool – signs of Stomach and Large Intestine insufficiency. There may be *sensations of fullness in the chest and lateral ribs* due to feeling full within the upper intestines and poor movement through the system.

> **Main Areas**—Epigastrium. Stomach.
> **Main Functions**—Harmonises the Stomach. Descends rebellious Qi. Alleviates pain.

KI 21   Youmen

Hidden Gate

幽門

Intersection of the Chong Mai on the Kidney channel

Myotome	T7–T12
Dermatome	T6/T7

Location

6 cun above the umbilicus, 0.5 cun lateral to the anterior midline.

To aid location, it is level with CV 14 and ST 19.

Alternative location

A number of sources place the points KI 18 to KI 21 further laterally, at a distance of 1.5 cun from the anterior midline.

Needling

0.5 to 1 cun perpendicular insertion. Be aware of the position of the liver on the right side and the peritoneum on the left – consider your client's constitution.

Actions and indications

KI 21 aids with *digestive disorders involving the Spleen and Stomach*. It is considered a good point for *pain in the region of the lower ribs and breast* and helps *resolve Liver Qi stagnation*. Resolves abdominal pain, nausea and vomiting.

It is said to help *distention under the diaphragm* with a *lack of desire to eat* as already feeing full.

> **Main Areas**—Epigastrium. Chest.
> **Main Functions**—Harmonises the Stomach. Clears Heat.

KI 22   Bulang

Stepping Upward

步廊

Myotome	C5–C8, T1
Dermatome	T5

Location

In the fifth intercostal space, 2 cun lateral to the anterior midline. Level with CV 16, approximately.

To aid location, the 2 cun line is halfway between the anterior midline and the infra-mammary line. KI 22 is three intercostal spaces below KI 25.

Needling

0.3 to 0.5 perpendicular insertion.
0.5 to 1 cun transverse insertion, laterally along the intercostal space.

Avoid deep perpendicular needling may puncture the lung or liver.

Actions and indications

Although KI 22 is not a very commonly used point, it can be helpful to regulate Qi in the chest, dispel stagnation and descend rebellious Lung and Stomach Qi.

> **Main Areas**—Chest. Epigastrium.
> **Main Functions**—Regulates Qi. Descends rebellious Qi.

KI 23 Shenfeng
Shen Manor

Myotome	C5–C8, T1
Dermatome	T4

Location
In the fourth intercostal space, 2 cun lateral to the anterior midline. Level with CV 17, approximately.

Needling
0.5 to 1 cun directed outward laterally and NOT perpendicularly. Beware the lung.

Actions and indications
In common with KI 22, CV 17 and other adjacent points, KI 23 can be helpful to regulate chest Qi, dispel stagnation and descend rebellious Lung and Stomach Qi.

KI 23 is also especially indicated for disorders of the breast, including painful swelling of the breast, palpable masses, fibrocystic breast disease, mastitis and difficulty with lactation.

> **Main Areas**—Chest. Lungs. Breast. Stomach.
> **Main Functions**—Descends rebellious Qi. Opens and relaxes the chest. Benefits the breast.

KI 24 Lingxu
Heart Mound

Myotome	C5–C8, T1
Dermatome	T3

Location
Situated in the third intercostal space, 2 cun lateral to the anterior midline. Level with CV 18, approximately.

Needling
0.5 to 1 cun directed outward laterally and NOT perpendicularly. Beware the lung.

Actions and indications
KI 24 can be helpful to regulate chest Qi, dispel stagnation and descend rebellious Lung and Stomach Qi. It can aid in clearing breast discomfort and fullness.

> **Main Areas**—Chest. Lungs. Breast.
> **Main Functions**—Descends rebellious Qi. Opens and relaxes the chest. Benefits the breast.

KI 25 Shencang
Shen Storehouse

Myotome	C5–C8, T1
Dermatome	T2

Location
In the second intercostal space, 2 cun lateral to the anterior midline (CV 19).

To aid location, locate the sternal angle, which is level with the second rib; palpate the second rib and drop your finger into the intercostal space below it.

Needling
0.3 to 0.5 cun perpendicular insertion.
0.5 to 1 cun transverse insertion, laterally along the intercostal space.

Deep needling may puncture the lung.

Actions and indications
KI 25 is an important point to *treat disorders of the chest and thorax, including rebellious Qi.*
It is particularly indicated for: shortness of breath,

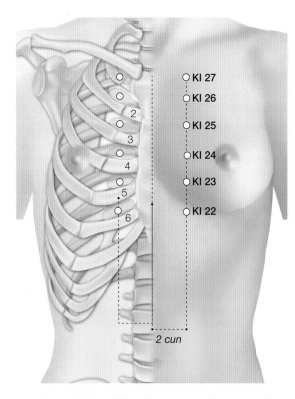

KI 27
KI 26
KI 25
KI 24
KI 23
KI 22

2
3
4
5
6

2 cun

Location

Directly below KI 27, in the first intercostal space, 2 cun lateral to the anterior midline.

To aid location, it is level with CV 14 and ST 19.

Needling

0.3 to 0.5 cun perpendicular insertion.
0.5 to 1 cun transverse insertion, laterally along the intercostal space.

Avoid deep needling otherwise this may puncture the lung.

Actions and indications

KI 26 can be used to help loosen the chest and resolve phlegm. Used for conditions effecting the Lungs and Stomach in addition to benefitting distension in the breasts.

> **Main Areas**—Epigastrium. Chest.
> **Main Functions**—Harmonises the Stomach. Clears Heat.

chronic weak breathing, dyspnoea, asthma, cough, palpitations, hiccup, and tightness and pain of the chest.

KI 25 *harmonises the Kidneys, Lungs and Heart and can help calm the mind and increase psychological confidence.*

> **Main Areas**—Chest. Lungs. Heart.
> **Main Functions**—Benefits respiration. Regulates chest Qi.

KI 27   Shufu
Shu Mansion

Myotome	C5/C6 and facial nerve through platysma
Dermatome	C4

Location

In the depression inferior to the medial end of the clavicle.

To aid location, it is 2 cun lateral to CV 21.

Needling

0.3 to 0.4 cun perpendicular insertion.
0.5 to 1 cun transverse-oblique insertion, laterally along the inferior border of the clavicle.

Deep needling may puncture the lung.

KI 26   Yuzhong
Refined Chest

Myotome	C5–C8, T1 and facial nerve through platysma
Dermatome	C4

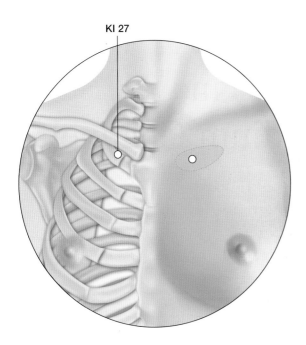

KI 27

Actions and indications

KI 27 is an important point to *treat disorders of the upper thorax and respiratory tract*. It is particularly indicated for: tightness and constriction of the chest and throat, sore or swollen throat, goitre, cough, dyspnoea, and asthma.

It has also been traditionally employed to harmonise the Stomach, descend rebellious Qi and treat nausea, vomiting, lack of appetite and abdominal distension.

> **Main Areas**—Chest. Throat.
> **Main Functions**—Descends rebellious Qi.
> Regulates chest Qi.

16 Points of the Arm Jue Yin Pericardium Channel

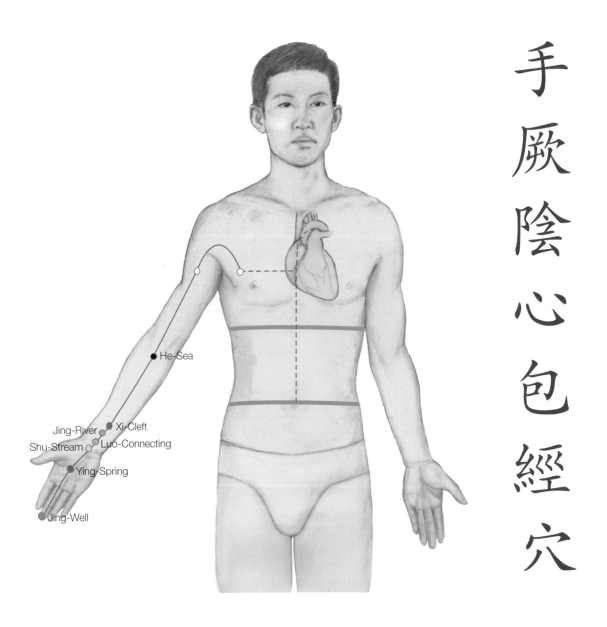

He-Sea

Jing-River   Xi-Cleft
Shu-Stream   Luo-Connecting
Ying-Spring

Jing-Well

手厥陰心包經穴

General	Starting in the middle of the chest, with a close relationship with the Heart, the Pericardium channel passes down the anteromedial aspect of the arm, crossing the elbow medial to the biceps tendon. From here it continues down the forearm in a straight line, over the centre of the palm, to finish at the tip of the middle finger. The channel has 9 points. It is grouped with the Triple Energizer under the Fire element in five-element theory.
More specifically	The main channel emerges 1 cun lateral to the nipple and travels up over the lower part of the axilla, to continue down the anteromedial aspect of the arm, following the biceps brachii. At the cubital crease, it lies next to the biceps tendon and then passes onto the flexor aspect of the forearm. Markers here are the palmaris longus (if present) and the flexor carpi radialis, with the channel travelling between them. At the palm it crosses the flexor retinaculum centrally, continuing to PC 8, which is a point in the very centre of the palm. (Found easily by getting the client to curl their fingertips down to their palm: PC 8 is where the tip of the middle finger contacts the palm.) The channel continues to the tip of the middle finger, although some sources also quote a branch from PC 8 to the radial side of the ring finger. The origin of the channel in the chest surrounds the Heart and then descends the abdomen, passing through the diaphragm centrally and connecting all the divisions of the Triple Energizer (its Yang partner).
Area covered	Chest. Diaphragm. Upper arm. Forearm. Wrist.
Areas affected with treatment	Conditions such as CTS, wrist flexor tension (can be associated with tennis elbow), elbow and chest tension. Diaphragm – PC 6 is the most researched point to have an anti-emetic response and settling of anxiety/chest tension. Often used when there is stress and tension, which causes stomach and chest tightness and symptoms.
Key points	PC 3, PC 5, PC 6, PC 8, PC 9.

PC 1   Tianchi
Heavenly Pool

天池

Intersection of the Gallbladder, Triple Energizer and Liver on the Pericardium channel
Window of the Sky point

Myotome	T4
Dermatome	T4

Location
Approximately 1 cun lateral and superior to the nipple, in the fourth intercostal space. It should be treated at a minimum distance of 0.5 cun lateral to the edge of the areola.

To aid location, it should be treated over the fourth intercostal space and under the mammary glands, regardless of the actual location of the nipple (it varies depending on the shape and size of the mammary glands).

In cases where the mammary glands are very enlarged, this site cannot be accessed, making treatment only applicable in the area supralateral to it.

Needling
0.2 to 0.5 cun oblique supralateral insertion.

Do not puncture the mammary glands.

Do not needle deeply because this poses a considerable risk of injuring the lung and causing a pneumothorax.

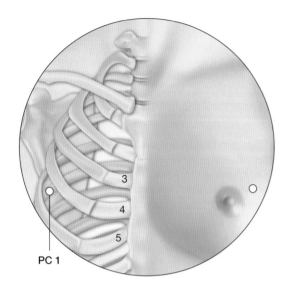

PC 1

Location

On the anterior aspect of the upper arm, 2 cun inferior to the end of the axillary fold, in the distinct trough of the channel pathway formed between the two heads of the biceps brachii muscle. Additionally, sometimes more reactive points can be found further down the channel (see blue shaded area).

Needling

0.5 to 1 cun perpendicular insertion.
0.5 to 2 cun oblique or slanted distal insertion.

Actions and indications

Although PC 2 is not a commonly used point, it is very effective to regulate Qi and Blood along the course of the channel pathway and dissipate stagnation from the chest. It is an especially responsive point, even to gentle manual pressure, and it is immediately noticeable that it dynamically opens and spreads the Qi.

Indications include: heaviness, tightness and pain of the chest, swelling, palpable masses or pain in the breast or axilla, tightness and pain of the shoulder or upper back, weakness of the arm, difficulty flexing the elbow, arm pain along the course of the channel, and as a distant point it can be helpful in CTS.

Other traditional indications include: mental agitation, cardiac pain radiating towards the arm or shoulder, palpitations and cough.

Carefully applied palm or finger pressure elicits a Qi sensation more easily compared to needling which can be quite tricky at this site.

Actions and indications

PC 1 is primarily used to treat *disorders of the breasts and chest*, particularly when there is *Qi and Blood stagnation or phlegm* accumulation.

Indications include: pain, swelling and palpable masses in the breast; insufficient lactation, swollen glands and nodules in the axilla; pain and difficulty lifting the arm; intercostal pain; and tightness and fullness of the chest. It has also been employed to treat: coughing, dyspnoea, palpitations, angina pectoris, headaches, and blurred vision.

> **Main Areas**—Breast. Chest. Ribs. Heart.
> **Main Functions**—Regulates Qi. Dispels stasis and unbinds the chest. Benefits the breast.

> **Main Areas**—Chest. Breast. Arm.
> **Main Functions**—Regulates Qi and Blood and alleviates pain. Dissipates stasis and unbinds the chest. Benefits the breast.

PC 2   Tianquan
Heavenly Spring

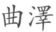

Myotome	None – superficial tissue between heads of biceps brachii
Dermatome	At junction of C5/T2

PC 3   Quze
Marsh at the Bend

He-Sea point, Water point

Myotome	None – superficial tissue adjacent to biceps tendon in cubital crease
Dermatome	C8/T1

Location

On the transverse cubital crease, in the depression on the medial (ulnar) side of the tendon of biceps brachii.

Flex the elbow against resistance to define the biceps tendon.

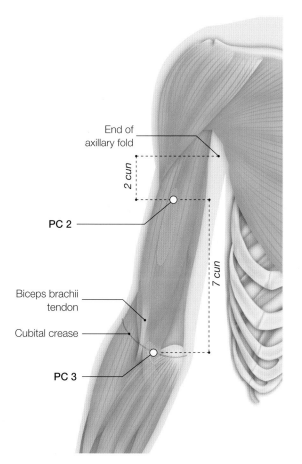

End of axillary fold

2 cun

PC 2

7 cun

Biceps brachii tendon

Cubital crease

PC 3

Needling

0.5 to 1 cun perpendicular insertion.
Prick to bleed.
Beware its deep position – the brachial artery and vein, and the median nerve.

Actions and indications

PC 3 is a powerful point to *clear heat* and *cool Blood, dispel stasis and open the chest*. It is also useful to descend rebellious Qi and harmonise the middle jiao/energizer.

Indications include: fullness or pain of the chest, palpitations, tachycardia, arrhythmia, dyspnoea, cough, nausea, vomiting, epigastric pain, haemoptysis, skin rashes, insomnia, headache, thirst, excessive menstrual bleeding, convulsions, fevers, heat stroke, and febrile diseases.

As a *local point*, PC 3 can be used to treat pain, stiffness and impaired mobility of the arm and elbow.

Note: PC 3 seems to reflect BL 40 on the upper limb because it has a similar anatomical location and also shares some of the same functions.

> **Main Areas**—Chest. Heart. Stomach. Elbow.
> **Main Functions**—Clears heat. Dispels stasis. Descends rebellious Qi.

PC 4   Ximen
Cleft Gate

Xi-Cleft point

Myotome	C7/C8
Dermatome	C6–C8

Location

On the anterior aspect of the forearm, 5 cun proximal to the transverse wrist crease, in the depression between the tendons of the palmaris longus and flexor carpi radialis muscles, on the line joining PC 7 with PC 3.

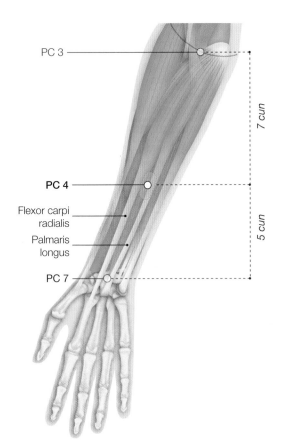

As a *local point*, PC 4 is useful in cases of: pain, stiffness or hypertonicity of the forearm, and impaired mobility of the wrist and fingers.

> **Main Areas**—Heart. Mind. Forearm.
> **Main Functions**—Cools Blood. Dispels stasis. Regulates Heart Qi. Calms the mind.

PC 5   Jianshi   間使
Intermediary Messenger

Jing-River point, Metal point

Myotome	C7/C8
Dermatome	C6–C8

Location

On the anterior aspect of the forearm, 3 cun proximal to the transverse wrist crease, between

To aid location, if the palmaris longus muscle is absent, locate PC 4 on the ulnar side of the flexor carpi radialis tendon.

Needling

0.5 to 1 cun perpendicular insertion.

Actions and indications

PC 4 *cools Blood, dispels stasis and alleviates pain, regulates Heart Qi* and *calms the mind.*

It is widely employed in such cases as: acute or chronic chest or cardiac pain, angina pectoris, arrhythmia, palpitations, vomiting, skin diseases due to heat and Blood stasis, epistaxis and coughing blood.

On psychological level it can help treat insomnia and fear, fright or depression due to weakness of the Heart Qi.

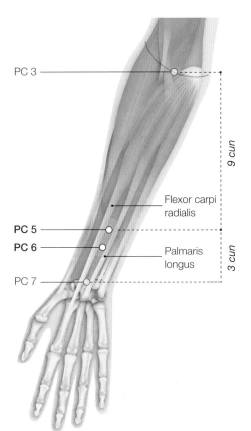

the tendons of the palmaris longus and flexor carpi radialis muscles, on the line joining PC 7 with PC 3.

To aid location, it is one quarter of the distance between the transverse wrist crease at PC 7 and the cubital crease at PC 3. If the palmaris longus muscle is absent, locate PC 5 on the ulnar side of the flexor carpi radialis tendon.

Needling
0.5 to 1 cun perpendicular insertion.

Actions and indications
PC 5 is a major point to *regulate chest Qi, resolve phlegm, clear heat, cool Blood* and *calm the mind.* In common with other Pericardium points, it also *descends rebellious Qi and harmonises the Stomach.*

Indications include: chest pain, palpitations, cough, stomach ache, vomiting, tidal fever, convulsions, epilepsy, insomnia, tongue ulcers, psychosis, and hysteria.

PC 5 has also been used to *regulate menstruation* and is indicated for dysmenorrhoea, irregular cycle, retention of the lochia, and leucorrhoea.

As a *local point,* PC 5 is useful to treat pain and stiffness of the forearm, wrist and fingers.

> **Main Areas**—Chest. Wrist. Heart. Stomach.
> **Main Functions**—Regulates chest Qi.
> Resolves phlegm. Calms the mind.
> Descends rebellious Qi.

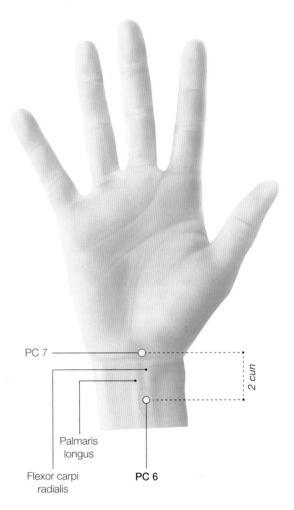

PC 7 — Palmaris longus — Flexor carpi radialis — **PC 6** — 2 cun

PC 6　Neiguan
Inner Gate

内關

Luo-Connecting point
Command point of the chest (thorax)
Opening point of the Yin Wei Mai

Myotome	C8/T1
Dermatome	C6–C8

Location
2 cun proximal to the transverse wrist crease, between the tendons of the palmaris longus and flexor carpi radialis muscles.

To aid location, PC 6 is located opposite TE 5. If the palmaris longus muscle is absent, locate PC 6 on the ulnar side of the flexor carpi radialis tendon.

Needling
0.2 to 0.5 cun perpendicular insertion.
1 to 1.5 cun perpendicular insertion to join with TE 5 on the posterior aspect of the forearm.
0.3 to 1.5 cun oblique insertion distally or proximally along the channel, depending on the area to be treated (deqi sensation should vary accordingly).

If there are visible vessels at the superficial location of PC 6, these are easily moved out of the way by stretching the skin slightly, or using the guide tube, if using one, to manouvre the vessels to the side.

If a strong electric sensation is felt on initial needle insertion at very superficial needling depths (as little as 3mm), it means that the needle tip may be touching the palmar cutaneous branch of the median nerve. If the sensation is very strong, do not manipulate the needle at all. If it is excessive and does not settle within 10 seconds, remove the needle.

PC 6 can be very painful and engender an electric deqi sensation. This means the needle tip may be touching the nerve(s) deep to the point. Do not manipulate strongly.

Actions and indications

PC 6 is one of the top most commonly used points for a wide variety of conditions. Its primary functions are to *dispel stasis and regulate the circulation of Qi and Blood throughout the three jiao. It has a particularly powerful effect on opening and relaxing the chest*; it also *clears heat and has a nourishing effect on the Blood and Yin*. All these functions are intimately connected to the *Yin Wei Mai* and the *luo-connecting channel* of the Pericardium, which are activated by treatment at PC 6.

Indications include: fullness and constriction of the chest, thoracic and cardiac pain, palpitations, arrhythmia, dyspnoea, cough, plum stone throat, pain or swelling of the throat, goitre, lymphadenopathy, phlegm nodules, fever, headache, migraine, hypochondrial and abdominal pain, and neck pain.

Needling PC 6 has been shown to *relax the coronary arteries* and increase blood supply to the myocardium. PC 6 has also been needled for *first aid following or during myocardial infarction*, and has been shown to minimise damage to the myocardium.

PC 6 also effectively *descends rebellious Qi and harmonises the Stomach and middle jiao*. It is an extremely important and widely used point in the treatment of many digestive disorders, including:

epigastric pain, acid reflux, heartburn, hiccup, oesophagitis, gastritis, nausea, vomiting, morning sickness during pregnancy, and other digestive disorders.

PC 6 is *extremely important to calm the mind* in the treatment of *emotional and psychosomatic complaints* such as insomnia, anxiety, irritability, emotional upset, propensity to crying, mood swings and depression.

It is particularly indicated for women with emotionally related *gynaecological complaints* such as premenstrual syndrome, breast pain, fibrocystic breast disease, mastitis, breast abscess, dysmenorrhoea, irregular menstruation, oligomenorrhoea, infertility, and postpartum dizziness or depression.

PC 6 also has an *analgesic effect* and thus it can be used for *post-operative pain* as well as *pain caused by injury*. Also, it can be used in anaesthesia (in conjunction with LI 4, LR 3 and ear points).

PC 6 is very effective to *open the orifices, resuscitate consciousness* and *clear the mind* in cases of diminished concentration, mental exhaustion, poor memory, amnesia, dizziness, vertigo, and symptoms following wind stroke.

It is very important as a *local point* for pain and restricted movement of the forearm, wrist and fingers, particularly if there is hypertonicity and tightness of the wrist flexors due to Qi and Blood stasis along the channel pathway. It is particularly indicated for CTS.

PC 6 has also been traditionally used for a variety of other disorders, including: tidal fevers, malaria, convulsions, spitting or vomiting blood, blood in the stools, prolapse of the rectum, jaundice, dysuria, epilepsy, loss of consciousness, coma, and even insanity.

Main Areas—Chest. Heart. Mind. Stomach. Wrist. Forearm. Neck.
Main Functions—Regulates Qi and Blood. Dispels stasis. Relaxes the chest. Benefits the breasts. Calms the mind. Descends rebellious Qi. Harmonises the Stomach.

PC 7   Daling
Great Mound

Shu-Stream point, Earth point
Yuan-Source point, Fourth Ghost point

Myotome	None – superficial tissue over wrist crease
Dermatome	C7

Location
In the middle of the transverse wrist crease, in the depression between the tendons of the palmaris longus and flexor carpi radialis muscles.

To aid location it is between the base of the thenar and hypothenar eminence (usually at the end of the crease formed between the two eminences, also known as the 'life line' in palmistry).

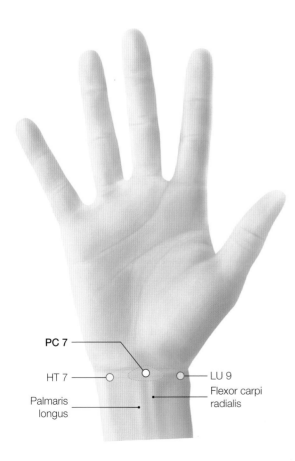

PC 7
HT 7
Palmaris longus
LU 9
Flexor carpi radialis

It is approximately midway between HT 7 and LU 9. If the palmaris longus muscle is absent, locate this point on the ulnar side of the flexor carpi radialis tendon.

Needling
0.3 to 0.5 cun perpendicular insertion.
0.5 to 1 cun oblique distal insertion into the carpal tunnel.

PC 7 can be very painful and engender electric deqi sensation. This means that the needle tip may be touching the median nerve deep to the point. Do not manipulate strongly.

Actions and indications
Although PC 7 was traditionally considered to be the yuan-source point of the Heart and have similar functions to HT 7, it is not as commonly used as the latter. It is, however, effective to *regulate Qi and Blood, cool the Heart, open the chest and calm the mind. It descends rebellious Qi and harmonises the Stomach.*

Indications include: pain and tightness of the chest, angina pectoris, palpitations, arrhythmia, tachycardia, fever, epigastric pain, nausea, vomiting, gastritis, epilepsy, depression, emotional upset, anxiety, and panic attacks.

As a *local point*, it is very effective to treat CTS and pain or stiffness of the wrist.

> **Main Areas**—Wrist. Chest. Heart. Stomach.
> **Main Functions**—Regulates Qi and Blood. Alleviates pain. Relaxes the chest. Calms the mind. Descends rebellious Qi.

PC 8   Laogong
Palace of Toil

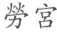

Ying-Spring point, Fire point
Ninth Ghost point

Myotome	C8/T1
Dermatome	C7

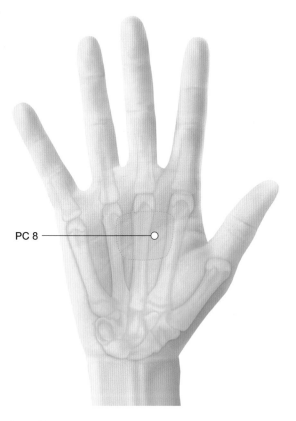

PC 8

Location
At the centre of the palm, in the depression between the second and third metacarpal bones, on the radial side of the third metacarpal.

To aid location, if the fist is clenched lightly, PC 8 is at the point where the tip of the middle finger touches the palm.

Needling
0.3 to 0.5 cun perpendicular insertion.

Use a thicker needle if the palmar skin is thick or hard. In practice, needling PC 8 is usually only employed to treat channel disorders because it is often very painful.

Actions and indications
PC 8 *strongly clears heat and fire from the Heart, subdues wind, restores consciousness and calms the mind.* Furthermore, it *descends rebellious Qi.*

Indications include: excessive sweating, fever, loss of consciousness, wind stroke, convulsions,

epistaxis, ulceration of the mouth and tongue, glossitis, swelling of the throat, halitosis, excessive thirst, nausea, gastritis, abdominal pain and hardness, blood in the stools, depression, mental agitation, delirium, palpitations, arrhythmia, angina pectoris, and chest pain.

PC 8 is also *extensively used in Qigong* and Eastern bodywork methods as a point to focus and strengthen the Qi, which then transmits to the patient during treatment. PC 8 can be combined with KI 1 for mental focus exercises.

> **Main Areas**—Palm. Chest. Heart. Mind.
> **Main Functions**—Clears heat. Restores consciousness. Calms the mind. Descends rebellious Qi. Focuses Qi in Qigong therapy.

PC 9   Zhongchong
Central Surge

Jing-Well point, Wood point

Myotome	None – superficial tissue at tip of finger
Dermatome	C8

Location
At the centre of the tip of the middle finger, approximately 0.1 cun distal to the end of the nail.

Alternative location
Located 0.1 cun proximal to the corner of the nail on the radial side of the middle finger, at the intersection of two lines following the radial border of the nail and the base of the nail.

Needling
0.1 to 0.3 cun perpendicular insertion.

Actions and indications
PC 9 has comparable functions to the other jing-well points, including *clearing heat, sedating interior wind, opening the orifices and restoring consciousness.* It is, however, considered

PC 9

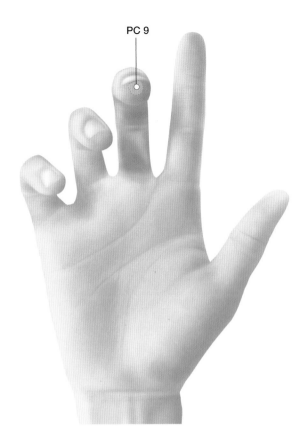

more powerful, and the Qi here is seen to be surging rather than still and small like a 'well'. Anatomically, the middle finger is the strongest of the four fingers, and the flesh at the tip of the finger is deeper than that situated at the corners of the nails.

Thus, PC 9 is one of the strongest points to *restore consciousness* and *stimulate the heart* in cases of loss of consciousness, syncope, coma, shock, convulsions, fever and delirium.

Because of its powerful effect as a *Heart tonic*, PC 9 is used in *Qigong therapy*, similarly to PC 8, to project Qi for healing or martial applications.

> **Main Areas**—Heart. Mind.
> **Main Functions**—Restores consciousness. Opens the orifices. Opens the chest.

17 Points of the Arm Shao Yang Triple Energizer Channel

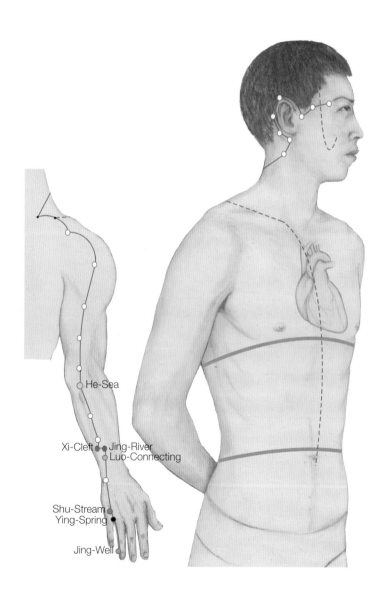

He-Sea

Xi-Cleft　Jing-River
Luo-Connecting

Shu-Stream
Ying-Spring

Jing-Well

手少陽三焦經穴

(Alternative names: historically, this channel and its associated organ is called the Sanjiao, which means 'three divisions' or 'three areas'; san – three, jiao – area/space).

Other names found in the literature include: Triple Burner, Triple Warmer and Triple Heater.

General	The various names for the Triple Energizer give clues as to the function of this organ, which is key in the Chinese medical model for the balance of body fluids/ oedema/ temperature regulation and smooth digestive function. It is difficult to find correlations within Western medicine, but the concept of the fluid movement within the interstitium and lymphatic systems goes part of the way to helping create a more structured vision. It is more about function than a specific pathway. The channel arises at the ring finger and travels up the back of the forearm and arm to the shoulder, crossing the posterior aspect of the elbow. At the shoulder TE 14 sits closely related to the subacromial space and then travels across the trapezius and up into the neck, closely hugging the outer ear. It finishes just forward of the temple, on the lateral end of the eyebrow ridge. The channel has 23 points. It is grouped with the Pericardium under the Fire element in five-element theory.
More specifically	Starting at the medial edge of the nail of the ring finger, the channel passes back over the hand, over the fourth and fifth metacarpal bones, and crosses the wrist just lateral to the tendon of the extensor digitorum. From here it travels directly up the posterior forearm, crossing the olecranon at a level 3 cun from the wrist crease with two points, TE 6 and TE 7, in line here. It passes over the posterior of the lateral condyle of the humerus, near the olecranon, and up through the triceps to meet the scapula/shoulder at TE 14, just posterior and inferior to the acromion. From here the channel moves medially over the trapezius, turning just above the medial end of the suprascapular fossa to travel up the lateral side of the cervical spine to the indent anterior to the mastoid process and situated over the transverse process of C1. Hugging the posterior auricle, the channel winds around the ear to TE 21, in front of the tragus of the ear and just above SI 19. The channel finishes forward of this point, crossing the temple and ending at TE 23 on the lateral edge of the eyebrow ridge, closely associated with GB 1. In the neck and shoulder region the channel has strong links to SI 12, GB 21, GV 14 and BL 11. Its primary internal links are found at GV 14, ST 12, CV 12 and CV 17.
Area covered	Hand and wrist. Elbow. Shoulder. Neck. Ear. Temple. Stomach/Spleen – middle jiao.
Areas affected with treatment	Digestion. Heat conditions in skin and blood. Temperature regulation issues. Ear – tinnitus/deafness. Locally, arm, shoulder and neck.
Key points	TE 5, TE 6, TE 8, TE 14, TE 15, TE 17, TE 23.

TE 1   Guanchong

Surge Gate

關衝

Jing-Well point, Metal point

Myotome	None – superficial tissue
Dermatome	C7

Location
On the ulnar side of the fourth (ring) finger, 0.1 cun proximal to the corner of the nail. At the intersection of two lines following the ulnar border of the nail and the base of the nail.

Needling
0.1 cun perpendicular insertion.

Actions and indications
TE 1 is mainly used to *clear exterior heat and wind* causing symptoms such as earache and sore throat.

In common with the other jing-well points, TE 1 will help restore consciousness in cases of coma or fainting.

Additionally, it opens the *Triple Energizer tendino-muscular meridian and treats pain* along the meridian pathway.

> **Main Areas**—Mind. Ears. Triple Energizer channel.
> **Main Functions**—Clears heat. Benefits the ears. Resuscitates consciousness.

TE 2   Yemen

Fluid Gate

液門

Ying-Spring point, Water point

Myotome	None – superficial tissue
Dermatome	C7

Location
0.5 cun proximal to the margin of the web between the fourth and fifth fingers, distal to the MCP joint.

To aid location, the hand should be in a loose fist and the fingers relaxed.

Needling
0.3 to 0.5 perpendicular insertion.

Actions and indications
The key use for this point is in cases of *sudden deafness, earache and tinnitus*. Also if these symptoms are associated with *redness in the face and headache* this can be a useful point.

Locally it can be used for arthritic and soft tissue injuries of the fifth MCP joint.

> **Main Areas**—Ears. MCP joint.
> **Main Functions**—Dissipates wind and clears heat. Benefits the ears. Alleviates pain.

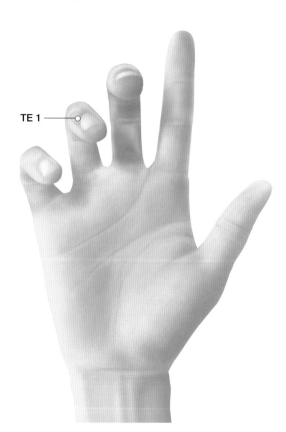

TE 1

TE 3   Zhongzhu
Central Islet

Shu-Stream point, Wood point

Myotome	C8/T1
Dermatome	C7

Location
On the dorsum of the hand, in the depression proximal to the MCP joints between the fourth and fifth metacarpal bones.

To aid location, the patient should make a loose fist. Also, TE 3 is opposite HT 8, which is situated on the palmar surface.

Needling
0.3 to 0.5 cun perpendicular insertion, or join with HT 8.

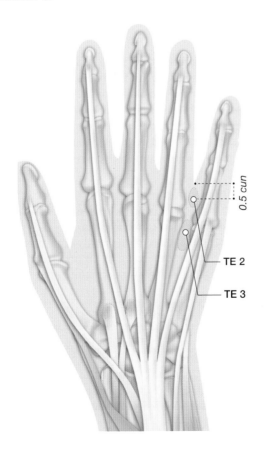

Actions and indications
Both TE 2 and TE 3 are useful points to *dissipate wind, clear heat and fire, regulate Qi and Blood* and *dispel stasis*, particularly from the *head and ears*.

Common indications include: ear infections, tinnitus, deafness, inflammation of the eyes, and headache.

TE 2 and TE 3 can also be used for *regional disorders*, including pain or stiffness of the fingers, elbow and arm.

> **Main Areas**—MCP joints. Triple Energizer channel. Ears.
> **Main Functions**—Clears heat. Dissipates wind. Benefits the ears. Regulates Qi and Blood. Alleviates pain.

TE 4   Yangchi
Yang Pool

Yuan-Source point

Myotome	None – superficial tissue
Dermatome	C7

Location
On the posterior aspect of the wrist, between the ulna and carpal bones, in the depression between the tendons of the extensor digitorum communis and extensor digiti minimi muscles.

To aid location, emphasise the tendon of the extensor digitorum communis muscle by asking the patient to extend the fingers.

Needling
0.3 to 0.5 cun perpendicular insertion between the junction of the triquetrum and lunate bones with the ulna. (Superficial needling may be as effective here.) 0.5 to 1 cun transverse insertion radially, under the tendon sheath.

It is also considered to *reinforce the Chong Mai and Kidney* and improve *fluid transformation*. Indications include: chronic tiredness, weakness and exhaustion, wasting syndromes, infertility, amenorrhoea, profuse urination, anuria, fluid retention, and oedema.

> **Main Areas**—Wrist. Triple Energizer channel. Ears.
> **Main Functions**—Regulates the Triple Energizer. Alleviates pain. Tonifies yuan Qi.

TE 5   Waiguan

Outer Gate

Luo-Connecting point
Opening point of the Yang Wei Mai

Myotome	C7/C8
Dermatome	C7

Location
Between the radius and the ulna, 2 cun above TE 4, on the radial edge of the extensor digitorum communis, close to the radial border. Situated in the extensor pollicis brevis muscle.

To aid location, it is approximately three finger-widths proximal to the transverse wrist crease.

Needling
0.3 to 1.5 cun perpendicular insertion as far as PC 6, on the anterior aspect of the forearm.
0.5 to 2 cun oblique insertion distally or proximally along the channel, depending on the area to be treated (sensation should vary accordingly).

Actions and indications
TE 5 is one of the *most important and commonly used points*. Its primary functions are to *release the exterior, dispel wind, clear both exterior and interior heat, dissipate Qi stagnation and smooth the Liver*. Furthermore, it is extensively employed to *descend excessive Yang, clear the head,*

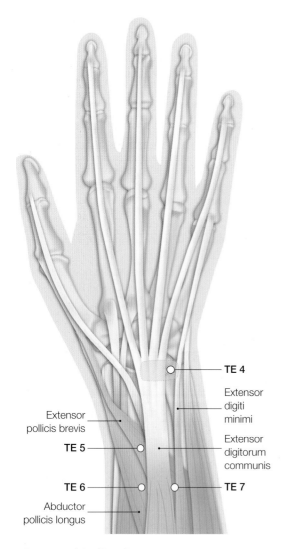

Extensor pollicis brevis

TE 5

TE 6

Abductor pollicis longus

TE 4

Extensor digiti minimi

Extensor digitorum communis

TE 7

Actions and indications
Although TE 4 is the yuan-source point of the Triple Energizer channel, in clinical practice it is primarily used to treat *regional disorders, particularly of the wrist*. It is particularly effective for pain, restricted movement or swelling of the wrist, hand and arm.

Additionally, it *clears exterior and interior heat* and treats *inflammation of the ears, eyes and throat*, including tonsillitis, otitis, fever, and thirst.

TE 4 has been *extensively employed to tonify the yuan Qi and augment the Qi of the entire body*, particularly in Japanese acupuncture traditions.

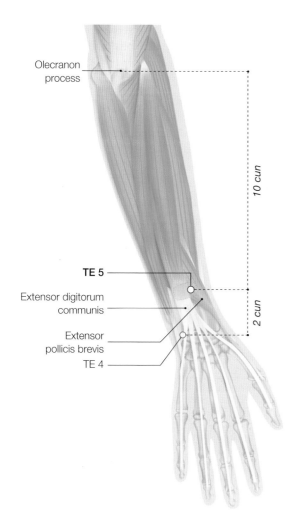

stiffness and pain of the arm, wrist, shoulder and neck.

> **Main Areas**—Lungs. Liver. Ears. Head. Eyes. Forearm and wrist. Triple Energizer channel.
> **Main Functions**—Releases the exterior and dispels wind. Dispels stasis and smooths the Liver. Clears interior and exterior heat. Descends excessive Yang. Alleviates pain.

TE 6   Zhigou   支溝
Branch Ditch

Jing-River point, Fire point

Myotome	C7/C8
Dermatome	C7

Location
In the depression 3 cun proximal to TE 4, between the radial side of the extensor digitorum communis muscle and the radius. Situated in the abductor pollicis longus muscle.

To aid location, TE 6 is approximately one hand-width proximal to TE 4. One quarter of the distance between TE 4 and the lateral epicondyle of the humerus or the tip of the olecranon process.

Needling
0.5 to 1 cun perpendicular insertion. Occasionally, due to anatomy, the point may be needled slightly obliquely medially.

Actions and indications
TE 6 is *widely used to clear heat, dissipate stagnation and smooth the flow of Qi in all three Jiao*, although it is particularly indicated for *disorders of the chest, sides and abdomen.*

In the Lower Jiao it *purges the Large Intestine* and is commonly used for acute and chronic constipation with abdominal pain. Furthermore, it can be helpful for gynaecological pain.

sharpen eyesight and hearing and regulate the Yang Wei Mai.

Indications include: fever with or without chills due to febrile diseases or Qi stagnation, upper respiratory tract infections, colds and flu, sore throat, headache, migraine, tinnitus, deafness, pain and inflammation of the ears or eyes, epistaxis, toothache, hypertension, dizziness, and hemiplegia.

TE 5 also successfully treats other manifestations of *Liver Qi stagnation*, including: irritability, mood swings, depression, hypochondrial distension or pain, vomiting, epigastric pain, abdominal distension and pain, and constipation.

TE 5 is also *important in the treatment of channel disorders* and is indicated for atrophy, paralysis,

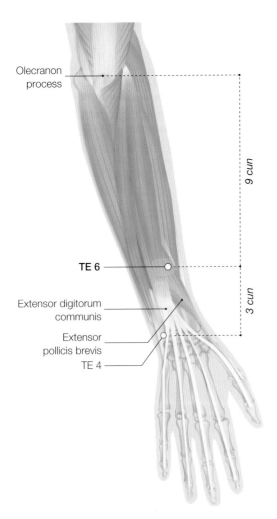

Olecranon process

9 cun

TE 6

3 cun

Extensor digitorum communis

Extensor pollicis brevis

TE 4

As a *local point*, TE 6 can be successfully employed in the treatment of pain, tightness or atrophy of the forearm and wrist.

> **Main Areas**—Chest. Sides. Abdomen. Large Intestine. Ears. Throat.
> **Main Functions**—Clears heat. Dispels stasis. Releases the exterior.

TE 7   Huizong   會宗
Convergence and Gathering

Xi-Cleft point

Myotome	None – superficial tissue
Dermatome	C6–C8 border

Location
3 cun proximal to TE 4, about one finger's width and on the ulnar aspect of TE 6, on the radial side of the ulna. Situated in the depression between the extensor digitorum communis muscle and the ulna.

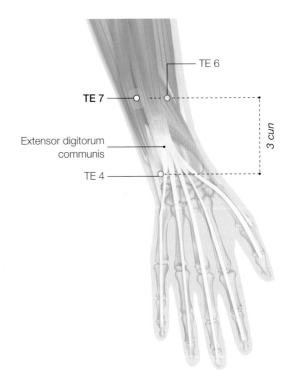

TE 6

TE 7

3 cun

Extensor digitorum communis

TE 4

In the Middle Jiao it *regulates the flow of Liver Qi* and treats symptoms of stagnation, including: nausea and vomiting and fullness, distension and pain of the epigastrium, abdomen, hypochondrium or chest.

In the Upper Jiao it unblocks the channel pathway and releases *exterior heat and wind*, treating pain and inflammation of the throat, ear, eye, arm, axilla and skin, including: tinnitus and deafness, headache, redness of the eyes, sudden loss of voice, oppression and heaviness of the chest, herpes zoster, intercostal neuralgia, urticaria and other skin diseases.

As a *jing-river point* it is useful in aiding diagnosis with regard to fascial tension throughout the tendino-muscular meridian.

Needling

0.5 to 1.5 cun slightly obliquely towards the ulnar aspect.
0.5 to 1 cun obliquely proximal or distal from point

Actions and indications

TE 7 is useful to *clear the channel pathway and alleviate pain*, particularly in the shoulder, arm, forearm and wrist. It is also useful for *disorders of the ears* such as tinnitus and deafness.

It has been traditionally used to treat a wide range of other disorders, including: fevers, dizziness, blurred vision, epilepsy, fright, and even insanity.

> **Main Areas**—Upper limb. Ears.
> **Main Functions**—Dispels stasis and alleviates pain. Clears heat.

TE 8   Sanyangluo   三陽絡
Three Yang Connection

Myotome	C7/C8
Dermatome	C6/C7

Location

4 cun proximal to the wrist joint space, 1 cun proximal to TE 6, between the radius and ulna, on the radial side of the extensor digitorum communis muscle.

To aid location, it is one third of the distance along the line joining TE 4 and the lateral epicondyle.

Alternatively, find the dip for TE 5, which is 2 cun above the wrist crease, and double it.

Needling

0.5 to 1 cun perpendicular insertion.

Actions and indications

In some texts this is contraindicated for needling. However, in Western medical practice it has proved

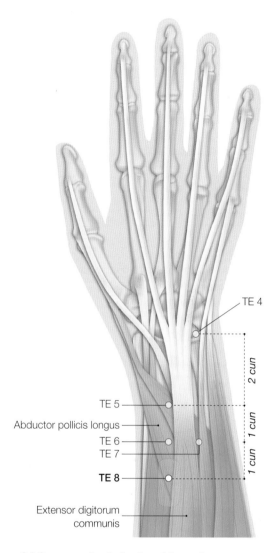

TE 4

2 cun

1 cun

TE 5

Abductor pollicis longus

TE 6
TE 7

1 cun

TE 8

Extensor digitorum communis

useful for musculo-skeletal problems. Its name suggests the Three Yang meridians of the forearm meet at this place (much like Sanyinjiao [SP 6] in the leg).

It can be very effective to help *regulate Qi and blood and alleviate stiffness and pain along the course of the channel pathway. Indications include: pain, stiffness or weakness of the arm, forearm, wrist, or fingers.*

TE 8 also releases the exterior and can be used for chills and fever and other related symptoms, notably sudden loss of voice or hearing for which it is traditionally indicated.

> **Main Areas**—Forearm. Arm. Ears. Throat.
> **Main Functions**—Alleviates stiffness and pain.
> Releases the exterior.

TE 9 Sidu 四渎
Four Rivers

Myotome	C6/C7
Dermatome	C6

Location
A little more than halfway up the posterior aspect of the forearm, 7 cun proximal to TE 4, in a depression between the radius and ulna.

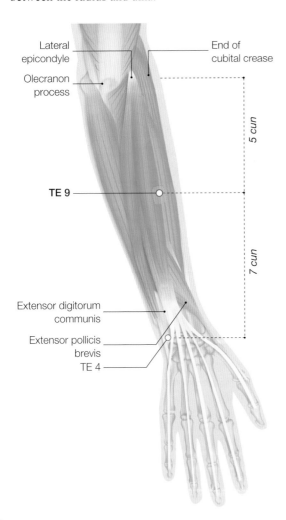

To aid location, it is on the line connecting TE 4 and the lateral epicondyle of the humerus, on the radial side of the extensor digitorum communis muscle.

Needling
1 cun perpendicular insertion.

Actions and indications
Whilst TE 9 has similar traditional indications to TE 8 in so far as it clears the exterior, it not often used in such cases.

Its actions are mainly regional, and it can be a particularly effective adjacent point in the treatment of extensor tendinitis.

> **Main Areas**—Forearm. Elbow.
> **Main Functions**—Alleviates stiffness and pain.
> Releases the exterior.

TE 10 Tianjing 天井
Upper Well

He-Sea point, Earth point

Myotome	None – superficial tissue
Dermatome	C7

Location
On the elbow, in the depression of the olecranon fossa, approximately 1 cun proximal to the tip of the olecranon process when the elbow is flexed.

Needling
0.5 to 1 cun perpendicular insertion.

Actions and indications
TE 10 is primarily used to *activate Qi and Blood circulation and dispel wind and dampness from the Triple Energizer channel.*

Symptoms include: pain and stiffness of the elbow, arm and shoulder and difficulty in flexing or extending the elbow.

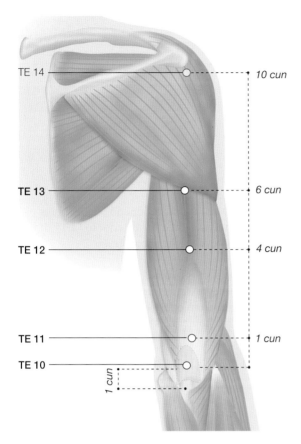

TE 14 ———————○———— 10 cun

TE 13 ———————○———— 6 cun

TE 12 ———————○———— 4 cun

TE 11 ———————○———— 1 cun

TE 10 ———————○————

1 cun

Location
1 cun proximal to TE 10, at the centre of the triceps brachii tendon.

Needling
0.5 to 1 cun perpendicular insertion

Actions and indications
In common with TE 10, TE 11 is traditionally indicated as a *cooling point* and to *clear damp heat*; however, it is most commonly used in regional disorders, particularly if there is difficulty flexing or extending the elbow joint.

> **Main Areas**—Elbow. Arm. Triple Energizer channel.
> **Main Functions**—Regulates Qi and Blood. Alleviates pain and swelling. Clears heat.

TE 12   Xiaoluo
Draining Marsh

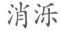

Myotome	C6–C8
Dermatome	C5–T1

Location
At the centre of the posterior aspect of the upper arm, 4 cun proximal to TE 10, in a depression between the lateral and long head of the triceps brachii muscle.

To aid location, palpate the channel between the two heads of the triceps (extend the elbow against resistance to contract the muscle bellies).

Needling
0.4 to 1 cun perpendicular insertion.
0.5 to 2 cun oblique insertion, usually in a distal direction.

Actions and indications
Although TE 12 is traditionally indicated for treating swelling due to its ascribed effect on draining excess fluids from the body, it is seldom used for this purpose in the modern day practice.

However, it has been traditionally employed to *transform phlegm and dissipate stagnation, descend rebellious Qi and calm the mind.*

Symptoms include: nodular swellings in the neck, goitre, productive cough, coughing blood, sore throat, headache, deafness, chest or flank pain, cardiac pain, chills and fever, malaria, urticaria, epilepsy, and even insanity.

> **Main Areas**—Elbow. Arm. Triple Energizer channel.
> **Main Functions**—Regulates Qi and Blood. Alleviates pain and swelling.

TE 11   Qinglengyuan
Cooling Deep Pool

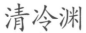

Myotome	C6–C8
Dermatome	C7

TE 12 can be a useful adjacent or local point in the treatment of regional disorders of the upper limb, particularly involving impaired movement, stiffness or pain of the elbow or shoulder, and weakness, atrophy or tightness of the triceps brachii muscle.

> **Main Areas**—Upper arm, shoulder and elbow. Triceps brachii muscle.
> **Main Functions**—Alleviates stiffness and pain. Drains dampness and treats swelling.

TE 13   Naohui

消泺

Upper Arm Intersection

Intersection of the Yang Wei Mai on the Triple Energizer channel

Myotome	C6–C8
Dermatome	C5–T1

Location
On the posterior aspect of the upper arm, just below the lower border of the deltoid muscle, approximately 6 cun proximal to TE 10, or 4 cun distal to TE 14.

To aid location, contract the posterior deltoid by extending the arm backwards against resistance and find the point just below its lower border, between the two heads of the triceps brachii muscle.

Needling
Perpendicular or oblique distal insertion 0.6 to 2 cun.

Actions and indications
Really useful point for *shoulder problems*, particularly involving *loss of lateral rotation and extension*, as is seen in *capsulitis and frozen shoulder*. Combined with SI 9 and SI 11 it forms a neat line of three points covering infraspinatus and teres major.

> **Main Area**—Upper arm and shoulder.
> **Main Function**—Alleviates stiffness and pain.

TE 14   Jianliao

肩髎

Shoulder Bone Hole

Myotome	C4–C6
Dermatome	C4

Location
On the posterolateral aspect of the shoulder, in the depression directly inferior to the acromion process, between the posterior and middle fibres of the deltoid muscle, directly posterior to LI 15. It is the posterior 'eye' of the shoulder.

To aid location, it is situated in the posterior of the two distinct depressions formed between the inferior border of the acromion process and the greater tubercle of the humerus. These depressions are

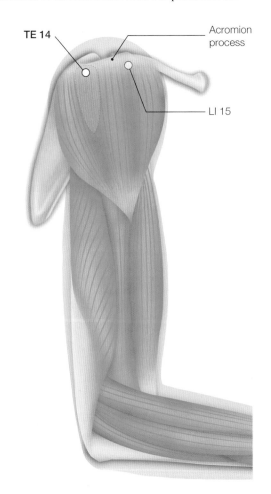

TE 14

Acromion process

LI 15

usually visible when the patient's arm is passively abducted to 90 degrees.

Needling

With the arm down by the side, 0.5 to 1.5 cun perpendicular insertion. The needle should enter the space between the subacromial bursa and the acromion process.

With the arm down by the side, 0.5 to 2 cun oblique or transverse insertion distally along the channel, between the posterior and medial fibres of the deltoid.

With the arm abducted (raised), 1 to 3 cun perpendicular insertion, directed towards HT 1 at the centre of the axilla. With the arm abducted (raised), 0.5 to 2 cun transverse oblique insertion into the deltoid fibres, directed distally down the arm. Anterior transverse insertion to join with LI 15.

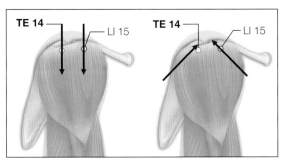

Needling direction

Actions and indications

TE 14 is a *very useful point for many types of shoulder and arm disorders* manifesting along the Triple Energizer channel pathway. It effectively *treats weakness, pain and stiffness of the shoulder*, especially if there is difficulty in lifting the arm and moving it backwards (abduction and extension).

It is particularly indicated for supraspinatus tendinitis, periarthritis of the shoulder, frozen shoulder, and spasticity, atrophy or paralysis of the upper limb.

> **Main Area**—Shoulder.
> **Main Functions**—Regulates Qi and Blood. Alleviates pain and reduces stiffness.

TE 15　Tianliao　
Upper Bone Hole

Intersection of the Yang Wei Mai and Triple Energizer

Myotome	C3–C6 and accessory nerve
Dermatome	C4

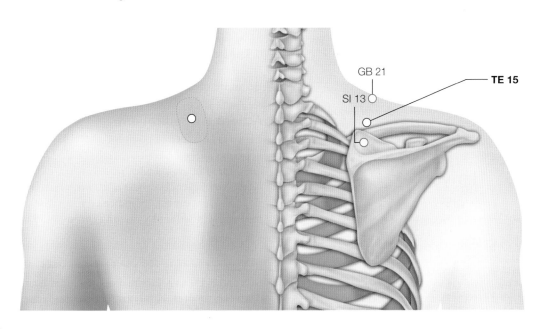

Location

On the posterior aspect of the shoulder, approximately 1 cun posterior and slightly medial to GB 21, midway between GB 21 and SI 13.

Needling

0.3 to 1 cun perpendicular insertion.

A very effective method to noticeably release trapezius tightness causing shoulder or neck pain or stiffness, is to needle TE 15 and GB 21 simultaneously so that the two needles are inserted at 90 degrees to each other and ideally the tips actually meet at the centre of the trapezius muscle belly. That way the strongest deqi can be achieved. Should this not be effective, use SI 12 instead of TE 15 to join with GB 21.

Actions and indications

TE 15 has *similar functions to GB 21*, albeit not as powerful. It helps *dispel wind and dampness and moderates pain*. Additionally, it *relaxes the chest and regulates Qi*.

It is primarily used as a *local point* in the treatment of pain and stiffness of the shoulder and back, and disorders of the cervical spine. Beyond trapezius lies the inferior attachments of levator scapulae.

It has also been traditionally used for a variety of other symptoms, including: fullness, tightness or pain in the chest, chills and fever, insomnia, and mental restlessness.

> **Main Areas**—Shoulder. Chest.
> **Main Functions**—Regulates Qi and Blood. Alleviates pain and stiffness.

TE 16   Tianyou
Sky Window

天牖

Window of the Sky point

Myotome	C1–C5 and accessory nerve
Dermatome	C3

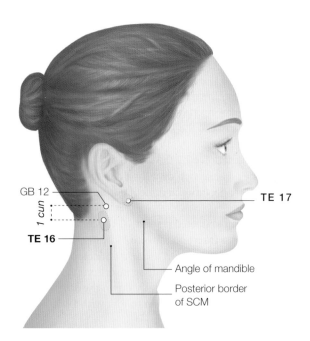

GB 12 · 1 cun · TE 17 · TE 16 · Angle of mandible · Posterior border of SCM

Location

On the posterior border of the SCM muscle, level with the angle of the mandible, approximately 1 cun posterior and inferior to the tip of the mastoid process.

To aid location, it is directly inferior to GB 12 and level with SI 17.

Needling

0.3 to 1 cun oblique inferior insertion into the SCM fibres.
0.3 to 1 cun perpendicular insertion.

Be aware of anatomy in this region

Actions and indications

TE 16 is an effective point for *disorders of the ears, neck and entire head*. It *activates Qi and Blood circulation* in the channel, *dispels wind, clears heat, transforms dampness and phlegm and reduces swelling*. It is especially indicated for *stiffness of the neck* with difficulty rotating and side-flexing the cervical spine.

Indications include: pain and inflammation of the ears and eyes, easy lacrimation, impaired hearing, deafness, tinnitus, nasal obstruction, headache, dizziness, swelling of the face, sore throat, phlegm nodules, and swollen glands.

Furthermore, it has been employed to treat a variety of other disorders, including: sudden deafness or loss of sight, loss of sense of smell, swelling of the breasts, tidal fevers, and mental confusion.

> **Main Areas**—Throat and neck. Ears.
> **Main Functions**—Regulates Qi and Blood. Alleviates pain. Transforms dampness and reduces swelling. Dispels wind and clears heat.

TE 17 Yifeng
Wind Screen

Intersection of the Gallbladder on the Triple Energizer channel

Myotome	None – superficial tissue
Dermatome	C2/C3

Location
Directly behind the ear lobe, at the centre of the deep depression formed between the mastoid process and the mandibular ramus.

To aid location, it is at the most tender spot, superior to the transverse process of the atlas.

Needling
0.5 to 1 cun perpendicular insertion.
1 to 1.5 cun oblique downward medial insertion.

Do <u>not</u> needle deeper. Posteriorly directed insertion can be dangerous with arterial and venous anatomy.

Actions and indications
TE 17 may be *the most important point for disorders of the ear* due to its powerful action on *clearing the channel pathway. It effectively dispels stagnation of any type and is especially indicated to clear heat* and *dissipate wind* of *exterior* or *interior origin*.

It is effectively used in a wide variety of conditions affecting the ear, including: tinnitus, diminished hearing, deafness, earache, acute or chronic otitis, and itching, discharge or other inflammatory disorders of the ear.

Due to the fact that TE 17 also *subdues interior wind and descends Yang from the head*, it may treat stubborn and difficult conditions such as Ménière's disease, dizziness, loss of balance, vertigo, blurred vision, stiffness of the jaw, sore throat, headache, sudden deafness, and extreme ear pain or tinnitus with dizziness and nausea due to *Liver Yang or phlegm-fire rising upward*.

TE 17 also may be the most important point for treating *disorders of the facial nerve* such as paralysis of the eye, mouth, tongue or submandibular muscles.

> **Main Areas**—Ears. Face. Throat. Neck.
> **Main Functions**—Benefits the ear. Alleviates pain. Clears heat. Dispels wind. Treats the facial nerve.

TE 18 Chimai
Convulsions Vessel

Myotome	Facial nerve
Dermatome	C2/C3

Location
Posterior to the helix of the ear, in a shallow depression, one third of the distance from TE 17 to TE 20. In the auricularis posterior muscle.

To aid location, find the palpable crevice-like depression on the posterior aspect of the mastoid process.

Needling
0.3 to 0.5 cun subcutaneously along the course of the channel.

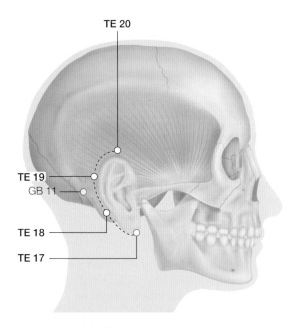

TE 20
TE 19
GB 11
TE 18
TE 17

Actions and indications

Although TE 18 is not very commonly used, it can be an effective ancillary point in the treatment of earache, tinnitus and other disorders of the ear. It is also traditionally indicated for more severe symptoms such as dizziness and epileptic convulsions caused by interior wind.

However, TE 18 is usually only ever used in regional pain disorders such as headache, migraine and neuralgia, and its treatment is especially recommended if it is sensitive on pressure palpation. In these cases, it usually also has an immediate calming effect on the mind.

> Main Areas—Ear. Mastoid area. Head.
> Main Functions—Benefits the ears. Dredges the channel and alleviates pain. Dispels exterior wind. Subdues interior wind. Calms the mind.

TE 19　Luxi　
Head's Tranquility

Myotome	Trigeminal nerve
Dermatome	C2/C3

Location
Posterior to the helix of the ear, in a distinct shallow depression, within temporalis, one third of the distance from TE 20 to TE 17.

To aid location, find GB 11 a little posterior and inferior to TE 19, and palpate them simultaneously to determine which one is most reactive to pressure palpation.

Needling
0.3 to 0.5 cun subcutaneously along the course of the channel.

Actions and indications
Although TE 19 is not a very commonly used point it can be effective to *relax and calm the mind*, for which it is traditionally indicated.

TE 19 can be a particularly effective local or adjacent point in the treatment of ear problems, headaches and other pain disorders.

It is also indicated in a range of other cases such as, disorders of the eyes and nose, epilepsy, convulsions, dizziness and other symptoms of interior wind.

> Main Areas—Head. Brain. Temple.
> Main Functions—Calms the mind. Dredges the channels and alleviates pain.

TE 20　Jiaosun　
Angle Vertex

Intersection of the Gallbladder and Small Intestine on the Triple Energizer channel

Myotome	Trigeminal nerve
Dermatome	C2/C3 but also crossover to trigeminal nerve

Location
In the shallow depression directly above the apex of the ear, within temporalis, just within the hairline.

To aid location, fold the ear forwards to locate the apex.

Needling

0.3 to 1.5 cun subcutaneous insertion in the direction of the area being treated, or join with adjacent points, e.g. GB 8 and GB 5.

Actions and indications

Although TE 20 is not a very commonly used point, it can be effective in the treatment of *regional pain and disorders of the ear and mouth*. Indications include: earache, tinnitus, discharge from the ear and toothache. It has also been employed in a variety of other cases, including sudden loss of vision, dryness of the lips and heat rash.

> **Main Areas**—Ear. Mouth.
> **Main Functions**—Regulates Qi and Blood. Alleviates pain and swelling.

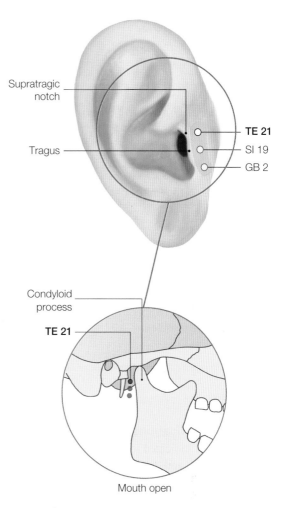

TE 21   Ermen
Ear Gate

耳門

Myotome	None – superficial tissue
Dermatome	Trigeminal nerve

Location

In the depression anterior to the supratragic notch and posterior to the condyloid process of the mandible, in line with SI 19 and GB 2.

To aid location, when the patient opens their mouth, the condyloid process of the mandible slides forwards to reveal the depression.

Needling

0.5 to 1 cun perpendicular needling, directed slightly posteriorly. Insert the needle with the patient's mouth open. After insertion the patient can close the mouth.

Actions and indications

TE 21 *is important in the treatment of disorders of the ear*, including: otitis, tinnitus, deafness, and Ménière's disease.

It is also effective for other disorders of the local area, including: stiffness of the jaw, temporal headache, toothache, facial pain, and inflammation of the eyes (see also GB 2 and SI 19).

> **Main Areas**—Ears. Temple. Jaw.
> **Main Functions**—Improves hearing and benefits the ears. Regulates Qi and Blood. Alleviates pain. Clears heat.

TE 22 Erheliao 耳和髎

Ear Harmonising
Foramen

Intersection of the Small Intestine and Gallbladder on the Triple Energizer channel

Myotome	Trigeminal nerve
Dermatome	Trigeminal nerve

Location

Approximately 0.5 cun anterior to base of the helix of the ear, at the posterior border of the temporal hairline. Situated in a depression formed superior to the zygomatic process and posterior to the main palpable mass of the temporalis muscle (clench the jaw to define the muscle).

Needling

Subcutaneous needling in direction of condition being treated.

Actions and indications

TE 20 is mainly indicated for disorders of the ear, including tinnitus and deafness, but also for tooth problems when pertaining to the teeth of the top jaw and the TMJ.

> **Main Area**—Ears.
> **Main Functions**—Dredges the channels and alleviates pain. Dispels wind. Benefits the ears.

TE 23 Sizhukong 絲竹空

Silken Bamboo Hollow

Myotome	Facial nerve
Dermatome	Trigeminal nerve

Location

At the lateral end of the eyebrow.

To aid location, palpate gently with the tip of the finger along the end of the eyebrow, to locate the depression in the bony cleft formed just superior to the supraorbital ridge.

Needling

0.2 to 0.4 cun transverse insertion posteriorly.

Actions and indications

TE 23 is primarily used to *dispel wind, clear heat, alleviate pain* and *benefit the eyes*. Its indications are similar to those of GB 1.

> **Main Areas**—Eyes. Temple.
> **Main Functions**—Regulates Qi and Blood. Alleviates pain. Dispels wind and clears heat. Clears the eyes.

TE 22   TE 23

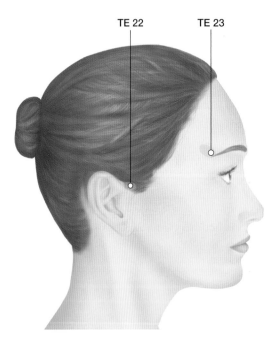

18 Points of the Leg Shao Yang Gallbladder Channel

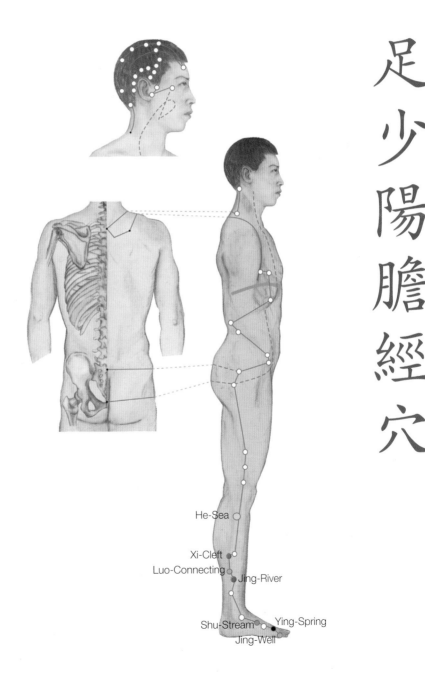

足少陽膽經穴

He-Sea

Xi-Cleft

Luo-Connecting

Jing-River

Ying-Spring

Shu-Stream

Jing-Well

| General | The Gallbladder channel is one of the longest and most far-reaching channels, especially in the world of musculo-skeletal medicine, because it covers so many key joints.

Starting at the lateral edge of the orbit, the channel travels obliquely backwards towards the ear, and then upwards to traverse the temporalis muscle before rounding the ear and reaching just behind the mastoid process at GB 12. From here it goes across the head once more, to the anterior, to the middle of the forehead at GB 14, and then back again, over the scalp to GB 20 in the dip between the trapezius and the SCM at the level of the upper cervical vertebrae.

Crossing the trapezius, the channel winds around the anterior aspect of the shoulder, like a holster, and then crisscrosses down across the rib cage. A key point is GB 25 at the end of the twelfth rib as a marker. From here it descends over the anterior spine of the pelvis and then diverts backwards into the gluteal muscles and onwards down the lateral leg, all the way to the mid-shin. Here, there is a side-step before it continues down the lateral side of the foot, crossing the anterolateral ankle, and finishing on the nail of the fourth toe.

The channel has 44 points. It is grouped with the Liver under the Wood element in five-element theory. |
|---|---|
| More specifically | Starting at a key small depression on the lateral side of the bony orbit of the eye, the channel heads posteriorly from GB 1 to GB 2, which sits in front of the tragus of the ear, directly beneath SI 19. From here, the channel goes upwards (another marker is that GB 3 sits in a line with ST 7 to aid location), to traverse the whole of the temporalis muscle. It then turns posteriorly at GB 7, following the shape of the ear (the Triple Energizer channel being inside the line of the GB channel) to the posterior edge of the mastoid process.

The channel then lurches forwards once more and goes across the scalp, to the middle of the forehead, directly above the eye at GB 14.

Reversing once more and going backwards over the top of the head, the channel finally leaves the head at GB 20. This is situated in between the muscle bulks of the upper trapezius and the posterior edge of the SCM, and the level of the suboccipital muscles of C1/2 and the skull. Crossing the upper fibres of the trapezius, and sited within them, is GB 21, which has inner channel links to GV 14 and ST 12 and can affect the eye and chest.

The key channel moves inferiorly, passing anteriorly over the shoulder, to the region between the ribs at the fifth intercostal space, the mid-axillary line. Coming forwards around the body, GB 24 lies in the seventh intercostal space, directly under the breast and situated close to LR 14. Next, the channel moves posteriorly to the end of the twelfth rib, before returning anteriorly to just inside the ASIS on the ilium but within the abdominals.

It is possible to see that because of the crisscrossing nature of this channel in the trunk it has widespread use. At GB 28 the channel becomes key for treating issues in the hip, crossing the gluteus medius and minimus, before turning at GB 30 in the gluteus maximus to travel down the lateral thigh – following the ITB. The next key station is GB 34, just anterior and inferior to the head of the fibula, and in general the channel runs down the lateral leg, across the anterolateral ankle and finishes on the lateral edge of the nail of the fourth toe. |

Area covered	Head and temples. Neck, shoulders, chest/breast, abdomen and pelvis, hip, thigh, knee, ankle.
Areas affected with treatment	Head in particular. Migraine, with or without aura. Stress and tension in the muscle system – locally and globally. Irritability. Rib cage, breasts. Lower abdominals, hip, knee, ankle.
Key points	GB 8, GB 9, GB 12, GB 20, GB 21, GB 25, GB 30, GB 34, GB 39, GB 40, GB 41.

GB 1   Tongziliao   瞳子髎
Pupil Bone Hole

Intersection of the Triple Energizer and Small Intestine on the Gallbladder channel

Myotome	Facial nerve
Dermatome	Trigeminal nerve

Location
In the small crevice-like depression, on the lateral margin of the orbit, approximately 0.5 cun lateral to the outer canthus. Situated in the orbicularis oculi muscle.

To aid location, palpate the lateral orbital margin gently with the pad of the index finger, to locate the narrow vertical crevice.

Alternative location
Alternatively, treat GB 1 further posteriorly in the temporal fossa, behind the posterior border of the lateral orbital margin, in the temporalis muscle.

Needling
0.2 to 0.4 cun transverse insertion posteriorly. 0.5 to 1 cun transverse insertion towards Taiyang (Ex HN 5).

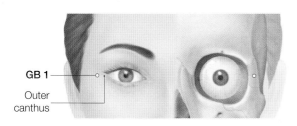

GB 1

Outer canthus

Insert the needle carefully and apply very little manipulation, or none at all. Apply pressure to the point after removing the needle. During needle retention, the patient should avoid unnecessary blinking.

This point can bruise easily. If any slight swelling of the skin is observed remove the needle immediately and apply pressure, plus a cold compress.

Actions and indications
GB 1 is an important point to *clear wind and heat from the eyes*, *promote Qi and Blood circulation*, *alleviate pain* and *improve vision*.

Indications include: pain, redness, swelling, itching and inflammation of the eye, sclera, eyelids and outer canthus, conjunctivitis, pain extending to the ear, trigeminal neuralgia, temporal headache, migraine, facial paralysis, deviation of the eye or cheek, glaucoma, night blindness, short-sightedness, cataract, and diminishing vision.

> **Main Areas**—Eyes. Outer canthus.
> **Main Functions**—Benefits the eyes and improves vision. Dispels wind and heat. Regulates Qi and Blood.

GB 2   Tinghui   聽會
Hearing Convergence

Myotome	None – superficial tissue
Dermatome	Trigeminal nerve

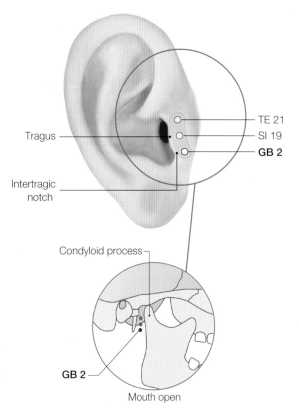

Tragus

TE 21
SI 19
GB 2

Intertragic
notch

Condyloid process

GB 2

Mouth open

Location

In the depression anterior to the intertragic notch, directly below SI 19, posterior to the condyloid process of the mandible.

To aid location, when the patient opens their mouth, the condyloid process of the mandible slides forwards to reveal the depression.

GB 2 is often chosen instead of, or in addition to, SI 19 and TE 21, and vice versa. Use pressure palpation in order to ascertain which point is most reactive.

Needling

0.5 to 1 cun perpendicular needling, directed slightly posteriorly. Insert the needle with the patient's mouth open. After insertion, the patient can close the mouth.

Actions and indications

GB 2 is an important point to *improve hearing* and treat a *variety of ear disorders.* It effectively dispels *wind and clears heat, promotes Qi and Blood circulation, dispels stagnation, relieves swelling* and *alleviates pain.*

Indications include: *acute or chronic inflammatory conditions of the ear*, itching, pain, swelling or discharge from the ear, diminished hearing, tinnitus, deafness, deviation of the eye or mouth, facial paralysis, facial pain, trigeminal neuralgia, migraine, headache, toothache, TMJ syndrome, and stiffness or injury of the jaw.

Furthermore, treatment applied to GB 2 is effective for other *disorders of the face and head*, including temporal headache, toothache and inflammation of the eyes.

> **Main Areas**—Ears. Temple. Jaw.
> **Main Functions**—Improves hearing and benefits the ears. Regulates Qi and Blood. Alleviates pain. Dispels wind and clears heat.

GB 3   Shangguan   上關
Above the Arch

Intersection of the Triple Energizer and Stomach on the Gallbladder channel

Myotome	Trigeminal nerve
Dermatome	Trigeminal nerve

Location

In the depression above the superior border of the zygomatic arch, directly above ST 7.

Contraindications

According to some classical texts, needling GB 3 is contraindicated. This may be due to the observation that puncturing vessels at this location can cause internal bleeding and lead to deafness or even death. Use of points GB 4 to GB 9 is much more common.

Needling

0.2 to 0.4 cun perpendicular insertion.

Do not needle deeper. Be aware of a lot of delicate anatomy in this region.

Actions and indications

Although GB 3 is not very commonly used, it can be remarkably effective to *promote Qi and Blood circulation, dissipate stasis and alleviate pain from the jaw, TMJ, sides of the face and ears.* Furthermore it helps *dispel wind and clear heat.*

Indications include: earache, acute or chronic inflammatory conditions of the ear, tinnitus, deafness, facial paralysis and pain, trigeminal neuralgia, migraine, toothache, stiffness of the jaw, TMJ syndrome, headache, parotitis, and swelling of the side of the face.

> **Main Areas**—Temple. Jaw. Ears.
> **Main Functions**—Regulates Qi and Blood. Alleviates pain. Clears heat. Improves hearing.

GB 4   Hanyan
Forehead Fullness
頷厭

Intersection of the Triple Energizer and Stomach on the Gallbladder channel

Myotome	Trigeminal nerve
Dermatome	Trigeminal nerve

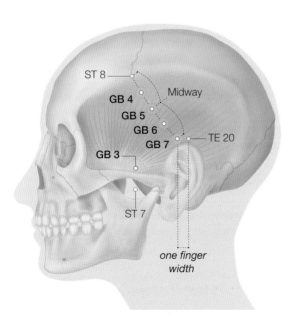

Location

In a shallow depression within the temporal hairline, below ST 8, one quarter of the distance between ST 8 and GB 7.

To aid location, it is just superior to a bulge in the temporal muscle appearing when the jaw is closed tight.

Needling

0.3 to 1.5 cun subcutaneous insertion in the direction of the area being treated. Join with adjacent points.

Pick up the cutaneous tissue of the scalp (pinch the scalp) and insert the needle subcutaneously, under the galea aponeurotica parallel to the bone. If the scalp is very tight, this may be difficult; therefore, needle perpendicularly 0.2 to 0.3 cun.

Actions and indications

GB 4 is used mainly as a *local point* in the treatment of headache and pain on the lateral aspect of the face and temple.

Indications include: migraine, trigeminal neuralgia, toothache, earache, tinnitus, and pain or inflammation of the eyes, particularly at the lateral aspect.

It has also been traditionally employed in a variety of other cases, including dizziness, convulsions, epilepsy, and stiffness of the neck. It is very close to a matching trigger point in the region that refers pain to the teeth.

> **Main Areas**—Temple. Jaw. Ears.
> **Main Functions**—Regulates Qi and Blood. Alleviates pain.

GB 5   Xuanlu
Suspended Skull
懸顱

Intersection of the Triple Energizer, Stomach and Large Intestine on the Gallbladder channel

Myotome	Trigeminal nerve
Dermatome	Trigeminal nerve

Location

In a shallow depression within the temporal hairline, below GB 4 and midway between ST 8 and GB 7.

Needling

0.3 to 1.5 cun subcutaneous insertion in the direction of the area being treated.

Actions and indications

GB 5 is used mainly as a *local point* in the treatment of headache and pain on the lateral aspect of the face and temple. Used with GB 4.

Indications include: migraine, trigeminal neuralgia, toothache, earache, tinnitus, and pain or inflammation of the eyes, particularly at the lateral aspect.

> **Main Areas**—Temple. Jaw. Ears.
> **Main Functions**—Regulates Qi and Blood. Alleviates pain.

GB 6   Xuanli
Suspended Tuft

Intersection of the Triple Energizer, Stomach and Large Intestine on the Gallbladder channel

Myotome	Trigeminal nerve
Dermatome	Trigeminal nerve

Location

In a shallow depression within the temporal hairline, midway between GB 5 and GB 7 (one quarter of the distance between GB 7 and ST 8).

Needling

0.3 to 1.5 cun subcutaneous insertion in the direction of the area being treated.

Actions and indications

GB 6 is another useful point for *one-sided headache* and *expels wind and clears heat.* Wind could give rise to tinnitus as a symptom.

> **Main Areas**—Temple. Jaw. Ears.
> **Main Functions**—Regulates Qi and Blood. Alleviates pain.

GB 7   Qubin
Temporal Hairline Curve

Intersection of the Bladder on the Gallbladder channel

Myotome	Trigeminal nerve
Dermatome	Trigeminal nerve

Location

On the temple, approximately one finger-width anterior to TE 20, level with the apex of the auricle.

To aid location, the shallow depression is easier to ascertain if the patient opens and closes the jaw.

Needling

0.3 to 1.5 cun subcutaneous insertion in the direction of the area being treated, or join with adjacent points, e.g. GB 8, TE 20 and GB 6.

Actions and indications

In common with TE 20, GB 7 can be effective in the treatment of regional pain, including temporal headache, migraine, swelling and pain of the cheek and submandibular region, stiffness and pain of the jaw and neck, earache, toothache, and trigeminal neuralgia.

> **Main Areas**—Temple. Ear. Cheek.
> **Main Functions**—Regulates Qi and Blood. Alleviates pain.

GB 8   Shuaigu
Leading Valley

率谷

> **Main Areas**—Temple. Ear. Brain.
> **Main Functions**—Regulates Qi and Blood.
> Alleviates pain. Relieves poisoning.

Intersection of the Bladder on the Gallbladder channel

Myotome	Trigeminal nerve
Dermatome	Trigeminal nerve, C2/C3

Location
In the shallow depression superior to the apex of the auricle, approximately 1.5 cun within the hairline and 1 cun directly above TE 20.

Needling
0.3 to 1.5 cun subcutaneous insertion in the direction of the area being treated, or join with adjacent points.

Actions and indications
In common with GB 7 and TE 20, GB 8 is primarily used in *regional pain and disorders of the ear and temple.* It has also been extensively employed to treat nausea, vomiting, headache and symptoms of alcohol poisoning.

GB 9   Tianchong
Upper Surge

天衝

Intersection of the Bladder on the Gallbladder channel

Myotome	Trigeminal nerve
Dermatome	C2/C3

Location
In the shallow depression approximately 0.5 cun posterior to GB 8.

Needling
0.3 to 1.5 cun subcutaneous insertion in the direction of the area being treated, or join with adjacent points.

Actions and indications
Similar to GB 8 and other adjacent points. GB 9 has additionally been employed to treat *psychological disturbances*, anxiety, agitation, panic attacks, fright and shock, epilepsy and even insanity.

> **Main Areas**—Head. Brain. Mind. Ear.
> **Main Functions**—Regulates Qi and Blood.
> Alleviates pain. Calms the mind.

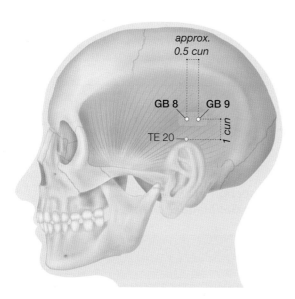

approx. 0.5 cun

GB 8   GB 9

TE 20   1 cun

GB 10   Fubai
Floating Bright

浮白

Intersection of the Bladder on the Gallbladder channel

Myotome	Trigeminal nerve
Dermatome	C2/C3

Location

In a shallow depression one third of the distance along the curved line joining GB 9 and GB 12.

To aid location, it is along the inferior temporal line.

Needling

0.3 to 1.5 cun subcutaneous insertion in the direction of the area being treated, or join with adjacent points.

Actions and indications

In common with other adjacent points, GB 10 can be used in *regional disorders* and *pain.* Although it is not a very commonly used point, it can be effective to *clear the head, benefit the ears, relax the neck* and *calm the mind.*

It has also been traditionally employed in a range of other disorders including toothache, inflammation of the eyes, cough, goitre, stiffness of the shoulder and weakness of the lower limbs.

> **Main Areas**—Side of head. Ear. Brain.
> **Main Functions**—Regulates Qi and Blood. Alleviates pain.

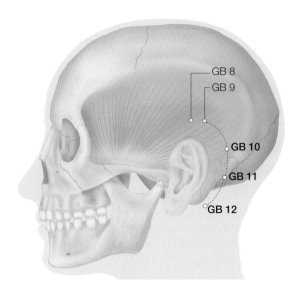

GB 11 Touqiaoyin 頭竅陰
Head Yin Openings

Intersection of the Bladder on the Gallbladder channel

Myotome	C2/C3 dorsal rami
Dermatome	C2/C3

Location

In a depression two thirds of the distance along the curved line joining GB 9 and GB 12. See also TE 19.

Needling

0.3 to 1.5 cun subcutaneous insertion in the direction of the area being treated. Join with adjacent points.

Pick up the cutaneous tissue of the scalp (pinch the scalp) and insert the needle subcutaneously, under the galea aponeurotica parallel to the bone. If the scalp is very tight, this may be difficult; therefore, needle perpendicularly 0.2 to 0.3 cun.

Actions and indications

Treats one sided headache, neck pain and stiffness and helps brighten the sense organs. Similar to GB 10, TE 19 and other adjacent points. GB 11 is traditionally indicated for disorders of the five sense organs, particularly the eyes and the ears.

> **Main Areas**—Side of head. Eye. Ear. Brain.
> **Main Functions**—Regulates Qi and Blood. Alleviates pain.

GB 12 Wangu 完骨
Mastoid Process

Intersection of the Bladder on the Gallbladder channel

Myotome	Accessory nerve and posterior rami of C2/C3
Dermatome	C2/C3

Location

In a small depression just posterior to the tip of the mastoid process. Situated superficially in the SCM muscle and more deeply, in the splenius capitis and longissimus capitis muscles. In its deep position, and depending on the angle and depth of needling or manual pressure, the digastric muscle can be accessed.

To aid location, slide a fingertip in a posterior direction from the tip of the mastoid process to find the small crevice-like depression between the bone and muscle. This crevice can be further defined between the fibres of the SCM and digastric muscle posterior belly attachment on the mastoid bone.

Needling

0.3 to 1 cun oblique inferior insertion into the SCM fibres.

Do not insert deeply, however this is a very useful point and should be included in many headache and other treatments.

Actions and indications

The functions of GB 12 are closely related to those of adjacent points at the base of the cranium, particularly GV 15, BL 10, GB 20 and Anmian (Ex-HN-54). All these points tend to *strongly relax the patient* by *balancing the nervous system* and *regulating the ascending and descending of Qi* from the head. They are therefore all useful in cases of *excessive rising Yang* or deficiency of the marrow causing *disorders of the brain and sense organs.*

Note that Anmian, located next to GB 12, has been named the *Peaceful Sleep*, reflecting the relaxing properties of the acupoints in this area. GB 12, however, is primarily used as a *local point* to treat regional disorders, particularly pain, stiffness and swelling.

It is a notable point of attachment for many channels such as BL, SI, GB, in fascial trains treatment. Self-pressure for the patient can be an aid to performance of exercises.

Indications include: pain or stiffness of the neck or jaw, earache, toothache, lymphadenopathy, facial paralysis, difficulty swallowing and painful swelling of the throat, cheeks and submandibular region.

Additionally, it has been employed to treat *interior symptoms of Gallbladder imbalance* such as headache, insomnia and sensations of heat.

> **Main Areas**—Neck. Head. Ears. Throat.
> **Main Functions**—Relaxes the body and calms the mind. Dissipates stasis and relieves swelling. Alleviates pain. Benefits the throat.

GB 13　Benshen
Shen Root

Intersection of the Yang Wei Mai on the Gallbladder channel

Myotome	Facial nerve
Dermatome	Trigeminal nerve

Location

In the shallow depression 0.5 cun within the anterior hairline, directly above the outer canthus.

To aid location, it is approximately two thirds of the distance between GV 24 and ST 8. The distance of two thirds is 3 cun.

Needling

0.3 to 1 cun transverse insertion posteriorly, or in other directions, depending on the desired result. Join with adjacent points such as ST 8 or GB 15.

Actions and indications

GB 13 is primarily used as a *local point in the treatment of pain* and headache. Furthermore, it has been employed to treat eye disorders, stiffness of the neck, dizziness, epilepsy, and psychological or emotional restlessness, agitation or anxiety.

> **Main Areas**—Head. Mind.
> **Main Functions**—Regulates Qi and Blood. Alleviates pain. Calms the mind.

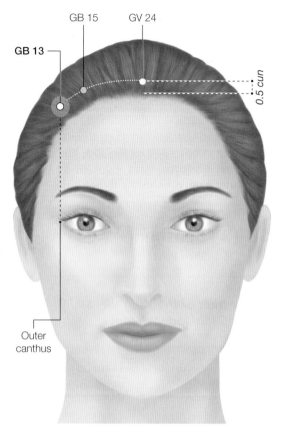

GB 13

GB 15   GV 24

0.5 cun

Outer
canthus

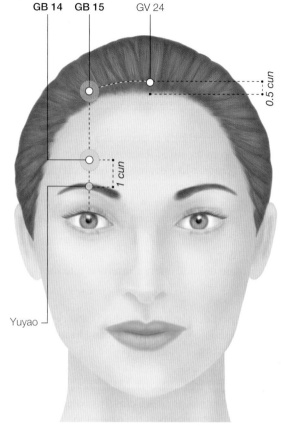

GB 14   GB 15   GV 24

0.5 cun

1 cun

Yuyao

GB 14   Yangbai
Yang Bright

陽白

*Intersection of the Yang Wei Mai, Stomach,
Large Intestine and Triple Energizer on the
Gallbladder channel*

Myotome	Facial nerve
Dermatome	Trigeminal nerve

Location
On the forehead, in a shallow depression
approximately 1 cun above the midpoint of the
eyebrow, one third of the distance from the eyebrow
to the anterior hairline.

To aid location, the small pulse of the supraorbital
artery should be felt on gentle palpation with the pad
of the finger. The midpoint of the eyebrow is level
with the pupil when the gaze is fixed straight ahead.

Needling
0.3 to 1 cun subcutaneous insertion in an inferior
direction towards Yuyao. Pick up the skin to insert
the needle subcutaneously, parallel to the bone.

Apply pressure to the point after removing the
needle.

Actions and indications
GB 14 is very important and widely used to *relax
the forehead, calm the mind* and *brighten the eyes*.
It *dispels wind* and *clears heat, regulates Qi and
Blood, dissipates stasis* and *alleviates pain*.

Indications include: headache, dizziness, pain
of the forehead, itching or inflammation of the
eyes, excessive lacrimation, diminishing vision,

deviation of the eye or mouth, and paralysis, twitching or spasm of the eyelids. Treatment at this site causes immediate relaxation and is useful in cases of excessive worry, stress and insomnia.

GB 14 is also an important beauty point, used to smooth the forehead and brighten the eyes.

> **Main Areas**—Forehead. Eyes. Supraorbital area.
> **Main Functions**—Calms the mind and relaxes the body. Dispels wind and heat. Dispels stasis. Alleviates pain. Improves appearance.

GB 15   Toulinqi
Head Overlooking Tears   頭臨泣

Intersection of the Yang Wei Mai and the Bladder on the Gallbladder channel

Myotome	Facial nerve
Dermatome	Trigeminal nerve

Location
In a shallow depression 0.5 cun within the anterior hairline, directly above GB 14, midway between GV 24 and ST 8.

Needling
0.3 to 1.5 cun transverse insertion, either posteriorly along the course of the channel or in other directions depending on the area to be treated.

Actions and indications
Although GB 15 is not a very commonly used point, it can be useful in such cases as: headache, vertigo, dizziness, epilepsy, convulsions, coma, nasal obstruction, excessive lacrimation, and inflammation of the eyes.

> **Main Areas**—Head. Forehead. Eyes.
> **Main Functions**—Dissipates fullness. Regulates Qi and Blood.

GB 16   Muchuang
Eye Window   目窗

Intersection of the Yang Wei Mai on the Gallbladder channel

Myotome	Galea aponeurotica (structure linking anterior and posterior parts of occipitofrontalis), facial nerve
Dermatome	Trigeminal nerve

Location
In a shallow depression one third of the distance between GB 15 and GB 18, 2.25 cun lateral to the midline.

Needling
0.3 to 1.5 cun transverse insertion, either posteriorly along the course of the channel or in other directions depending on the area to be treated.

Actions and indications
Key functions *of benefitting the eyes in all kinds of eye conditions.* (As its name suggests) *Eliminates Wind and alleviates pain* in the region.

> **Main Areas**—Head. Brain. Eyes.
> **Main Functions**—Dredges the channel and dispels wind and heat. Alleviates pain.

GB 17   Zhengying
True Ying   正營

Intersection of the Yang Wei Mai on the Gallbladder channel

Myotome	Galea aponeurotica (structure linking anterior and posterior parts of occipitofrontalis), facial nerve
Dermatome	Trigeminal nerve

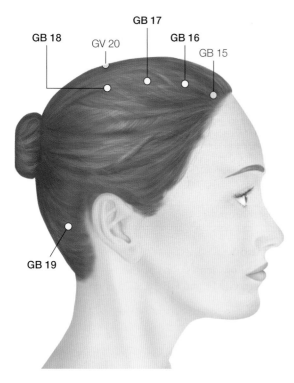

GB 18
GV 20
GB 17
GB 16
GB 15

GB 19

Location
In a shallow depression two thirds of the distance along the line connecting GB 15 and GB 18.

Needling
0.3 to 1.5 cun transverse insertion, either posteriorly along the course of the channel or in other directions depending on the area to be treated.

Actions and indications
Headache, one sided headache, pain in the jaw and teeth.

Main Areas—Head. Brain. Eyes.
Main Functions—Alleviates pain. Calms the mind.

GB 18   Chengling
Parietal Support

承靈

Intersection of the Yang Wei Mai on the Gallbladder channel

Myotome	Galea aponeurotica (structure linking anterior and posterior parts of occipitofrontalis), facial nerve
Dermatome	Trigeminal nerve, C2

Location
Directly lateral to GV 20, in line with GB 17, approximately 2.25 cun lateral to the midline.

Needling
0.3 to 1.5 cun transverse insertion, either posteriorly along the course of the channel or in other directions depending on the area to be treated.

Actions and indications
Headache, dizziness and eye pain – *benefits the head in general*. Specifically used for *nasal conditions* such as rhinitis and congestion.

Main Areas—Head. Brain. Nose. Eyes.
Main Functions—Regulates Qi and Blood. Calms the mind and opens the orifices.

GB 19   Naokong
Cranial Cavity

脑空

Intersection of the Yang Wei Mai on the Gallbladder channel

Myotome	Facial nerve
Dermatome	C2

Location

Directly above GB 20 and level with BL9 and GV 17, approximately 2.25 cun lateral to the midline.

Needling

0.3 to 1.5 cun transverse insertion, either posteriorly along the course of the channel or in other directions depending on the area to be treated.

Actions and indications

Another point that *benefits the head* and alleviates pain. *Opens the sense organs.*

> **Main Areas**—Head. Brain. Ear.
> **Main Functions**—Regulates Qi and Blood.

GB 20   Fengchi
Wind Pool

Intersection of the Yang Wei Mai, Yang Qiao Mai and Triple Energizer on the Gallbladder channel

Myotome	Posterior rami of adjacent cervical level
Dermatome	C2/C3

Location

At the centre of the sizeable depression directly below the occipital bone, within the posterior hairline. This depression is formed between the trapezius (medially), the SCM (laterally) and the splenius capitis (inferiorly). Situated superficially in the semispinalis capitis and, in its deep position, in the rectus capitis posterior major and the obliquus capitis superior on its lateral side.

To aid location, it is at the centre of the largest palpable depression at the base of the head. Also, it is approximately midway between GV 16 and the tip of the mastoid process.

Needling

0.5 to 1.2 cun perpendicular insertion, directed towards the opposite eye.

GB 20 is usually needled reasonably deeply in order to induce adequate deqi. The needle should be inserted at the level of the space between the occipital bone and transverse process of the atlas. It can go through the semispinalis capitis and reach a depth of 1.5–3cm close to the obliquus capitis and posterior rectus capitis muscles when needled by a competent practitioner.

If the needle is inserted even deeper it may injure the spinal cord, and in a superior direction even the medulla oblongata. Whilst this sounds traumatic it must be noted that this point is one of the most frequently used points for the head and is completely safe when following the correct direction. The target is muscle, not anything else.

Actions and indications

GB 20 is a very important point because it *effectively descends pathological Qi* from the head while at the same time *raising clear Qi* and *nourishing the Sea of Marrow*. It is possibly the most powerful point of the region and has been extensively employed to *clear heat, descend rising Yang, sedate interior wind* and treat symptoms of *wind stroke*. It is indicated for initial invasion of *exterior pathogenic factors at the Tai Yang stage.*

GB 20 has a marked effect on the head and brain and is important to *calm the mind* and *relax the body*. It is also widely used for *disorders of the sense organs*, and is especially indicated to *brighten the eyes* and *improve vision and hearing*. It also *dynamically activates Qi and Blood circulation* in the channel and is important to treat pain, stiffness, spasticity, atrophy and paralysis.

It has been extensively used in a *wide variety of disorders,* including: headache, migraine, pain and stiffness of the neck and shoulder, difficulty flexing the neck and turning or bending the head forwards, degenerative disorders of the cervical spine, postural hypotension, pain and inflammation of the eyes, tired eyes, excessive lacrimation, diminishing vision, earache, tinnitus, impaired hearing, disorders

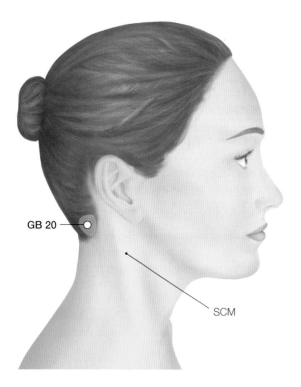

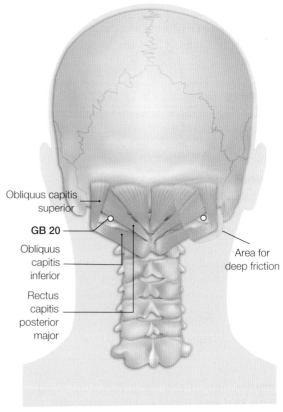

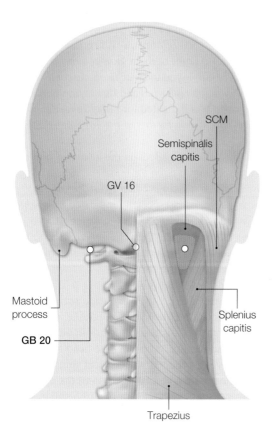

of the inner ear, Ménière's disease, facial paralysis, disorders of the jaw, TMJ syndrome, swelling and lumps on the neck, tidal fever, chills and fever, nasal obstruction, sinusitis, epistaxis, dizziness, vertigo, aphasia, hypertension, transient ischaemic attack, hemiplegia and other symptoms following wind stroke, epilepsy, convulsions, spasticity, tiredness, heavy feeling in the head, mental exhaustion, diminishing mental functions, amnesia, difficulty concentrating, poor memory, depression, premenstrual syndrome, insomnia, mental restlessness, irritability, and mood swings.

Main Areas—Head. Occiput. Neck. Eyes. Ears. Brain. Mind. Muscles. Entire body.
Main Functions—Calms the mind and relaxes the body. Descends rising Yang. Benefits the Sea of M arrow. Alleviates pain. Dispels wind and clears heat. Brightens the eyes. Benefits the ears.

GB 21   Jianjing
Shoulder Well

Intersection of the Yang Wei Mai, Stomach and Triple Energizer on the Gallbladder channel

Myotome	Accessory nerve, C2–C4
Dermatome	C4

Location
On the top of the shoulder, midway between the spinous process of C7 and the tip of the acromion process. On the highest point of the trapezius, where the muscle fibres separate on pressure palpation, directly posterior to ST 12.

To aid location, it is usually at the site of most tenderness. If the therapist places the base of each palm on the scapular spine with the thumbs touching the spinous process of C7 and the fingers resting on the upper portion of the trapezius, GB 21 lies below the tip of the middle finger if it is flexed slightly.

Do not treat GB 21 during pregnancy or in cases of severe deficiency or sinking Qi with manifestations such as excessive uterine bleeding, prolapse, diarrhoea, tiredness, dizziness, palpitations and very low blood pressure.

Needling
0.5 to 1.5 cun posterior oblique insertion into the trapezius muscle fibres.
0.3 to 0.5 cun perpendicular insertion.

Do not needle deeply and at a perpendicular angle. This, particularly in thin recipients, holds considerable risk of puncturing the apex of the lung and causing a pneumothorax.

Actions and indications
GB 21 is one of the *most commonly used and dynamic points* of the body and has been extensively employed in a wide variety of cases. It is one of the *strongest points to activate Qi and Blood circulation* and *dispel stasis.* Importantly, it also powerfully *descends Qi* and *clears heat.* It is extensively used to *treat pain* and *calm the mind,* as well as to *clear the head* and *open the sense organs.*

Indications include: headache, migraine, sinusitis, facial paralysis, TMJ syndrome, pain and inflammation of the eyes, earache, tinnitus, deafness, hypertension, fever, mental irritability or anxiety, depression, and insomnia.

GB 21 is probably the *strongest point of the region* and has been extensively used in the treatment of *disorders of the neck, shoulder and*

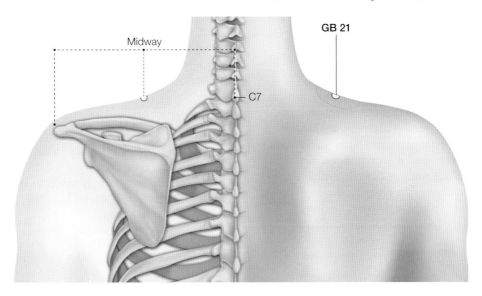

Midway

GB 21

C7

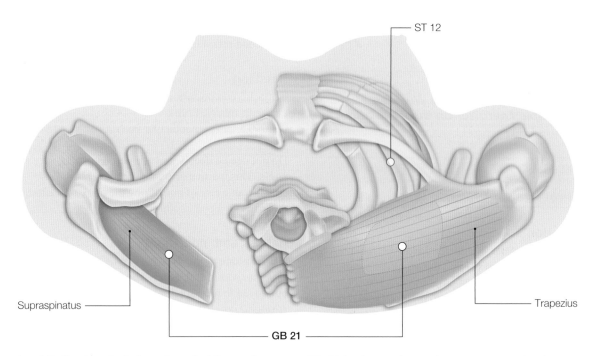

ST 12

Supraspinatus

Trapezius

GB 21

head. Indications include: pain and stiffness of the neck and shoulder, difficulty in turning the head, disorders of the cervical spine, spasm of the trapezius, tightness and pain of the upper back, frozen shoulder, periarthritis, difficulty raising the arm, and paralysis of the upper limb. It is also indicated for disorders of the throat, including: goitre, pain, swelling and palpable nodules or masses.

Furthermore, it effectively *dispels wind and cold* and is important to *open and relax the chest and alleviate dyspnoea and cough*. Indications include: pain and tightness of the chest, shortness of breath, asthma, respiratory diseases, chills and fever, headache, and sore or swollen throat.

GB 21 also descends the Qi dynamically through to the lower jiao, making it very effective for *gynaecological disorders* and *inducing labour* for which it is extensively employed. Indications include: amenorrhoea, dysmenorrhoea, abnormal uterine bleeding, prolonged labour, difficult delivery, retention of the placenta, uterine bleeding following miscarriage or delivery, swelling and pain of the breasts, mastitis, and difficult lactation.

GB 21 is also used to *sedate interior wind* and treat such cases as: dizziness, vertigo, Ménière's disease, epilepsy, wind stroke, hemiplegia, and other neurological disorders.

Diagnostically, spontaneous tenderness at GB 21, and the area posterior to it (including TE 15 and SI 12), may indicate referred pain from stomach disease on the left side and from the liver or gallbladder on the right. Moreover, chronic stiffness and tightness of the trapezius muscle surrounding GB 21 can indicate longstanding Liver Qi stagnation, interior cold or Blood deficiency.

It is also a *known trigger point* in the upper trapezius and needling here can send referred ache over the head, into the eye and around the bottom of the jaw.

> **Main Areas**—Neck. Shoulder. Upper back. Lungs. Chest. Breasts. Uterus. Head. Mind. Temple. Face. Eyes. Ears. Nose. Entire Body.
> **Main Functions**—Strongly descends Qi. Dispels stasis. Alleviates pain. Clears the chest. Induces menstruation and labour.

GB 22   Yuanye
Armpit Source

淵腋

Myotome	C5–C8
Dermatome	T5

Location
Approximately 3 cun below the centre of the axilla, on the mid-axillary line. Situated in the fifth intercostal space, approximately level with the nipple. To aid location, GB 22 is one hand-width inferior to the axilla, or one quarter of the distance between HT 1 and GB 26.

Needling
0.3 to 0.8 cun oblique insertion along the intercostal space towards GB 23.

Deep needling at the wrong angle poses considerable risk of puncturing the lung and causing a pneumothorax. Sensible knowledge of the layers of muscular anatomy is paramount.

Actions and indications
GB 22 and GB 23 are not very commonly used, although treatment at these sites can be very effective for *regional pain, stiffness* and *swelling*. It is especially useful for disorders of the axilla, mammary glands and shoulder, including swellings and nodules, intercostal neuralgia, herpes zoster and excessive sweating.

Additionally, both GB 22 and GB 23 help *open and relax the chest* and hypochondrial region and regulate Liver and Gallbladder Qi throughout the three jiao.

> **Main Areas**—Axilla. Breast. Ribs.
> **Main Functions**—Regulates Qi. Dissipates stasis and accumulation.

GB 23   Zhejin
Sinew Seat

輒筋

Intersection of the Bladder on the Gallbladder channel

Myotome	C5–C8
Dermatome	T5

Location
1 cun anterior and slightly inferior to GB 22, in the fifth intercostal space, approximately level with the nipple.

Needling
0.3 to 0.8 cun oblique insertion along the intercostal space.

Actions and indications
See GB 22.

Due to its location closer to the breast, GB 23 is more effective to treat *disorders of this area*. It is also indicated to descend rebellious Qi and clear stagnation causing symptoms such as heartburn, vomiting, hiccup, cough, excessive salivation, jaundice, insomnia and depression.

Furthermore, according to the *Great Compendium of Acupuncture and Moxibustion*, this is the front-mu

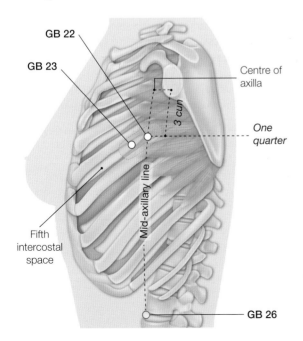

GB 22
GB 23
Centre of axilla
3 cun
One quarter
Mid-axillary line
Fifth intercostal space
GB 26

point of the Gallbladder. It is therefore indicated for similar disorders to those associated with GB 24.

GB 24   Riyue
Sun and Moon

日 月

Front-Mu point of the Gallbladder
Intersection of the Spleen, Yang Wei Mai
and Bladder on the Gallbladder channel

Myotome	T5–T12
Dermatome	T7

Location

Below the breast, in the seventh intercostal space, inferior and slightly lateral to LR 14.

To aid location, GB 24 is in the most medial palpable depression of the seventh intercostal space. It is often described as located on the mid-mamillary line. In practice, however, it is apparent that the shape of the costal cartilages varies in a large percentage of the population, placing this point slightly further laterally on most people.

Needling

0.3 to 1 cun oblique or transverse insertion, laterally along the intercostal space.

Deep needling poses considerable risk of puncturing the lung and causing a pneumothorax.

Actions and indications

GB 24, *particularly on the right side*, is an important point for *disorders of the gallbladder*. It regulates Liver and Gallbladder Qi and is very important to *transform dampness* and *clear heat* from these organs. It also effectively *descends rebellious Qi, harmonises the middle jiao* and benefits the hypochondrial region and ribs.

Indications include: nausea, vomiting, epigastric pain, heartburn, gastric ulceration, belching, hiccup, diarrhoea, abdominal rumbling, gastroenteritis, abdominal distension, hypochondrial pain and distension, jaundice, cholecystitis, acute or chronic hepatitis, pain and tightness of the chest, breast pain, mastitis, pain of the ribs, herpes zoster, and intercostal neuralgia.

GB 24 has also been traditionally employed to treat *psychosomatic disorders*, including frequent sighing, depression, propensity to sadness, indecisiveness, and lack of courage.

Spontaneous pain at GB 24 on the right side is a *diagnostic indication of disorders of the gallbladder.*

> **Main Areas**—Hypochondrium. Ribs. Gallbladder. Chest. Epigastrium. Abdomen.
> **Main Functions**—Regulates Gallbladder and Liver Qi. Alleviates pain. Dispels dampness and heat.

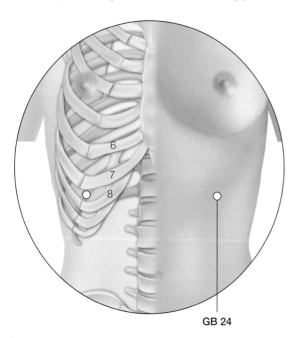

GB 24

GB 25 Jingmen

Capital Gate

京門

Front-Mu point of the Kidneys

Myotome	T5–T12
Dermatome	T8–T10

Location

On the lower back, at the inferior border of the free end of the twelfth rib.

To aid location, it is usually at the most tender site, ascertained by light palpation (it is a very sensitive point).

Alternative location

Locate GB 25 at the tip of the free end of the twelfth rib. This location may be better for manual techniques. Alternatively, palpate the entire area around the tip and under the free end of the rib and treat where it is most reactive during pressure palpation.

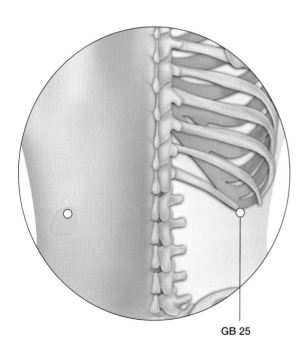

GB 25

Needling

0.3 to 1 cun oblique or transverse insertion, medially along the lower border of the twelfth rib.
0.3 to 0.5 cun perpendicular insertion.

Do not needle too deeply.

Actions and indications

Although GB 25 is not as commonly used as other front-mu points, it can be effective to *tonify the Kidneys* and *strengthen the lumbar area, dispel dampness* from the lower jiao and *open the water passages*, as well as *regulate the intestines*. It also *activates Qi and Blood circulation and alleviates pain.*

Indications include: acute or chronic lumbar pain, renal colic, frequent urination, dysuria, haematuria, cold lower back, hip pain, abdominal rumbling, diarrhoea, vomiting, intercostal neuralgia, and hypochondrial or abdominal distension and pain.

Spontaneous pain at this location on one or both sides may be a *diagnostic indication* of kidney disease.

> **Main Areas**—Kidneys. Lumbar area. Flank.
> **Main Functions**—Benefits the Kidneys. Transforms dampness and heat. Regulates Qi and Blood. Alleviates pain.

GB 26 Daimai

Girdle Vessel

帶脈

Intersection of the Dai Mai on the Gallbladder channel

Myotome	T7–T12
Dermatome	T10

Location

On the lateral aspect of the abdomen, below the free end of the eleventh rib, approximately on the mid-axillary line and level with the umbilicus.

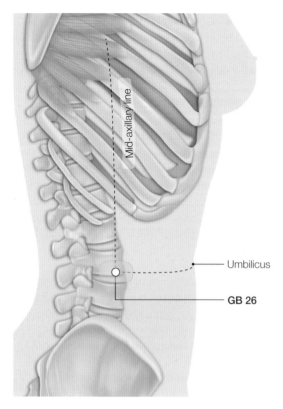

Mid-axillary line

Umbilicus

GB 26

It is a key point to consider when treating lumbar and low thoracic back pain.

> **Main Areas**—Abdomen. Sides. Lumbar area. Uterus. Girdle Vessel.
> **Main Functions**—Clears dampness and heat. Benefits the lower jiao. Regulates menstruation. Aids in weight loss.

GB 27　Wushu
Fifth Pivot

Intersection of the Dai Mai on the Gallbladder channel

Myotome	T7–T12
Dermatome	T11/T12

Needling
0.5 to 1 cun perpendicular insertion.

Do not needle too deeply.

Actions and indications
GB 26 is an important point to *activate Qi and Blood circulation* in the lower jiao and *regulate the Dai Mai*, from which it takes its name.

It is useful to *clear dampness and heat from the abdomen, harmonise the lower jiao* and *regulate menstruation.* .

Indications include: pain, distension, swelling or flaccidity of the abdomen, lumbar and girdle area, lower abdominal pain in women, irregular menstruation, amenorrhoea, chronic leucorrhoea, bloodstained discharge, hernia, diarrhoea, and abdominal rumbling.

Treatment at GB 26 is seemingly useful in *weight loss* programs because it helps *tonify the intestines and strengthen the abdominal wall*, helping to lose inches around the waist.

Location
On the lower abdomen in the depression just medial to the tip of the ASIS.

To aid location, it is approximately level with CV 4 and ST 28, 3 cun below the umbilicus.

Needling
0.5 to 1.5 cun perpendicular insertion.
1 to 2 cun oblique inferior insertion towards GB 28 and Zigong (Ex-CA-1).

Do not needle deeply.

Actions and indications
Both GB 27 and GB 28 help *activate Qi and Blood circulation in the Dai Mai* and *dispel stasis from the lower abdomen*. They can be very effective in the treatment of: pain and distension of the lower abdomen, hardness of the abdomen, acute abdominal pain, peritonitis, chronic appendicitis, testicular or hernia pain, testicular torsion, renal colic pain, hip pain, chronic constipation or diarrhoea, irritable bowel syndrome, irregular menstruation, uterine prolapse, and leucorrhoea.

GB 27 is generally considered more important for men's complaints, whereas GB 28 is more for women's complaints.

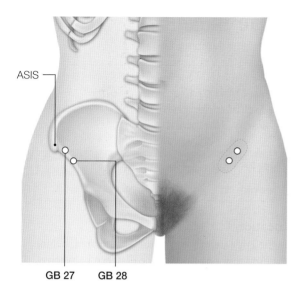

ASIS

GB 27   GB 28

> **Main Areas**—Lower abdomen. Uterus.
> Intestines. Testicles.
> **Main Functions**—Regulates the lower jiao.
> Alleviates pain.

GB 28   Weidao
Binding Channel
(Dai Mai Point)

維道

Intersection of the Dai Mai on the Gallbladder channel

Myotome	T7–T12
Dermatome	T11/T12

Location
On the lower abdomen in the depression just medial to the inferior border of the ASIS, 0.5 cun inferior and slightly medial to GB 27.

Needling
0.5 to 1.5 cun perpendicular insertion.
1 to 2 cun oblique inferior insertion towards GB 28 and Zigong (Ex-CA-1).

Do not needle deeply.

Actions and indications
Both GB 27 and GB 28 help *activate Qi and Blood circulation in the Dai Mai* and *dispel stasis from the lower abdomen.* They can be very effective in the treatment of: pain and distension of the lower abdomen, hardness of the abdomen, acute abdominal pain, peritonitis, chronic appendicitis, testicular or hernia pain, testicular torsion, renal colic pain, hip pain, chronic constipation or diarrhoea, irritable bowel syndrome, irregular menstruation, uterine prolapse, and leucorrhoea.

GB 27 is generally considered more important for men's complaints, whereas GB 28 is more for women's complaints.

> **Main Areas**—Lower abdomen. Uterus.
> Intestines. Testicles.
> **Main Functions**—Regulates the lower jiao.
> Alleviates pain.

GB 29   Juliao
Squatting Bone Hole

Intersection of the Yang Qiao Mai on the Gallbladder channel

Myotome	L4–S1
Dermatome	L1/L2

Location
Superior to the hip joint, at the centre of the large depression formed when the hip joint is flexed. Midway between the ASIS and the protuberance of the greater trochanter.

GB 29 is situated, superficially, in the tensor fasciae latae muscle and, more deeply, in the gluteus medius and minimus muscles. In its deep position lie the rectus femoris attachments.

Needling
1.0 to 3.0 cun perpendicular insertion.

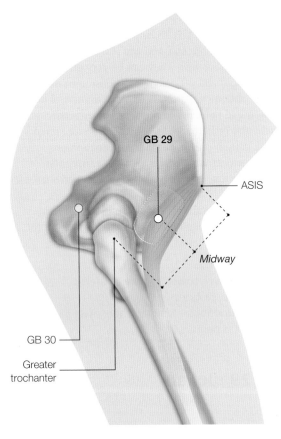

GB 29

ASIS

Midway

GB 30

Greater trochanter

Actions and indications

GB 29 is an extremely powerful and widely used point for many *disorders of the hip joint*. It *dispels wind, cold and dampness, regulates Qi and Blood and dispels stasis*.

It is probably the most important point for *pain at the lateral and anterior aspects of the hip and thigh* and helps restore mobility, even in chronic cases.

Also a point to consider when treating *tension in the ilio-tibial band* such as in *patella tracking* issues and subsequent knee problems.

> **Main Areas**—Hip. Thigh.
> **Main Functions**—Alleviates pain. Dispels stasis. Restores mobility to the hip.

GB 30 Huantiao

Jumping Circle

Intersection of the Bladder on the Gallbladder channel
Heavenly Star point

Myotome	L5–S2
Dermatome	L2 and S3 junction

Location

In the large depression of the gluteal area, behind the hip joint, one third of the distance between the prominence of the greater trochanter and the sacral hiatus. Locate with the thigh flexed. Situated, superficially, in the gluteus maximus muscle, and, more deeply, between the inferior margin of the piriformis and superior margin of the internal obturator. In its deep position lies the gemellus superior muscle.

To aid location, place the palm of the hand on the greater trochanter with the fingers facing the coccyx. The fingertips fall naturally into the wide depression behind the greater trochanter.

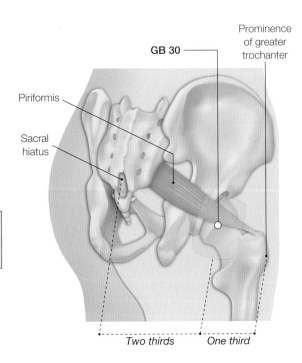

GB 30

Prominence of greater trochanter

Piriformis

Sacral hiatus

Two thirds   One third

Alternative locations
Locate the epicentre of GB 30 and then find four, eight or twelve points around it in a circle. Determine which is most reactive to pressure palpation.

Needling
1 to 4 cun perpendicular or slightly oblique insertion, in a direction down the leg, towards the clients opposite knee, when both knees are flexed. The oblique direction ensures there is less likelihood of catching the sciatic nerve, although anatomically it is unusual to do this.

Actions and indications
GB 30 is a very *dynamic point*, widely used for *many disorders of the hip*, thigh, entire lower limb, and gluteal and lower back areas. It effectively *strengthens the hips, pelvic area* and *lower jiao, tonifies Yang Qi and dissipates cold*. It is particularly indicated for: sciatica, pain of the hips, lower back, knees and legs, stiffness and restricted movement of the lower limbs, atrophy of the surrounding musculature, hemiplegia, and genital or gynaecological pain.

> **Main Areas**—Thigh. Entire lower limb. Lumbar area. Sciatic nerve.
> **Main Functions**—Dispels wind, cold and dampness. Regulates Qi and Blood. Alleviates pain. Strengthens the lower back.

GB 31   Fengshi
Wind Market

Myotome	L2–L4
Dermatome	L2

Location
On the midline of the lateral aspect of the thigh, 7 cun proximal to the popliteal crease, at the posterior border of the ITB. Situated in the vastus lateralis muscle.

To aid location, ask the patient to stand with the arms hanging relaxed by the sides. Find GB 31 at

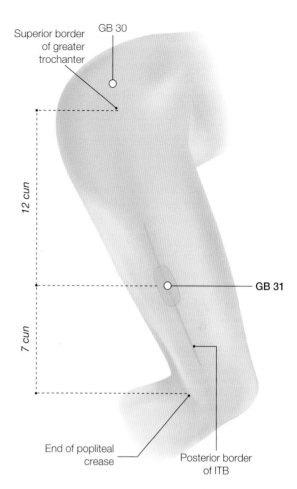

the point where the tip of the middle finger touches the thigh.

Needling
0.5 to 1.5 cun perpendicular insertion.
1 to 2 cun transverse insertion distally or proximally.

Actions and indications
GB 31 is a useful point in cases of *weakness, pain, sciatica, atrophy* and *paralysis of the lower limbs*. It has also been employed to *expel wind* causing swelling or itching of the skin on the legs or the whole body.

It is a good point to include in patella tracking and knee injuries where the ITB is tight.

> **Main Areas**—Thigh. Entire lower limb.
> **Main Functions**—Dispels wind and dampness. Regulates Qi. Alleviates pain.

GB 32 Zhongdu
Ditch Centre

Myotome	L2–L4
Dermatome	L2

Location
5 cun proximal to the popliteal crease, in the depression between the tendon of the biceps femoris muscle and the posterior border of the ITB, posterior to the shaft of the femur. It may pick up the lower border of vastus lateralis.

Note: Select GB 33 instead of GB 32 if it is more tender on pressure palpation.

Needling
0.5 to 1 cun perpendicular insertion.

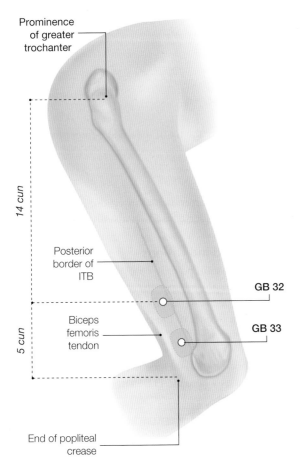

Prominence of greater trochanter

14 cun

5 cun

Posterior border of ITB

Biceps femoris tendon

GB 32

GB 33

End of popliteal crease

Actions and indications
In common with GB 31 and GB 33, GB 32 is used to *dispel wind, dampness and cold and stimulate the circulation of Qi and Blood in the channel.* Its primary function is to *alleviate regional pain.*

> **Main Area**—Lateral thigh.
> **Main Functions**—Dissipates wind and cold.
> Dispels stasis of Qi and Blood. Alleviates pain.

GB 33 Xiyangguan
Knee Yang Gate

Myotome	None – superficial tissue
Dermatome	L2

Location
At the centre of the large depression formed between the tendon of the biceps femoris muscle and the posterior border of the ITB, directly superior to the lateral condyle of the femur. Locate and treat with the knee flexed at an angle of 90 degrees.

To aid location, GB 33 is directly lateral to ST 35 when the knee is flexed, and approximately 3 cun proximal to GB 34.

Needling
0.5 to 1 cun perpendicular insertion, directed slightly posteriorly.

Actions and indications
Similarly to the previous two points, GB 33 also *dissipates wind, dampness and cold, regulates Qi* and *Blood in the channel and alleviates pain.*

It is an important *local point* for disorders of the lateral aspect of the knee and is particularly indicated for tightness and shortening of the soft tissues in this area.

> **Main Areas**—Knee. Lateral thigh.
> **Main Functions**—Dissipates wind and cold.
> Dispels stasis of Qi and Blood. Alleviates pain.

GB 34 Yanglingquan 陽陵泉
Yang Mound Spring

He-Sea point, Earth point
Influential point of the Sinews
Heavenly Star point

Myotome	L4–S1
Dermatome	L5

Location
In the palpable depression anterior and inferior to the head of the fibula. Approximately 1 cun lateral and superior to ST 36. Situated at the anterior border of the fibularis longus, in the extensor digitorum longus muscle. Locate with the knee flexed.

To aid location, place your fingertip on the prominence of the head of the fibula and slide the fingertip anteriorly and inferiorly until it slips into the depression.

Needling
0.5 to 1.5 cun perpendicular insertion.

Actions and indications
GB 34 is one of the top most commonly used points with a wide range of applications. It is one of the most significant points to *regulate Qi throughout the entire body, relieve stagnation* and *smooth the Gallbladder and Liver*, thus alleviating pain of both exterior and interior origin. GB 34 is also important to *clear dampness and heat from the Liver and Gallbladder.*

Common indications include hypochondrial distension and pain, jaundice, cholecystitis, cholelithiasis, bitter taste, chills and fever due to ShaoYang disharmony, hypertension, headaches, nausea, vomiting, abdominal distension and pain, diarrhoea, constipation, intercostal neuralgia, breast pain or swelling, dysmenorrhoea, premenstrual syndrome, irritability, and depression.

GB 34 is also an extremely important point for disorders of the *joints and sinews* and has a special effect on the *sides of the body, rib cage* and *breasts*. It is very important in the treatment of *musculo-skeletal disorders* affecting any part of the body, including: tendinitis, arthritis, cramps, spasm, tic, and stiffness, contraction, shortening and weakness or atrophy of the soft tissues. It is widely used to treat disorders of the neck, shoulder, arm, knee or hip, lumbar or thoracic pain, and sciatica, atrophy, paralysis or hemiplegia.

GB 34 is also useful as a general treatment to *strengthen and relax the musculo-skeletal system* in athletes and other professionals who place great demands on the body.

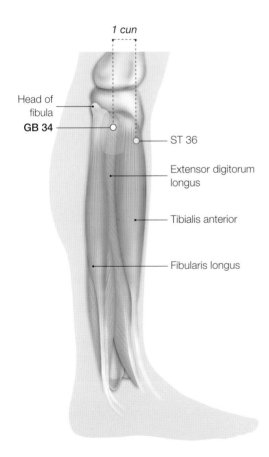

1 cun

Head of fibula

GB 34

ST 36

Extensor digitorum longus

Tibialis anterior

Fibularis longus

> **Main Areas**—Sinews (muscles, tendons, ligaments and other soft tissues). Joints. Flank. Hypochondrium. Gallbladder. Chest. Entire body.
> **Main Functions**—Regulates Qi. Smoothes the Gallbladder and Liver. Dissipates stagnation. Alleviates pain. Benefits the sinews.

GB 35 Yangjiao
Yang Intersection

陽交

Xi-Cleft point of the Yang Wei Mai

Myotome	L4/L5, S1
Dermatome	L5/S1

Location
In the depression at the posterior border of the fibula, 7 cun proximal to the prominence of the lateral malleolus, level with GB 36, ST 39 and BL 58.

Needling
0.5 to 1.5 cun perpendicular insertion.

Actions and indications
GB 35 is not very commonly used for interior disorders, because GB 34 and other points are considered more effective. It is, however, useful to treat pain at the lateral aspect of the lower leg, ankle and knee.

Nevertheless, it has been traditionally employed to treat *disorders of the Gallbladder and Yang Wei Mai*. Symptoms include: chills and fever, dyspnoea, sore throat, swelling of the face, palpitations, fright, anxiety, depression, and irritability.

> **Main Areas**—Leg. Yang Wei Mai.
> **Main Functions**—Regulates Qi. Dissipates stagnation. Alleviates pain. Benefits the Yang Wei Mai.

GB 36 Waiqiu
Outer Hill

外丘

Xi-Cleft point

Myotome	L4/L5, S1
Dermatome	L5/S1

Location
On the anterior border of the fibula, 7 cun proximal to the prominence of the lateral malleolus, anterior to GB 35.

To aid location, it is level with BL 58 and ST 39.

Needling
0.5 to 1.5 cun perpendicular insertion.

Actions and indications
GB 36 is not as commonly used as other points for interior disorders. It can, however, be useful in the treatment of pain or swelling at the lateral aspect of the leg or ankle.

Nevertheless, it has been traditionally used for *clearing heat and expelling poisons*. Indications include: irritability, depression, fullness of the chest and abdomen, and febrile diseases.

As a xi-cleft point it can indicate *acute conditions* within the gallbladder.

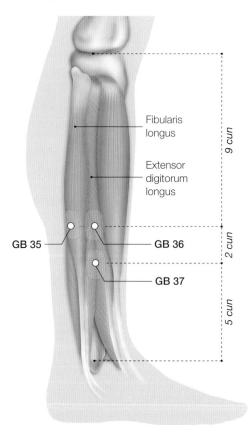

Main Areas—Leg. Gallbladder.
Main Functions—Alleviates pain. Clears the Gallbladder.

GB 37　Guangming　光明
Bright Light

Luo-Connecting point

Myotome	L4/L5, S1
Dermatome	S1

Location
At the anterior border of the fibula, 5 cun proximal to the prominence of the lateral malleolus, in the depression between the fibularis longus and brevis and the extensor digitorum longus muscles.

Needling
0.5 to 1.5 cun perpendicular insertion.

Actions and indications
GB 37 is an important point for treating *disorders of the eyes*. Indications include: pain, itching, inflammation, swelling and redness of the eyes, excessive lacrimation, migraine with aura, and glaucoma, keratitis, night blindness and failing vision.

It can also be effectively employed as a *local point* in the treatment of pain, stiffness or atrophy of the leg, in common with GB 34, GB 35 and GB 36.

Additionally, it has been traditionally used to treat *interior Gallbladder* and *Liver disorders*. Indications include: distension, fullness or pain of the hypochondrial area and chest, pain or swelling of the breast, and headache, grinding of the teeth, depression and irritability.

Main Area—Eyes.
Main Functions—Benefits eyesight and brightens the eyes. Regulates the Gallbladder.

GB 38　Yangfu　陽輔
Yang Assistance

Jing-River point, Fire point

Myotome	L4/L5, S1
Dermatome	S1

Location
In the depression 1 cun below GB 37, 4 cun proximal to the prominence of the lateral malleolus, on the anterior border of the fibula.

To aid location, it is one quarter of the distance between the lateral malleolus and the popliteal crease.

Needling
0.5 to 1.5 cun perpendicular insertion.

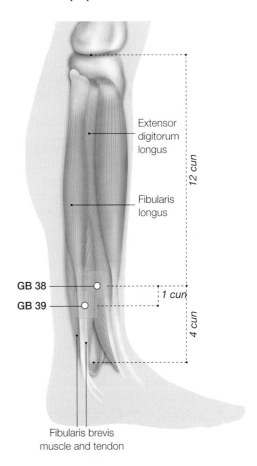

Extensor digitorum longus

Fibularis longus

12 cun

GB 38

GB 39

1 cun

4 cun

Fibularis brevis muscle and tendon

Actions and indications

GB 38 has been traditionally employed to *clear heat from the Gallbladder*, but in practice it is rarely used for this purpose. It can, however, be effective to treat pain of the lateral aspect of the leg. As a jing-river point it can indicate tightness in the entire lateral anatomy, including ipsilateral hip/trunk and shoulder.

> **Main Area**—Gallbladder fu and channel.
> **Main Functions**—Clears heat. Regulates Qi.

GB 39   Xuanzhong

Suspended Bell

Influential point for the Marrow

Myotome	L4/L5, S1
Dermatome	S1

Location

In the small depression 3 cun proximal to the prominence of the lateral malleolus, between the tendons of the fibularis longus and brevis muscles.

Alternative locations

GB 39 can also be located between the posterior border of the fibula and the tendon of the fibularis brevis muscle. In cases of extreme tightness of the fibularis muscles, or difficulty in inducing deqi at the above locations, treat it on the anterior border of the fibula, directly inferior to GB 38.

To aid location, it is one hand-width proximal to the prominence of the lateral malleolus.

Needling

0.5 to 1.5 cun perpendicular insertion.

Actions and indications

GB 39 is an important point to *benefit the sinews and bones and to strengthen the skeletal system*. Its primary functions are to *dispel wind and dampness* from the channel and *clear heat from*

the bones and Marrow. Marrow is akin to the nervous system in Western medicine. It is widely used to treat *disorders of the neurological system,* particularly weakness and chronic conditions, especially in the elderly (MS, Guillain-Barré syndrome, MND etc.).

It is indicated for disorders of the joints, spine and neck, although classical texts emphasise the latter. These include: osteoporosis, arthritis, spinal diseases, ankylosis, pain and stiffness of the joints, bone pain, heat in the bones, difficulty walking, sciatica, atrophy or paralysis of the lower limbs, and hemiplegia.

Additionally, GB 39 can treat other disorders of the Sea of Marrow (brain), such as chronic tiredness, dizziness, reduced concentration, diminishing mental faculties in the elderly, headache, chronic inflammatory diseases, and fever.

GB 39 clears *heat from the Gallbladder* and can be used to treat various manifestations of Gallbladder disharmony, including hypochondrial pain and distension, fullness of the chest, coughing, swelling of the axilla, anxiety, and irritability.

> **Main Areas**—Neck. Spine. Joints. Bones. Marrow. Sinews.
> **Main Functions**—Benefits the Marrow, Sinews and bones. Clears heat. Regulates the Gallbladder channel.

GB 40   Qiuxu

Between the Mounds

Yuan-Source point

Myotome	L5/S1
Dermatome	S1

Location

Aat the centre of the sizeable depression anterior and inferior to the lateral malleolus, lateral to the

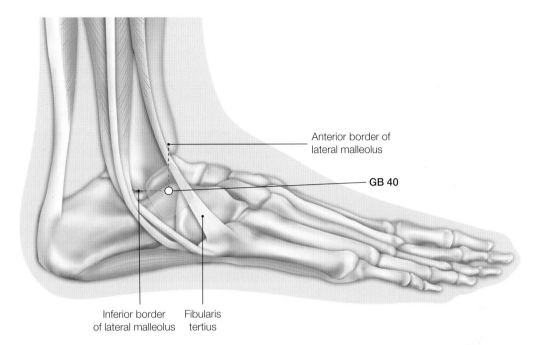

Anterior border of
lateral malleolus

GB 40

Inferior border
of lateral malleolus

Fibularis
tertius

tendon of the fibularis tertius muscle and distal to the inferior fibular retinaculum. Situated in the extensor digitorum brevis muscle.

To aid location, it is at the intersection of two lines following the anterior and the inferior border of the lateral malleolus.

Needling
0.5 to 1.5 cun perpendicular insertion.

Actions and indications
GB 40 is an important point to treat both *deficiency and excess disorders*. Its main functions are to *clear dampness and heat from the Gallbladder, promote Qi and Blood circulation and alleviate pain*.

Indications include: hypochondrial distension and pain, heartburn, nausea, vomiting, swelling of the axilla, frequent sighing, headache, neck pain, sciatica, and paralysis of the lower limb.

GB 40 is an important point for psychological disorders and is beneficial in cases of depression, mental irritability and inability to make decisions or act with courage.

As a local point, GB 40 can be useful in the treatment of injury and other disorders of the ankle and foot. Symptoms include: pain, swelling, stiffness, and cramping. It is one of the 'eyes' of the ankle, along with SP 5.

> **Main Areas**—Ankle. Foot. Gallbladder. Mind. Emotions.
> **Main Functions**—Regulates Qi. Clears dampness and heat.

GB 41 Zulinqi
Foot Governor of Tears

足臨泣

Shu-Stream point, Wood point
Opening point of the Dai Mai

Myotome	S1–S3
Dermatome	S1

Location
In the depression distal to the junction of the fourth and fifth metatarsal bones, between the tendons of the extensor digitorum longus of the little toe and the fibularis tertius.

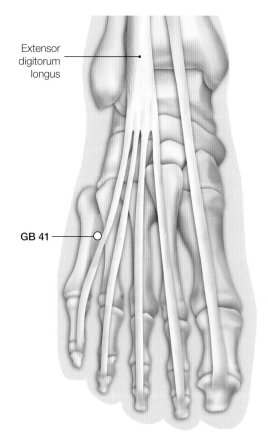

Extensor
digitorum
longus

GB 41

To aid location, lift the patient's little toe to define the tendon. Also, GB 41 may be located one hand-width distal to GB 40.

Alternatively, identify the tendon and then slide your nail back from the little toe, under the tendon and an obvious dip can be felt approximately half way up, inferiorly to the tendon.

Needling
0.3 to 0.5 cun perpendicular insertion.

Actions and indications
GB 41 is an important point with a wide range of indications. Its main function is to *regulate Liver Qi* and it is very important for *disorders of the Gallbladder channel, especially tightness, stiffness and pain*. It is possibly the most effective distal point to *release tension along the entire course of the Gallbladder channel*.

GB 41 is an absolute key point for migraine with eye involvement.

GB 41 is also effective to *clear dampness and heat and regulate the lower jiao. It transforms phlegm, opens and relaxes the chest and benefits the flanks and breasts*. It is also important to *clear the head and eyes, and balance the emotions.*

Indications include: abdominal distension and pain, stiffness and pain of the hip, lower backache, dysmenorrhoea, leucorrhoea, hypochondrial distension and pain, pain and swelling of the breasts or axilla, tightness of the chest, headache, migraine, dizziness, and disorders of the eyes and ears.

As the Opening point for the Dai Mai it can have a strong effect on back pain.

GB 41 has been employed to regulate menstruation and is beneficial during pregnancy for pain of the lower back or hips. As a *local point*, it is useful for disorders of the foot and toes.

Interesting is its segmental supply of S1/2 and the encouragement to use this in pregnancy, as opposed to SP 6, which has the same segmental supply but is contraindicated in pregnancy. Segmentally, there is no reason, but in terms of Chinese function of the two organs, they are radically different. The Spleen will 'relax', and possible miscarriage can result, whereas the Gallbladder is about 'tension' and so maintaining a pregnancy. A conundrum for the Western world!

> **Main Areas**—Gallbladder channel. Foot. Breast. Flanks. Abdomen. Dai Mai. Gallbladder. Head. Eyes. Mind.
> **Main Functions**—Regulates Qi. Clears dampness and heat. Regulates the Dai Mai.

GB 42 Diwuhui
Earth Fivefold
Convergence

Myotome	S1–S3
Dermatome	S1

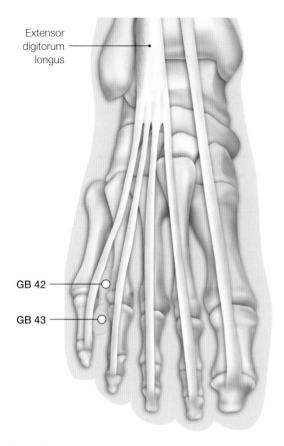

Extensor digitorum longus

GB 42

GB 43

Location

In the depression proximal to the heads of the fourth and fifth metatarsal bones, medial to the tendon of the extensor digitorum longus of the little toe.

Needling

0.3 to 0.4 cun perpendicular insertion.

Actions and indications

GB 42 can be used in cases of regional disorders of the foot, including pain, swelling and tendinitis. In clinical practice, however, this point is very seldom used for interior complaints.

> **Main Area**—Foot.
> **Main Functions**—Alleviates regional pain.

GB 43 Xiaxi

Narrow Stream

俠谿

Ying-Spring point, Water point

Myotome	None – superficial tissue
Dermatome	S1

Location

Situated on the dorsum of the foot, between the fourth and fifth toes, proximal to the margin of the web, level with the fourth MTP joint. Furthermore, GB 43 is also one of the Bafeng points.

Needling

0.3 to 0.5 cun oblique insertion between the fourth and fifth MTP joints.

Actions and indications

GB 43 is a useful point to *clear interior heat and descend rising Yang from the head, ears and eyes*. Indications include: fever, dizziness, hypertension, painful and swollen eyes, headache, migraine, and tinnitus.

As a *local point*, it can be employed in the treatment of pain, swelling and inflammation of the dorsum of the foot and the fourth and fifth toes.

According to the *Five Element* model, GB 43 is a *tonification point and can be used to strengthen the Gallbladder and Liver*.

> **Main Areas**—Gallbladder. Head. Eyes. Mind.
> **Main Functions**—Clears heat. Descends Yang. Clears the head, ears and eyes.

GB 44   Zuqiaoyin
Foot Yin Openings

Jing-Well point, Metal point

Myotome	None – superficial tissue
Dermatome	S1

Location
On the lateral side of the fourth toe, about 0.1 cun proximal to the corner of the nail.

To aid location, it is at the intersection of two lines following the lateral border and the base of the nail.

Needling
0.1 cun perpendicular insertion.

Actions and indications
In common with the other jing-well points, GB 44 *restores consciousness, drains heat and clears the head and brain.*

Additionally, GB 44 *benefits the eyes, the chest and the sides* of the body.

> **Main Areas**—Gallbladder channel. Head. Eyes. Mind.
> **Main Functions**—Restores consciousness. Clears the head and brain. Benefits the eyes.

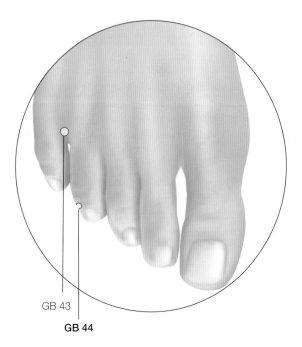

GB 43

GB 44

Points of the Foot Jue Yin Liver Channel

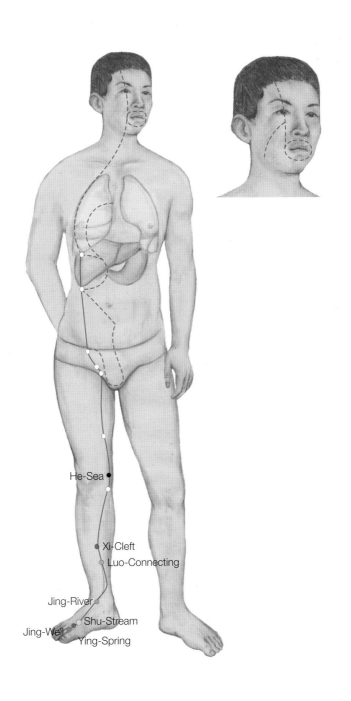

足厥陰肝經穴

He-Sea

Xi-Cleft
Luo-Connecting

Jing-River
Shu-Stream
Jing-Well
Ying-Spring

General	The Liver channel completes the cycle of the twelve main channels, finishing under the ribs, where the Lung channel – the first in the series – would then start as Qi flows round the circuit once more in the traditional Chinese medical model.
	LR 1 is at the lateral edge of the nail of the hallux, and the channel moves up through the first lumbrical of the foot and crosses the ankle on the anteromedial side. Its path takes it up to the medial side of the knee and then on upwards into the groin, crossing the hip joint anteriorly, closely connected to the Spleen channel. From here, one internal pathway surrounds the genitals and connects with the Conception Vessel in the lower pelvis. The channel then continues up to the lateral ribs, and the main channel finishes at LR 14 in the sixth intercostal space, in line with the nipple, 4 cun from the midline.
	The channel has 14 points. It is grouped with the Gallbladder under the Wood element in five-element theory.
More specifically	The jing-well point for the Liver starts at the lateral edge of the nail of the hallux, and as it crosses the first interosseous of the foot, it is here that we find LR 3, one of the most used acupuncture points. LR 4 is just medial to the tendon of the tibialis anterior as it crosses the ankle, and the channel continues upwards, sending a branch to SP 6. LR 8 at the knee is sited immediately over the middle of the medial collateral ligament of the knee, and LR 9 sits in a groove between the sartorius and the vastus medialis in the mid-thigh.
	As the channel crosses the front of the hip, it is closely associated with the Spleen channel, crossing it and the Stomach channel, which lies slightly lateral to it. Internal branches here surround the genitals, and this channel is often used for urogenital conditions. There is also a branch to the Conception Vessel and upwards towards the Gallbladder, through the diaphragm, with the channel diverging outwards and affecting the lateral costal margins and hypochondrium.
	A further internal branch continues upwards through the Lung, affecting the throat and also the eye, giving this channel one of its prime usages for migraine headaches with visual disturbance and emotional disturbances affecting the throat and head. This branch joins GV 20.
Area covered	Foot. Ankle. Medial knee/adductors/groin. Anterior hip. Lateral costal margins. Throat and head.
Areas affected with treatment	Emotions – especially those associated with anger and a build-up of frustration. Stress. Any propensity to physical violence. Head/migraine, throat constrictions, lateral lower ribs. Anterior hip, medial thigh/adductors. Medial knee, ankle and foot.
Key points	LR 3, LR 4, LR 8, LR 13.

LR 1   Dadun
Big Mound

Jing-Well point, Wood point

Myotome	None – superficial tissue
Dermatome	L5

Location
On the dorsum of the big toe, midway along the line connecting the lateral corner of the base of the nail and the centre of the IP crease.

LR 1 seems to cover a slightly larger area than the other jing-well points (with the exception of KI 1).

Alternative location
In common with the other jing-well points, LR 1 can be located 0.1 cun proximal to the lateral corner of the base of the nail.

Needling
Up to 0.3 cun perpendicularly.

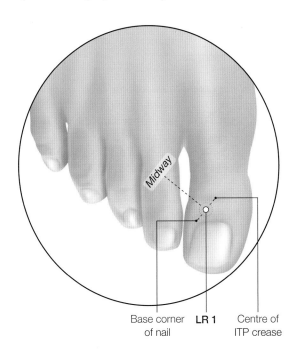

Base corner of nail   **LR 1**   Centre of ITP crease

Actions and indications
LR 1 is an important point used to *subdue interior wind*, *restore consciousness* and *calm the mind*.

Other traditional functions include regulating Liver Qi and harmonising the lower jiao and urogenital system.

In common with SP 1, LR 1 also helps dramatically *arrest bleeding*.

> **Main Areas**—Head. Nervous system. Uterus.
> **Main Functions**—Subdues interior wind. Calms the mind. Arrests bleeding.

LR 2   Xingjian
Passing Between

行間

Ying-Spring point, Fire point

Myotome	None – superficial tissue
Dermatome	L5

Location
On the dorsal aspect of the foot, on the web between the first and second toes, distal to the MTP joint.

To aid location, LR 2 is approximately 0.5 cun proximal to the margin of the web. Also, when the toes are closed together, LR 2 is situated at the end of the crease formed between the two toes.

Furthermore, LR 2 is also one of the Bafeng points (Ex-LE-10).

Needling
0.3 to 1 cun oblique insertion, directed towards the heel, between the first and second metatarsal bones. 0.3 to 0.5 cun perpendicular insertion.

Actions and indications
LR 2 is a powerful point to *soothe the Liver* and is primarily employed to *clear heat and drain fire*. It effectively *cools Blood, descends rising Yang* and *subdues interior wind*.

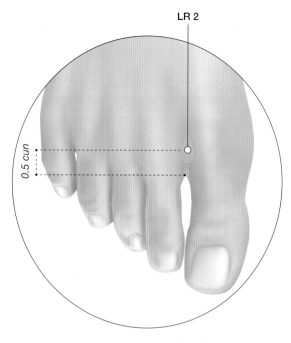

LR 2

0.5 cun

LR 3   Taichong

Great Surge

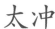

Yuan-Source point, Shu-Stream point
Earth point, Heavenly Star point

Myotome	L5/S1
Dermatome	L5

Location
In the depression distal to the junction of the first and second metatarsal bones. Situated in the dorsal interosseous muscle, lateral to the tendon of the extensor hallucis brevis.

To aid location, it is level with SP 3. Palpate for the tenderest spot.

Needling
0.3 to 1 cun perpendicular insertion. The needle should be angled in a slightly proximal-lateral direction, or 1.5 cun to join with KI 1.

Actions and indications
LR 3 is one of the top most commonly used points with a wide range of applications in both excess and deficiency disorders.

It is a *primary point to smooth the Liver, dispel stasis and improve circulation of Qi and Blood* throughout the three jiao. At the same time, LR 3 is extremely important to *nourish Yin and Blood and cool the Liver.* It effectively *clears interior heat, sedates excessive Yang and subdues interior wind.*

LR 3 has extremely *powerful Qi-moving qualities* and, alongside LI 4, is possibly the most *important point* to alleviate pain of any cause or location. LR 3 and LI 4 are known as the Four Gates, and combined are extensively used for pain relief and anaesthesia (see also LI 4).

Thus, LR 3 has a powerful *calming and soothing effect on the mind* and is important to *release blocked emotional states* causing mental restlessness, psychological instability, mood swings, depression, fear or irritability. It has

Clinical manifestations include: migraine, headache (notably with a sensation of heat in the head) painful and inflamed eyes, red eye, dizziness, hypertension, transient ischaemic attack, numbness of the face and limbs, convulsions, epilepsy, facial paralysis, fever, sore throat, soreness of the genital region, dysmenorrhoea, irregular menstruation, excessive or incessant menstruation, abnormal uterine bleeding, mental agitation, insomnia, and irritability.

LR 2 is also indicated for urinary disorders, including, dysuria, hot or turbid urine, urethritis, cystitis, urinary retention, and incontinence.

Other traditional indications include: hypochondrial pain caused by liver disease, soft stool diarrhoea, abdominal distension and pain, indigestion, hernia, retching, lower back pain and disorders of the chest area including palpitations, cardiac pain, spitting blood and shortness of breath.

Additionally, LR 2 is effective as a local point for disorders of the first and second MTP joints and is particularly indicated for inflammation and swelling.

Main Areas—Head. Eyes. Nervous system. Abdomen.
Main Functions—Clears heat and drains fire. Descends excessive Yang. Regulates Liver Qi.

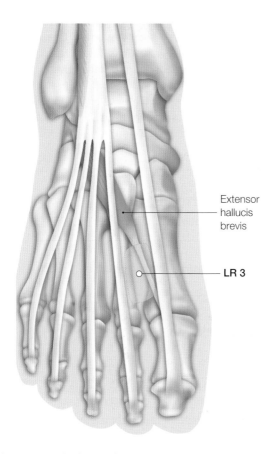

Extensor hallucis brevis

LR 3

In relation to the *cardiovascular system*, LR 3 has been used to treat a variety of conditions, including: hypertension, coronary heart disease, angina pectoris, tightness, heaviness or pain of the chest, palpitations, swelling of the legs, circulation and vascular disorders, varicose veins, cold feet, bleeding disorders, and anaemia.

LR 3 has also been successfully employed in the treatment of disorders of the *respiratory system* and throat. Indications include: cough, asthma, dyspnoea, tightness and constriction of the chest and throat, inflammation of the throat, pharyngitis, laryngitis, goitre, hyperthyroidism, and swelling of the glands.

In relation to the *liver, gallbladder and digestive system*, LR 3 has been extensively used to treat a variety of cases, including: liver and gallbladder disease, hepatitis, jaundice, gallstones, pancreatitis, hypochondrial distension and pain, epigastric pain, heartburn, indigestion, gastritis, oesophagitis, gastric ulceration, nausea, vomiting, abdominal distension and pain, abdominal rumbling, irritable bowel syndrome, diarrhoea, dysentery, blood in the stools, and constipation.

been extensively employed to treat a variety of *psychosomatic symptoms*, including: insomnia, dream-disturbed sleep, frequent sighing, constriction of the chest, plum stone throat as seen in depression, addiction disorders, and pain or other symptoms with no apparent medical cause.

LR 3 also has a particularly powerful effect on the *head, eyes and nervous system* because it *clears heat and descends excess Yang at the same time as nourishing and cooling the Liver Yin and Blood.*

Indications include: headache, migraine, dizziness, pain and inflammation of the eyes, dry or tired eyes, blurred or failing vision, glaucoma, Ménière's disease, and tinnitus.

In addition, LR 3 is commonly used to treat a variety of *neurological disorders*, including: symptoms following cerebrovascular accident, paralysis, atrophy, spasticity, neuritis, disorders of the cranial nerves, facial paralysis, transient ischaemic attack, tremor, tic, spasm, epilepsy, convulsions, dizziness, and vertigo.

LR 3 is very extensively used to help *regulate menstruation* and is extremely important in the treatment of many gynaecological disorders, including: dysmenorrhoea, premenstrual syndrome, breast swelling and pain, irregular or delayed menstruation, amenorrhoea, abnormal uterine bleeding, excessive or incessant menstruation, infertility, and leucorrhoea.

Treatment applied to LR 3 before and during labour helps the cervix dilate (combine with LR 5 and SP 6 for this purpose), but also offers pain relief and relaxation for the mind and body during labour (combine with LI 4 and Ear Shenmen for the latter functions). LR 3 has also been traditionally used to treat mastitis, insufficient lactation and uterine prolapse and to arrest severe sweating after childbirth.

It is also a significant point to *clear damp heat, harmonise the lower jiao and benefit the urogenital system.* Indications include: dysuria, cystitis, urethritis, urinary incontinence or retention, itching, inflammation or pain of the external genitals, impotence, and testicular pain, swelling or retraction.

LR 3 is important in the treatment of *musculo-skeletal disorders,* including: cramping, spasm tightness or contraction of the muscles, tics and tremors (contained pathogenic wind), tendinitis, pain, atrophy or weakness of the lower limbs, arthritis, and lumbar pain.

Also, because LR 3 increases Qi and Blood circulation, it can be used to help support the musculo-skeletal system in persons who physically overexert themselves, including athletes and labourers. Treatment can help relax tight sinews and muscles throughout the entire body and is also of benefit during intensive sports and/or flexibility training. For the latter purpose, combine LR 3 with GB 34, ST 36 and LI 4.

LR 3 has been employed to treat a variety of other symptoms and disorders, including: swelling and pain of the axilla, inflammation of the sweat glands, excessive sweating, cold feet, and umbilical pain.

As a local point, it effectively treats pain and swelling of the dorsum of the foot.

> **Main Areas**—Entire body. Abdomen. Digestive system. Reproductive systems. Chest. Head. Eyes. Nervous system. Muscles and sinews. Mind. Foot.
> **Main Functions**—Regulates Liver Qi. Dispels stasis. Alleviates pain. Nourishes Yin and Blood. Cools the Liver. Regulates menstruation. Calms the mind.

LR 4   Zhongfeng   中封
Between the Mounds

Jing-River point, Metal point

Myotome	None – superficial tissue
Dermatome	L5

Location
In the depression anterior to the prominence of the medial malleolus, medial to the tibialis anterior tendon when the foot is at right angles to the tibia. It is situated anterior to the great saphenous vein and posterior to the tendon of the tibialis anterior. In its deep position and laterally, lies the extensor hallucis longus muscle.

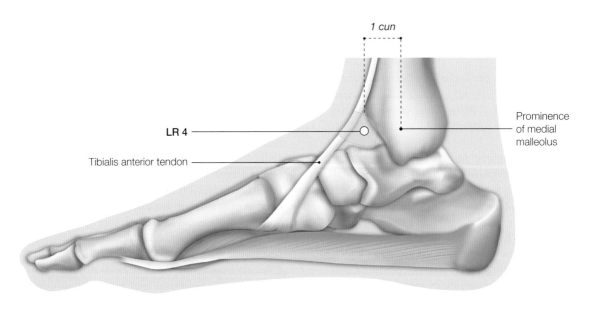

1 cun

LR 4

Tibialis anterior tendon

Prominence of medial malleolus

Needling

0.3 to 1 cun perpendicular insertion under the tibialis anterior tendon, towards ST 41.
0.5 to 1 cun oblique distal insertion in a slightly lateral direction under the tendon.

Note: Palpate the great saphenous vein and, if necessary, move it slightly posteriorly with the fingertip, so as to insert the needle anterior to it. This is an uncommon anatomical feature.

Actions and indications

LR 4 is not as commonly used as other Liver points for its interior functions that include *regulating Liver Qi* and *harmonising the lower jiao*. It does, however, effectively treat pain, swelling and stiffness of the ankle and medial aspect of the foot. It has a strong role to play in the musculo-skeletal treatment of this channel, as being a jing-river point it can aid in diagnostically determining the tension within the channel and line of fascia.

Other indications include gynaecological complaints, dysmenorrhoea, abdominal pain, genital pain, hernia, retraction of the testicles, dysuria, retention of urine, jaundice, and hepatitis.

> **Main Areas**—Ankle. Abdomen.
> **Main Functions**—Regulates Liver Qi. Harmonises the lower jiao. Alleviates swelling and pain.

LR 5   Ligou
Woodworm Channel

蠡溝

Luo-Connecting point

Myotome	S1/S2
Dermatome	L4

Location

5 cun above the medial malleolus, in a small depression just at the medial tibial border.

To aid location, LR 5 is one third of the distance between the prominence of the medial malleolus

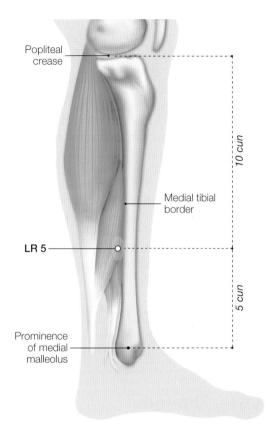

Popliteal crease

10 cun

Medial tibial border

LR 5

5 cun

Prominence of medial malleolus

and the popliteal (knee) crease. Also, a visible depression normally appears at LR 5 when the foot is dorsiflexed.

If gentle palpation is applied with the fingertip to the medial tibial border, the small hole, comparable to a 'channel' made by a woodworm, will be perceived.

Needling

0.5 to 1 cun perpendicular insertion.
0.5 to 1.5 cun oblique proximal insertion, following the posterior border of the tibia.

Actions and indications

LR 5 is an important point to *regulate Liver Qi* and clear dampness and heat. It is particularly indicated for *lower jiao disorders* affecting the *gynaecological and urogenital systems*.

Indications include: pain, itching and inflammation of the external genitals or urethra, lower abdominal pain, dysuria, leucorrhoea, irregular menstruation, dysmenorrhoea, insufficient dilation of the cervix during labour, prolapse of the uterus, inguinal or scrotal hernia, testicular pain, testicular retraction, prostatitis, excessive libido, priapism, and impotence.

It also effectively treats other symptoms of *Liver Qi stagnation* such as hypochondrial pain, tightness of the chest, plum stone throat, poor vision, mood swings and irritability.

LR 5 has a significant effect on the person's psycho-emotional state and can help release stuck emotions, particularly anger, depression and sadness.

LR 5 is also effective as a local point and can be used to treat pain, swelling or restricted mobility of the leg.

> **Main Areas**—Genitourinary system. Mind. Liver.
> **Main Functions**—Regulates Liver Qi. Benefits the genitals and uterus. Clears damp heat.

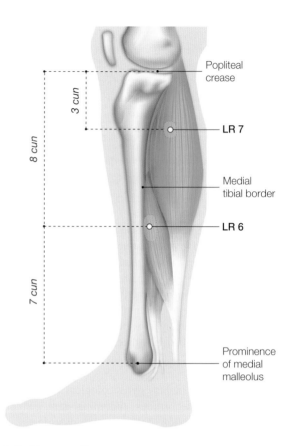

LR 6   Zhongdu
Central Confluence
中都

Xi-Cleft point

Myotome	S1/S2
Dermatome	L4

Location
7 cun above the medial malleolus, just posterior to the medial tibial border within soleus.

Actions and indications
LR 6 treats *acute pain* of the channel pathway as well as interior *Blood stasis* and heat, although it is not as commonly used as other Liver points. Indications include: abdominal pain, excessive menstruation, dysmenorrhoea, and pain or swelling of the leg.

> **Main Areas**—Leg. Liver.
> **Main Functions**—Dispels Blood stasis. Alleviates pain.

LR 7   Xiguan
Knee Joint
膝關

Myotome	S1/2
Dermatome	L4

Location
Situated on the medial aspect of the calf, in the upper portion of the medial head of the gastrocnemius muscle, 1 cun posterior to SP 9, level with the lower border of the medial tibial condyle.

Needling
0.5 to 1 cun perpendicular insertion.

Actions and indications
LR 7 is primarily used as a *local point* to dispel wind and dampness, reduce swelling and relax the sinews. It helps treat pain, swelling, and restricted mobility of the knee.

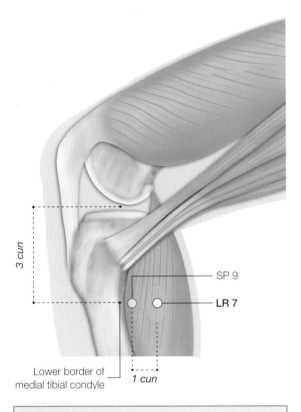

3 cun

SP 9

LR 7

Lower border of
medial tibial condyle

1 cun

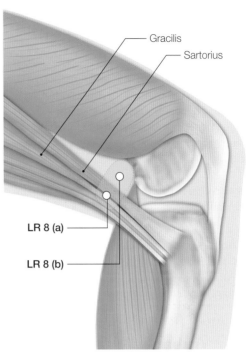

Gracilis

Sartorius

LR 8 (a)

LR 8 (b)

> **Main Area**—Knees.
> **Main Functions**—Dispels dampness. Alleviates swelling and pain.

LR 8   Ququan
Spring at the Bend   曲泉

He-Sea point, Water point

Myotome	L3/L4 in terms of between sartorius and gracilis
Dermatome	L3/L4

Location
At the medial aspect of the knee, in a small depression between the tendon of the gracilis and the posterior border of the sartorius muscle on, or slightly proximal to, the medial end of the popliteal (knee) crease illustrated as LR 8 (a). Locate with the knee flexed.

To aid location, grasp the flesh at the medial aspect of the knee, with the index finger placed on KI 10. The thumb will fall on LR 8.

Alternative locations
In cases where there is a lot of subcutaneous fat or the underlying muscles are either very flaccid or too tight, the small depression at the LR 8 (a) main location is not easily palpable. In these cases locate it further anteriorly, at the centre of the prominent depression formed between the sartorius muscle and the medial femoral condyle. See LR 8 (b).

To aid location, observe the large depression formed by the muscles attaching at the medial aspect of the knee and the medial femoral condyle, and locate LR 8 at its centre. If the depression is not visible due to swelling or excess fat, palpate gently with the palm to ascertain its centre.

Needling
0.5 to 1.5 cun perpendicular insertion.

Actions and indications
LR 8 is a major point to *nourish Liver Blood and Yin* and *cool the Liver*. It also effectively *dispels*

325

dampness, heat and Blood stasis from the lower jiao and benefits the Liver, Kidneys, uterus and urogenital system.

Indications include: itching and inflammation of the genitals, dysuria, turbid urine, cystitis, urethritis, leucorrhoea, dysmenorrhoea, endometriosis, ovarian cysts, oligomenorrhoea, amenorrhoea, abdominal distension and pain, impotence, diarrhoea and headache.

LR 8 is also *effective as a local point*, to treat pain, swelling and restricted mobility of the knee and leg.

> **Main Areas**—Lower jiao. Genitourinary system. Uterus. Knee.
> **Main Functions**—Nourishes Blood and Yin. Cools the Liver. Clears dampness and heat.

LR 9 Yinbao
Yin Receptacle (Uterus) 陰包

Myotome	L2–L4
Dermatome	L3

Location
On the medial aspect of the thigh, 4 cun proximal to the medial end of the popliteal (knee) crease, in the depression between the vastus medialis and sartorius muscles. To aid location, if the knee joint is extended and the foot dorsiflexed, a groove appears between the muscles.

Needling
0.5 to 1.5 cun perpendicular insertion.

Actions and indications
LR 9 is not a very commonly used point for its internal functions that include *regulating the lower jiao* and *benefiting menstruation*. However, it can be very useful in the treatment of *channel disorders*, including pain or swelling of the medial aspect of the knee, sciatica and thigh pain.

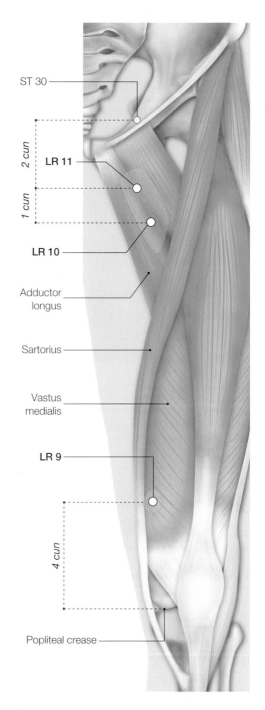

ST 30
2 cun
1 cun
LR 11
LR 10
Adductor longus
Sartorius
Vastus medialis
LR 9
4 cun
Popliteal crease

Other indications include: irregular menstruation, abdominal pain, lumbar pain, frequent urination, enuresis, incontinence, and urinary retention.

> **Main Areas**—Genitals. Uterus. Thigh.
> **Main Functions**—Regulates Qi. Benefits the lower jiao. Alleviates pain.

LR 10   Zuwuli
Leg Five Miles

足五里

Myotome	L2/L3
Dermatome	L1

Location
3 cun distal to ST 30, on the anterior border of the adductor longus muscle. Situated between the adductor longus and pectineus muscles. In its deep position lies the adductor brevis and, deeper still, the adductor minimus.

To aid location, it is approximately one hand-width distal to ST 30. Also, the adductor longus tendon is the most prominent tendon in the groin.

Choose between LR 10 and LR 11, depending on which is more reactive to pressure palpation (these points are used for similar purposes).

Do not apply any form of treatment to this area if thrombosis has not been excluded.

Needling
0.5 to 1.5 cun perpendicular insertion.
There is a lot of delicate anatomy to be aware of in this region.

Actions and indications
Although LR 10 and LR 11 are not very commonly used points, they can be effectively employed to treat *groin pain, hernia,* testicular pain or swelling, impotence, dysmenorrhoea, infertility, dysuria, and prostatitis.

As *local points*, LR 10 and LR 11 can be used to treat injury, spasm or inflammation of the adductors.

> **Main Areas**—Thigh. Groin. Genitals.
> **Main Functions**—Regulates Qi and dispels stasis. Dissipates cold from the Liver channel. Alleviates pain.

LR 11   Yinlian
Yin Corner

陰廉

Myotome	L3/L4
Dermatome	L1

Location
1 cun proximal to LR 10, on the anterior border of the adductor longus muscle.

Use pressure palpation to choose between LR 10 and LR 11.

Needling
0.5 to 1.5 cun perpendicular insertion.
There is a lot of delicate anatomy to be aware of in this region.

Actions and indications
LR 11 is used for similar purposes to LR 10, although its traditional indications emphasise *gynaecological disorders and infertility.*

> **Main Areas**—Thigh. Genitals. Uterus.
> **Main Function**—Dispels cold and pain.

LR 12   Jimai
Urgent Pulse

急脈

Myotome	L2–L4, but mostly superficial
Dermatome	L1

Location
On the inguinal groove, in the depression medial to the femoral artery and vein, approximately 2.5 cun lateral to the anterior midline, distal and slightly lateral to ST 30. Situated below the inguinal ligament in the depression of the saphenous hiatus. In its deep position lies the pectineus muscle.

To aid location, LR 12 is about one finger-width medial to the palpable femoral artery and approximately 1 cun medial to SP 12 (on the lateral side of the femoral artery).

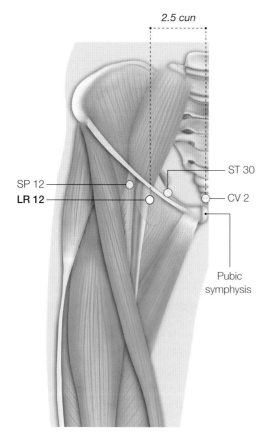

2.5 cun

SP 12

LR 12

ST 30

CV 2

Pubic symphysis

Needling

0.5 to 1 cun insertion medial to the femoral vein, in a perpendicular or slightly oblique and medial direction.

Be aware of a lot of delicate anatomy in this region.

Actions and indications

LR 12 is a very useful *local point* to treat *disorders of the groin area*, including: hernia, testicular pain or swelling, impotence, dysmenorrhoea, and uterine prolapse. In common with SP 12, it is useful in cases of poor circulation, vascular disorders and cold in the lower limbs.

Additionally, LR 12 can be used to treat *injury* and inflammation of the adductors and sciatica.

> **Main Areas**—Groin. Genitals. Blood vessels. Entire lower limb.
> **Main Functions**—Improves Qi and Blood circulation. Dispels cold. Alleviates pain.

LR 13   Zhangmen

Completion Gate

 章門

Front-Mu point of the Spleen
Influential point for the Yin organs (Zang)
Intersection of the Gallbladder on the
Liver channel

Myotome	T8–T12
Dermatome	T10/T11

Location

On the lateral side of the abdomen, below the free end of the eleventh rib, near the mid-axillary line and just superior to the level of the umbilicus. Situated in the oblique abdominal muscles.

To aid location, if the arm is bent at the elbow and held down by the side, the tip of the elbow approximately touches the free end of the eleventh rib.

Alternative locations

Locate LR 13 at the free end of the eleventh rib. This location may be better for manual techniques.

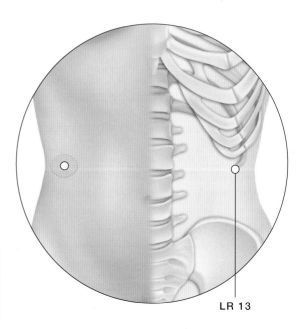

LR 13

Alternatively, palpate the entire area around the tip of and under the free end of the rib and treat where it is most reactive during pressure palpation.

Needling

0.3 to 1 cun perpendicular or slightly oblique insertion. However, in many cases there is a lot of subcutaneous fat requiring deeper needling to obtain deqi.
0.5 to 1.5 cun oblique inferior insertion.

Be aware of the anatomical position of the liver. The point is within the oblique muscles however, so deep needling should not be required.

Actions and indications

LR 13 is an extremely important point to *harmonise the middle jiao and Spleen*. Combined with CV 12 it opens the middle jiao.

It is effective to *boost Spleen Qi* and *regulate the Liver*, particularly in relation to the *digestive system* and has been extensively employed in a variety of such disorders. These include: abdominal or epigastric distension, swelling and pain, indigestion, abdominal rumbling, diminished appetite, belching, nausea, vomiting, hypochondrial distension and pain, jaundice, hepatitis, enlargement of the liver or spleen, gastroenteritis, flatulence, diarrhoea, loose or rough stools, undigested food in the stools, and constipation.

LR 13 also treats other manifestations of *Spleen and Liver disharmony*, including: distension, fullness and pain of the chest, and dyspnoea or coughing due to Qi stagnation or phlegm-damp accumulation in the chest and abdomen.

Additionally, LR 13 has been extensively used to treat a variety of other cases, including: chronic tiredness, weakness of the limbs and body, emaciation, mental agitation, fever, difficulty raising the arms due to contraction of the abdominal muscles, pain of the lumbar or thoracic spine, and difficulty rotating or side-flexing the trunk.

> **Main Areas**—Abdomen. Hypochondrium. Chest. Digestive system.
> **Main Functions**—Harmonises the Liver and Spleen. Boosts Spleen Qi.

LR 14 Qimen
Cycle Gate

期門

Front-Mu point of the Liver
Intersection of Yin Wei Mai and Spleen on the Liver channel

Myotome	T8–T12
Dermatome	T6

Location

Directly below the root of the breast on the mid-mamillary line in the sixth intercostal space, approximately 4 cun lateral to the anterior midline. Situated in the oblique abdominal muscles and, deeper, the intercostal muscles.

To aid location, palpate the intercostal space reasonably strongly to ascertain a small nodule, usually at the most tender spot.

Alternative location

'Lower Qimen' is located directly below the main LR 14 location, under the lower border of the costal cartilage, 4 cun lateral to the anterior midline.

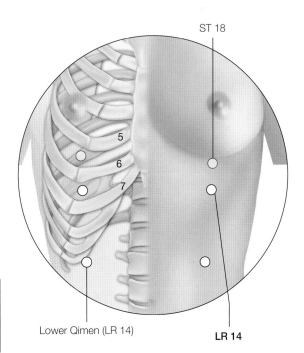

ST 18

5

6

7

Lower Qimen (LR 14)

LR 14

Needling

0.3 to 0.8 cun oblique insertion, directed laterally along the intercostal space.
Needling can also be applied in a medial direction along the intercostal space.

Do not needle deeply. This poses a considerable risk of puncturing the lung and inducing a pneumothorax.

Actions and indications

LR 14 is a very important and widely used point because it *effectively regulates Qi, dispels stasis, cools Blood* and *nourishes the Liver*. It has a range of applications in both excess and deficiency disorders and is particularly indicated for *diseases of the chest, hypochondrium and abdomen* caused by *Qi and Blood stasis.*

It has been extensively employed for disorders of the lungs, heart, breast and gynaecological system. Indications include: breast pain, mastitis, fibrocystic breast disease, premenstrual syndrome, excessive uterine bleeding, failure to discharge the placenta, tightness and pain of the chest, intercostal neuralgia, dyspnoea, coughing, angina pectoris, palpitations, depression, irritability, mood swings, and *frequent sighing as seen in stress conditions.*

LR 14 is also especially indicated to *harmonise the Liver and Stomach* and can be used for many digestive disorders, including: hypochondrial pain and distension, jaundice, hepatitis, gallstones, palpable abdominal masses, enlargement of the Liver or Spleen, stomach ache, heartburn, hiccup, indigestion, nausea, vomiting, gastritis, gastric ulceration and distension, and tightness or hardness of the epigastrium or abdomen.

Other traditional indications include tiredness, chills and fever, tidal fever, feeling of heat in the body, malaria, masses, swellings and nodules, stiffness and pain of the neck, and skin diseases with redness and heat.

Main Areas—Hypochondrium. Chest. Breast. Abdomen.
Main Functions—Regulates Liver Qi. Dispels stasis. Cools Blood.

---

20 Points of the Conception Vessel

(Alternative names: 'Ren Mai', 'Sea of Yin', 'Controlling Vessel' or 'Directing Vessel')

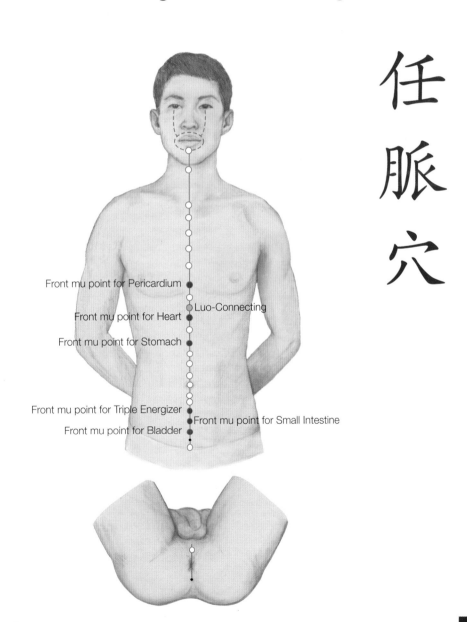

任脈穴

Front mu point for Pericardium

Luo-Connecting

Front mu point for Heart

Front mu point for Stomach

Front mu point for Triple Energizer

Front mu point for Small Intestine

Front mu point for Bladder

General	The Conception Vessel is one of the eight Extra Meridians, also called the Extraordinary Meridians. It is commonly used in practice and often appears, as it does in this book, in the section containing the twelve main meridians. Its paired meridian is the Governor Vessel (alternative name: Du Mai), and it has 24 points.
	The Conception Vessel is considered very Yin in its actions and the Governor Vessel very Yang. The pair create a balance around the whole body, from the perineum all the way through to the mouth, with one channel going up the anterior aspect of the body and the other, the posterior. Both channels are said to start from the region between the kidneys, and pass downwards to the perineum.
	The Conception Vessel in particular has a strong association with the uterus on its path downwards, and then CV 1 emerges onto the perineum. The channel then travels up the anterior midline of the body, passing through the umbilicus at CV 8 (forbidden to needle), and ends on the lower jaw, just under the mouth at CV 24.
More specifically	Historically, and in energetic terms, an individual's Qi begins in the region between the Kidneys, Ming Men, and travels downwards to the perineum, where it splits into the Conception Vessel and the Governor Vessel.
	Some texts have the Conception Vessel arising in the uterus, and the channel does indeed have very strong associations with the reproductive system, as its name indicates.
	CV 1 starts on the perineum, anterior to the anus, although both CV and GV channels are said to initially emerge at GV 1. The channel then travels upwards, over the area of the uterus and bladder in women and the bladder in men. It continues its ascent directly up the midline all the way to the lower jaw, just below the mouth, ending in a depression in the mentolabial groove on the mandible.
	CV 4 and CV 6 are two of the most commonly used points for constitutional weakness and deficiency, as they affect the lower jiao, which houses the Dantian – the store/core of baseline Qi. This area is also very important in all martial art, Qi Gong and Tai Chi practices.
	The channel passes through CV 8, the umbilicus, and it is forbidden to needle this point, although moxa can be applied for conditions where there is extreme energy loss. There are many front-mu points on this line, and the use of this channel in treatments can have a profound effect on many aspects of visceral health. This is one of its key uses.
	At the mouth there is a connection with the Governor Vessel at GV 28, so the mouth is surrounded by these two channels and interlinks with the LI and ST channels.
	A second aspect of this main branch also arises in the lower pelvis but travels backwards along the perineum and up through the spine, emerging in the suboccipital region, forwards towards the jaw.

Area covered	Pelvis, abdominal viscera, thoracic cavity viscera, throat, mouth.
Areas affected with treatment	Pelvic floor, pelvis and associated organs, urogenital conditions, reproductive system conditions for both men and women, all viscera through the PSNS and innervation via the anterior primary rami of the spinal nerves, fatigue and energy loss, anxiety, panic and heart conditions.
Key points	CV 1, CV 3, CV 4, CV 5, CV 6, CV 12, CV 14, CV 17.

CV 1   Huiyin
Meeting of Yin

Intersection of the Chong Mai and Governor Vessel on the Conception Vessel
Eleventh Ghost point

Myotome	S3/S4, but in fascia
Dermatome	S4

Location
At the centre of the perineum, midway between the posterior border of the genitals and the anus.

Needling
0.5 to 1 cun perpendicular insertion.

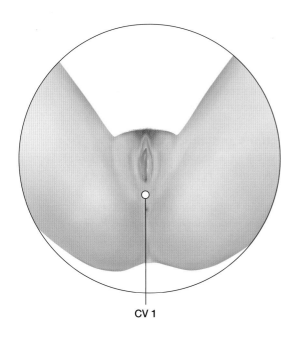

CV 1

Actions and indications
Traditional functions of CV 1 include *nourishing the Yin and benefiting the jing, and resolving dampness and heat from the lower jiao.* Additionally, it is considered as the *jing-well point of the Conception Vessel* and has been used to *calm the mind, clear the sense organs, treat epilepsy and restore consciousness* and is *traditionally indicated to resuscitate from drowning.*

In the clinic, however, needling CV 1 is used only in cases such as *paralysis of the perineum or lower limbs, uterine prolapse, incontinence,* testicular disorders including retraction, and inflammation of the skin surrounding the genitalia caused by severe herpes or other infections.

> **Main Areas**—Genitals. Mind. Entire body.
> **Main Functions**—Boosts the lower jiao.
> Lifts sinking Qi. Increases libido.

CV 2   Qugu
Curved Bone

Intersection of the Liver on the Conception Vessel

Myotome	None – superficial fascia
Dermatome	T5–T12

Location
Just above the superior border of the pubic symphysis on the anterior midline, 5 cun below the umbilicus.

Contraindicated during pregnancy.

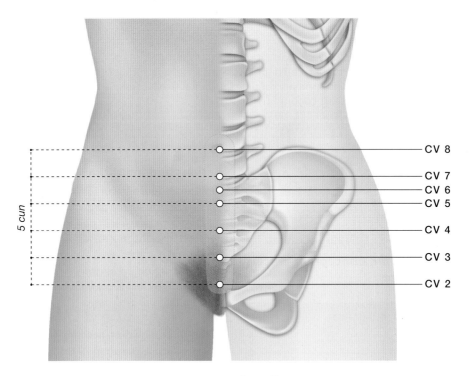

Needling

0.5 to 1 cun perpendicular insertion.

Beware full bladder. Ask client to empty their bladder before treatment in this region.

Actions and indications

Similar to CV 3. Use CV 2 instead of CV 3 if it is more reactive to pressure palpation.

> **Main Areas**—Bladder. Genitals. Uterus.
> **Main Function**—Benefits the genitourinary system and lower jiao.

CV 3   Zhongji
Middle Pole

中極

Front-Mu point of the Bladder
Intersection of the Spleen, Liver and
Kidney on the Conception Vessel

Myotome	None – superficial fascia
Dermatome	T5–T12

Location

On the anterior midline, 4 cun below the umbilicus, 1 cun superior to the upper border of the pubic symphysis.

Contraindicated during pregnancy. This site is often tender spontaneously or on pressure palpation if there is inflammation of the bladder.

Needling

0.5 to 1.5 cun perpendicular insertion.

Do not needle deeply. Do not puncture the peritoneum or a full bladder.

Actions and indications

CV 3 is an *important point for disorders of the urogenital and gynaecological systems*.

Its main functions include *regulating the transformation of Qi and fluids in the lower jiao, clearing dampness and heat, fortifying the Kidneys, and benefiting the genitourinary system and uterus.*

Common indications include: dysuria, frequent urination, urinary retention, incontinence, cystitis, urethritis, prostatitis, impotence, premature ejaculation, lower abdominal pain and distension, leucorrhoea, genital itching and pain, uterine prolapse, infertility, dysmenorrhoea, and irregular menstruation. Moxibustion effectively *dispels cold and warms the lower jiao.*

If deqi cannot be achieved at CV 3, use CV 2 or CV 4 instead.

> **Main Areas**—Bladder. Uterus. Lower jiao.
> **Main Functions**—Dispels dampness, heat and cold. Strengthens the genitourinary system.

CV 4   Guanyuan
Gate of Origin

Front-Mu point of the Small Intestine
Intersection of the Spleen, Liver and
Kidney on the Conception Vessel

Myotome	None – superficial fascia
Dermatome	T12

Location
On the anterior midline, 3 cun below the umbilicus.

Contraindicated during pregnancy.

Needling
0.5 to 1.5 cun perpendicular insertion.
0.5 to 2 cun oblique inferior insertion.

Actions and indications
CV 4 is an important point to *strengthen and regulate the three key Yin organs: Kidney, Liver and Spleen.* CV 4 is called the *Original Qi Gate* because it has a direct effect on the Kidney Qi and *strengthens the entire lower jiao.* It *nourishes Yin, Blood and Jing, and has a calming and grounding action on the mind* (it is often combined with SP 6 for this purpose). Furthermore, it is effective to *dispel dampness, cold and heat from the lower jiao.*

Common indications include irregular menstruation, amenorrhoea, infertility, uterine fibroids, polycystic ovarian syndrome, endometriosis, dysmenorrhoea, excessive menstruation, postpartum haemorrhage, leucorrhoea, genital itching, dysuria, frequent urination, urinary tract infections, incontinence, impotence, prostatitis, abdominal distension and pain, irritable bowel syndrome, constipation, anxiety, restlessness, insomnia, palpitations, sore throat, tinnitus, diminishing vision and hearing, heat due to Yin deficiency, emaciation, lumbar pain, and chronic tiredness, weakness and exhaustion.

> **Main Areas**—Entire body. Abdomen.
> Small Intestine. Bladder. Uterus.
> **Main Functions**—Augments yuan Qi. Nourishes Yin and Blood. Calms the mind. Reinforces the Kidneys. Regulates Qi and Blood. Strengthens the lower jiao. Benefits the Small Intestine.

CV 5   Shimen
Stone Gate

Front-Mu point of the Triple Energizer

Myotome	None – superficial fascia
Dermatome	T10

Location
On the anterior midline, 2 cun below the umbilicus, 3 cun superior to the pubic symphysis.

Contraindicated during pregnancy.

Needling
0.5 to 1 cun perpendicular insertion.

Actions and indications
As the front-mu point for the Triple Energizer, this point is often include in treatments which involve fluid movement, or lack of it. The Triple Energizer as an organ function is all to do with regulation of tissue and body fluid movement. Conditions such a poor *bladder control, painful urinary conditions, distension and bloating in the lower abdomen.*

It is strongly *advised against using this point in treatments for female reproductive disorders*, with one text giving an alternative name for this point of Jueyun, which means 'infertility'. The premise being repeated in further traditional texts, that needling this point could result in infertility for the woman.

> **Main Areas**—Abdomen. Uterus.
> **Main Functions**—Mobilises yuan Qi.
> Warms and strengthens the lower jiao.

CV 6   (Xia) Qihai   (下)氣海
(Lower) Sea of Qi

Myotome	None – superficial fascia
Dermatome	T10

Location
On the anterior midline, 1.5 cun below the umbilicus, in a small depression at the lower border of the fleshy bulge formed by the subcutaneous fat deposit under the umbilicus (visible on most people, but more prominent on women).

To aid location, place the middle finger in the umbilicus and grasp the fleshy bulge under the umbilicus with the thumb. The tip of the thumb should locate CV 6. This fleshy bulge is formed by the subcutaneous fat cells deposited in a slightly thicker layer around the umbilicus in a U shape.

According to certain Japanese hara (abdominal) diagnosis models, this is the Kidney diagnostic area. CV 6 lies close to the lower border of the Kidney diagnostic area.

Contraindicated during pregnancy.

Needling
0.5 to 1.5 cun perpendicular insertion.
0.5 to 2 cun oblique or transverse inferior insertion.

CV 6 may bruise easily because the superficial veins (particularly the paraumbilical vein) are very delicate in this area.

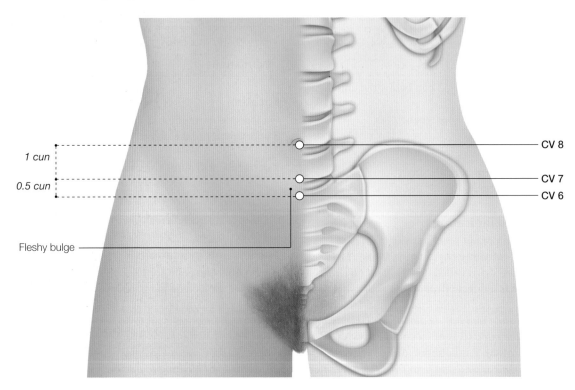

1 cun
0.5 cun
Fleshy bulge
CV 8
CV 7
CV 6

Actions and indications

CV 6 is a *hugely important point to tonify and lift Qi, warm and restore Yang* (with moxibustion) and *fortify the Kidneys*. (Compared with CV 4, CV 6 is all about generating Yang and Qi, whereas CV 4 is about generating Yin and Blood).

It is a major point to *boost energy* and *is considered vital in the treatment of deficiency conditions* such as chronic tiredness, weakness, debility, exhaustion, old age or weakened immunity. It can be employed in *many chronic or serious diseases to help the general health and enliven the patient.*

It also effectively *regulates the abdominal Qi and dispels dampness, particularly from the lower jiao*. It is an important point to *treat disorders of the abdomen and pelvis, including digestive, gynaecological and urogenital conditions.*

Indications include: abdominal distension and pain, bloating, irritable bowel syndrome, diarrhoea, constipation, dysmenorrhoea, amenorrhoea, irregular menstruation, leucorrhoea, prolapse of abdominal or pelvic organs, frequent urination, male and female fertility disorders, impotence, and frigidity.

> **Main Areas**—Entire body. Lower jiao. Abdomen.
> **Main Functions**—Tonifies and warms Yang. Lifts sinking Qi. Warms the abdomen. Regulates Qi in the lower jiao.

CV 7   Yinjiao
Yin Intersection

Intersection of the Kidney and Chong Mai on the Conception Vessel

Myotome	None – superficial fascia
Dermatome	T9/T10

Location
On the anterior midline, 1 cun below the umbilicus.

Needling
0.5 to 1.5 cun perpendicular insertion.

Actions and indications

Although CV 7 is not as commonly employed as the previous Conception Vessel points, it can be employed for similar purposes, including *regulating menstruation and Qi in the abdomen.*

Indications include: abdominal distension and pain, leucorrhoea, infertility, excessive or irregular menstruation, well as testicular retraction.

As a *local point*, CV 7 is useful in cases of periumbilical pain and hernia.

> **Main Areas**—Abdomen. Umbilicus. Uterus.
> **Main Functions**—Regulates Qi in the lower jiao. Alleviates pain.

CV 8   Shenque
Spirit Palace Gate

Myotome	None – superficial fascia
Dermatome	T9

Location
On the anterior midline, at the centre of the umbilicus.

Contraindications
Needling is contraindicated.

Needling
Moxa can be applied via a barrier such as salt or a slice of ginger in traditional treatments but needling is forbidden. It can be useful to advise the client to use heat, in the form of a warm water bottle or wheat-bag, over this area if they are very deficient in energy and to use it on a regular basis. Heat equals energy, so even if feeling relatively well, it can be adding a reservoir of energy to the system if used regularly.

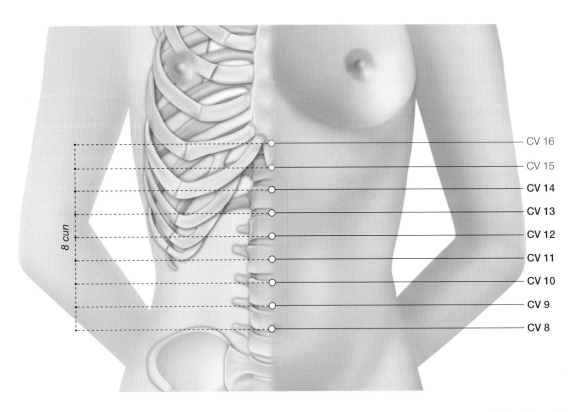

Actions and indications

The application of moxibustion to CV 8 is considered *very important to restore collapsed Yang and raise sinking Qi*. It also effectively regulates the flow of Qi in the abdomen.

Indications include: chronic or severe diarrhoea, abdominal swelling and oedema, abdominal pain, periumbilical pain, various prolapses, generalised weakness, loss of consciousness, wind stroke, arrhythmia, cardiac failure, cyanosis, profuse sweating, and hypothermia.

Lightly applied indirect moxibustion over and around the navel is also useful for *infantile diarrhoea and colic*.

Traditionally, *burning large moxa cones on the umbilicus was used after all other treatment failed, in cases where imminent death was apparent.* The navel is considered the site where the spirit enters and leaves the body, hence its name 'Spirit Palace Gate'.

> **Main Areas**—Navel. Abdomen. Entire body.
> **Main Functions**—Tonifies, warms, lifts and revives Yang. Regulates Qi in the abdomen.

CV 9   Shuifen
Water Separation

Myotome	None – superficial fascia
Dermatome	T8

Location
On the anterior midline, 1 cun above the umbilicus.

Needling
0.5 to 1.5 cun perpendicular insertion.

Actions and indications
CV 9 is primarily used to promote and regulate *fluid transformation* as its name suggests.

Indications include: oedema, swelling and pain of the abdomen; diarrhoea, profuse urination, and leucorrhoea.

> **Main Areas**—Abdomen. Entire body.
> **Main Function**—Reduces oedema.

CV 10 Xiawan
Lower Stomach

Intersection of the Spleen on the Conception Vessel

Myotome	None – superficial fascia
Dermatome	T8

Location
On the anterior midline, 2 cun above the umbilicus.

Needling
0.5 to 1.5 cun perpendicular insertion.

Actions and indications
CV 10 is an important point to *descend rebellious Stomach Qi*. It is specifically indicated for disorders of *the lower part of the stomach*, therefore relieving food retention. CV 10 also *tonifies the Spleen Qi*.

Indications include: indigestion, nausea, heartburn, hiccup, fullness of the epigastrium and abdomen, abdominal rumbling, foul breath, and belching.

> **Main Areas**—Stomach. Abdomen.
> **Main Functions**—Descends rebellious Qi.
> Relieves food stagnation.

CV 11 Jianli
Strengthen the Interior

Myotome	None – superficial fascia
Dermatome	T7/T8

Location
On the anterior midline, 3 cun above the umbilicus.

Needling
0.5 to 1 cun perpendicular insertion.

Actions and indications
CV 11 *harmonises the middle jiao* and *regulates Qi* in a similar way to CV 10 and CV 12. It should be chosen instead of the latter points if it is found to be more reactive to gentle pressure palpation.

> **Main Areas**—Stomach. Middle jiao.
> **Main Function**—Harmonises the middle jiao.

CV 12 Zhongwan
Middle Cavity

**Front-Mu point of the Stomach
Influential point for the Yang organs (Fu)
Intersection of the Small Intestine, Triple Energizer and Stomach on the Conception Vessel**

Myotome	None – superficial fascia
Dermatome	T7

Location
On the anterior midline, 4 cun above the umbilicus.

To aid location, CV 12 is midway between the umbilicus and the xiphisternal junction (the junction of the xiphoid process with the body of the sternum). It is usually found along one of the horizontal creases on the epigastrium, defined when the patient bends the trunk forwards.

Needling

0.5 to 1.5 cun perpendicular insertion.

Actions and indications

CV 12 is a *very important point to tonify the middle jiao*. It is used in many conditions caused by *deficiency of the Stomach and Spleen* and also helps *transform dampness and phlegm*. It is specifically indicated for disorders of the *middle part of the stomach and also descends rebellious Qi.*

Indications include: poor appetite and digestion, nausea, morning sickness during pregnancy, loss of taste, fullness and heaviness of the epigastrium, stomach ache, gastritis, gastric ulceration, heartburn, hiatus hernia, abdominal pain, abdominal rumbling, loose stools, dry stools, difficult defecation, jaundice, productive cough, poor concentration, and tiredness.

CV 12 is also very important to *nourish Yin and body fluids*. Symptoms include: thirst, dry mouth, dark and scanty urine, dry skin, and mental restlessness.

Additionally, CV 12 helps to *calm the heart and ease stress and tension*. Indications include: mental restlessness, anxiety, cardiac pain, and palpitations. It is important for digestive disorders caused by stress.

Used with LR 13 bilaterally it can open the middle jiao, which is helpful in digestive dysfunction.

> **Main Areas**—Middle jiao. Epigastrium. Stomach. Abdomen. Entire body.
> **Main Functions**—Tonifies the Stomach and Spleen. Transforms dampness. Dispels cold. Harmonises the middle jiao and descends rebellious Qi. Nourishes fluids and Yin. Soothes the Heart and calms the mind.

CV 13   Shangwan
Upper Cavity

Intersection of the Small Intestine and Stomach on the Conception Vessel

Myotome	None – superficial fascia
Dermatome	T7

Location

On the anterior midline, 5 cun above the umbilicus, and 3 cun below the xiphisternal junction.

Needling

0.5 to 1.5 cun perpendicular insertion.

Actions and indications

Similar to CV 12. However, CV 13 is specifically indicated for disorders of the *upper part of the stomach* and *more for acute cases*, particularly nausea and vomiting.

> **Main Area**—Stomach.
> **Main Function**—Harmonises the Stomach.

CV 14   Juque
Great Gateway

Front-Mu point of the Heart

Myotome	None – superficial fascia
Dermatome	T6/T7

Location

On the anterior midline, 6 cun above the umbilicus.

Needling

0.5 to 1 cun perpendicular insertion.
1 to 1.5 cun oblique inferior insertion.

Do not needle in an upward direction.

Actions and indications

CV 14 is used to treat *symptoms of heat and stagnation in the Heart and chest*, including: palpitations, dyspnoea, coughing, pain and constriction of the chest and epigastrium, *insomnia, anxiety, and emotional disturbances in general.*

It is a key point to be used in conditions involving feelings of panic. CV 14 also *descends rebellious Stomach Qi* in cases of heartburn, nausea and vomiting.

> **Main Areas**—Heart. Chest. Epigastrium.
> **Main Functions**—Soothes the Heart and calms the mind. Harmonises the Heart and Stomach.

CV 15   Jiuwei

Turtledove Tail

(Xiphoid Process)

Luo-Connecting point of the Conception Vessel

Myotome	None – superficial fascia
Dermatome	T6

Location

On the anterior midline, 7 cun above the umbilicus, at the tip of the xiphoid process.

To aid location, if the xiphoid process is very long, find CV 15 further inferiorly. It is always at the tip of the xiphoid process.

Needling

0.5 to 1 cun oblique inferior insertion just below the tip of the xiphoid process.

Do not needle deeper or upward. This poses considerable risk of puncturing the liver or an enlarged heart.

Actions and indications

CV 15 is effective to *free up the entire abdomen when there is Qi blockage*. It is *particularly*

indicated for psychosomatic disorders, as well as diseases of the Heart, Lungs and chest.

Indications include: abdominal swelling or pain, itching or pain of the skin of the abdomen, difficulty swallowing, indigestion, heartburn, palpitations, cardiac pain, fullness of the chest, dyspnoea, coughing, haemoptysis, mental agitation, fright, abnormal behaviour, psychological disorders, and epilepsy.

CV 15 *augments the functions of the Yin organs and boosts original (yuan) Qi.*

> **Main Areas**—Chest. Abdomen.
> **Main Functions**—Regulates Qi and dispels stasis. Calms and balances the mind.

CV 16   Zhongting

Central Court

Myotome	None – superficial fascia
Dermatome	T5

Location

On the midline of the sternum, at the xiphisternal junction. To aid location, the xiphisternal junction is a distinct depression, visible on thin patients. Slide the fingertip down the midline of the sternum and it will drop in to the depression naturally.

Needling

0.5 cun transverse inferior insertion.

Actions and indications

CV 16 is not as commonly used as other adjacent points. It can, however, help *relax the chest, harmonise the Stomach and descend rebellious Qi.* Indications include: fullness and heaviness of the chest, heartburn, difficulty swallowing, nausea, vomiting, and epigastric pain.

> **Main Areas**—Chest. Abdomen.
> **Main Functions**—Regulates Qi and dispels stasis. Calms and balances the mind.

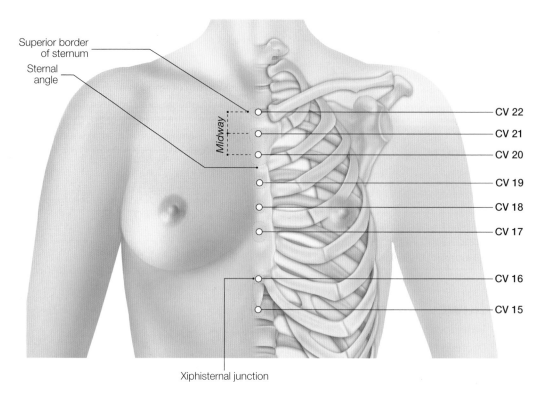

Superior border of sternum
Sternal angle
Midway

Xiphisternal junction

CV 22
CV 21
CV 20
CV 19
CV 18
CV 17
CV 16
CV 15

CV 17 Shanzhong

膻中

Chest Centre

Influential point of Qi, Sea of Qi point
Front-Mu point of the Pericardium
Intersection of the Spleen, Kidney, Small
Intestine and Triple Energizer on the
Conception Vessel

Myotome	None – superficial fascia
Dermatome	T4

Location

At the centre of the chest on the sternal midline, level with the fourth intercostal space, between the nipples.

Needling

0.3 to 1 cun transverse inferior or superior insertion.

Do NOT needle perpendicularly.

Actions and indications

CV 17 is a *major point to tonify and regulate chest Qi* and is widely used for disorders of this area.

Common indications include: constriction, tightness, pain or heaviness of the chest, cardiac pain, palpitations, frequent sighing, plum stone throat, shortness of breath, dyspnoea, wheeze, cough, insufficient lactation, and breast pain.

CV 17 may also be thought of as the *front-mu point for the Shen (mind)* because it is used to treat many *psycho-emotional disorders*, including: depression, propensity for crying, sadness, hysteria, and insomnia.

Additionally, CV 17 is useful in chronic or serious diseases to enliven the Qi throughout the body.

> **Main Areas**—Heart. Lungs. Chest. Breast. Entire body.
> **Main Functions**—Regulates Qi and dispels stasis. Tonifies Qi. Calms and balances the mind. Benefits the chest.

CV 18 Yutang
Jade Hall

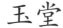

Myotome	None – superficial fascia
Dermatome	T3

Location
On the sternal midline, level with the third intercostal space.

Needling
0.3 to 1 cun transverse inferior or superior insertion.

Do NOT needle perpendicularly.

Actions and indications
Similar to CV 17. However, CV 18 is more indicated for imbalances that manifest along the external and internal course of the channel, particularly in relation to *inflammation or spasm of the throat, bronchi or oesophagus.*

Symptoms include sternal or retrosternal pain, heartburn, nausea, difficulty swallowing, sore throat, cough, bronchitis, dyspnoea, asthma as well as pain, swelling or other disorders of the anterior aspect of the chest and breasts.

> **Main Areas**—Sternum. Chest. Lungs. Heart. Breast.
> **Main Functions**—Regulates Qi, dissipates stasis and alleviates pain. Calms and balances the mind. Benefits the chest.

CV 19 Zigong
Purple Palace

Myotome	None – superficial fascia
Dermatome	T2

Location
On the sternal midline, level with the second intercostal space.

Needling
0.3 to 1 cun transverse inferior or superior insertion.

Do NOT needle perpendicularly.

Actions and indications
This point helps with *tightness and pain in the chest.* Also useful for conditions involving *vomiting with bitter regurgitation* and difficulty in eating.

> **Main Areas**—Sternum. Chest. Lungs. Heart. Breast.
> **Main Functions**—Regulates Qi, dissipates stasis and alleviates pain. Calms and balances the mind. Benefits the chest.

CV 20 Huagai
Splendid Covering

Myotome	None – superficial fascia
Dermatome	C4–T2

Location
On the midline of the manubrium, just superior to the sternal angle, level with the first intercostal space.

To aid location, the sternal angle is palpable as the small bump of the manubrosternal articulation. CV 20 is in the first palpable depression superior to the sternal angle.

Needling
0.3 to 0.5 cun transverse inferior or superior insertion.

Actions and indications

In common with other adjacent points, CV 20 regulates Qi, descends rebellious Qi and helps relax the chest. It is used in such cases as cough, asthma, dyspnoea, pain and fullness of the chest, and angina pectoris.

> **Main Areas**—Heart. Lungs. Chest.
> **Main Functions**—Regulates Qi. Relaxes the chest.

CV 21   Xuanji
Pivot of Rotation

Myotome	None – superficial fascia
Dermatome	C4

Location

In the shallow depression slightly superior to the centre of the manubrium, about 1 cun inferior CV 22.

To aid location, it is midway between CV 20 and CV 22.

Needling

0.5 to 1 cun inferiorly directed insertion.

Actions and indications

Although CV 21 is not very commonly used, it can help *descend rebellious Qi, relax the chest and benefit the throat*. Indications include: sore throat, cough, dyspnoea, asthma, chest pain, epigastric fullness, nausea, and vomiting.

> **Main Areas**—Chest. Throat.
> **Main Functions**—Relaxes the chest. Descends rebellious Qi.

CV 22   Tiantu
Celestial Chimney/
Heavenly Prominence

Intersection of the Yin Wei Mai on the Conception Vessel
Window of the Sky point

Myotome	None – superficial fascia
Dermatome	C3

Location

On the anterior midline, just superior to the suprasternal (jugular) notch.

Needling

0.3 cun perpendicular insertion.
0.5 to 1 cun inferior retrosternal insertion. Insert the needle perpendicularly about 0.3 cun and then direct it downward along the posterior border of the manubrium 0.5 to 1 cun.

Do not needle deeper perpendicularly, because this holds substantial risk of injuring sensitive anatomy.

Actions and indications

CV 22 is primarily used to *descend rebellious Qi, alleviate cough and benefit the throat and voice*.

Indications include: acute dyspnoea, (in cases of an asthma attack, as example) acute coughing, wheeze or asthma, hoarseness or loss of voice, tightness, pain and swelling of the throat, and goitre. Furthermore, it has been used to treat heartburn, nausea and vomiting.

> **Main Areas**—Throat. Chest.
> **Main Functions**—Descends rebellious Qi. Alleviates dyspnoea and cough. Treats asthma.

CV 23　Lianquan

Fountain at the Angle

(Tongue Root)

Intersection of the Yin Wei Mai on the Conception Vessel

Myotome	None – superficial fascia
Dermatome	C3

Location

On the anterior midline, just superior to the hyoid bone.

To aid location, it is where the chin joins with the throat, midway between the tip of the chin and the laryngeal prominence. Palpate gently superior to the hyoid bone to find the small depression.

Needling

0.5 to 1.2 cun oblique insertion towards the base of the tongue.

Actions and indications

CV 23 is a *useful point for disorders of the tongue, throat and submandibular glands.*

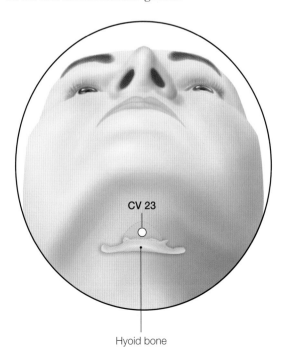

CV 23

Hyoid bone

Indications include: swelling and inflammation of the submandibular glands, goitre, paralysis or rigidity of the tongue, drooling, speech disorders, loss of voice, soreness or swelling of the throat, snoring, and sleep apnoea.

Furthermore, according to classical texts, it is indicated for thirst and diabetes mellitus.

> **Main Areas**—Tongue. Submandibular area. Throat.
> **Main Functions**—Resolves phlegm and clears heat. Descends rebellious Qi.

CV 24　Chengjiang

Saliva Receptacle

Intersection of the Governor Vessel, Stomach and Large Intestine on the Conception Vessel
Eighth Ghost point

Myotome	None – superficial fascia
Dermatome	Trigeminal nerve

Location

On the anterior midline, in the depression at the centre of the mentolabial groove, approximately midway between the lower lip and the tip of the chin.

To aid location, palpate the mentolabial groove for the small, but distinct, depression between the orbicularis oris and mentalis muscles.

Needling

0.2 to 0.3 cun upward oblique insertion. Transverse horizontal insertion along the mentolabial groove towards Jiachengjiang.

Actions and indications

CV 24 is an effective point to treat *various disorders of the region, including: facial paralysis,* deviation of the mouth, facial pain, trigeminal neuralgia, swelling of the face, and *disorders of the gums,*

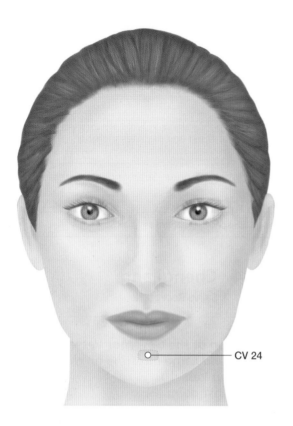

CV 24

salivary glands and teeth. Clears and brightens the eyes.

Additionally, CV 24 is an *important beauty point to improve appearance*. Needling horizontally into, or applying pressure across, the wrinkle of the mentolabial groove is effective.

CV 24 helps *release tension* from the entire chin area and cheeks. It is also a useful point to *clear heat from the face* and treat acne, distended capillaries and red blotchy skin.

> **Main Areas**—Chin. Face.
> **Main Functions**—Dispels wind and clears heat. Treats paralysis. Alleviates pain. Improves appearance.

Points of the Governor Vessel

(Alternative names: 'Du Mai', 'Governing Vessel')

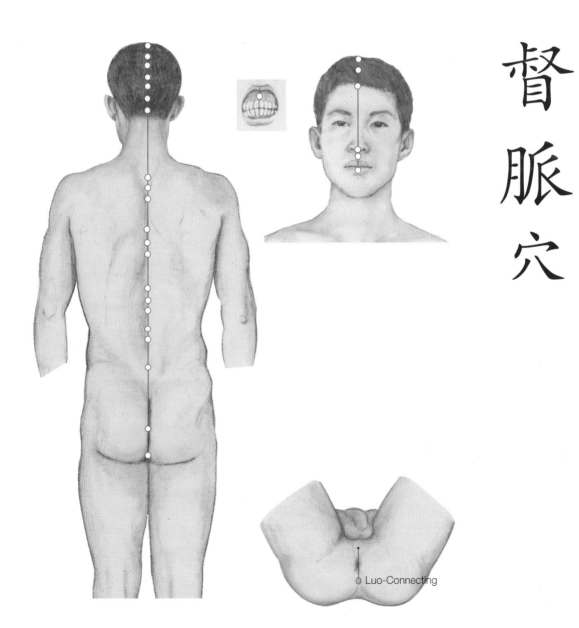

○ Luo-Connecting

督
脈
穴

General	The Governor Vessel is one of the eight Extra Meridians (or Extraordinary Meridians). It is commonly used in practice and often appears, as it does in this book, in the section containing the twelve main meridians. Its paired meridian is the Conception Vessel, and it has 28 points. The Governor Vessel is considered very Yang in its actions and the Conception Vessel very Yin. The pair create a balance around the whole body, from the perineum all the way through to the mouth, with one channel going up the anterior aspect of the body and the other, the posterior. Both channels are said to start from the region between the kidneys, and pass downwards to the perineum. GV 1 starts on the perineum, and the channel ascends the posterior surface of the body, straight up the midline, over the spinous processes of the coccyx, sacrum and all vertebrae. At the skull it continues in the midline to the apex of the head, at GV 20, and then forwards, between the eyebrows, over the nose and down over the upper lip. It finishes inside the mouth, on the inside of the upper lip.
More specifically	Historically, and in energetic terms, an individual's Qi begins in the region between the Kidneys, Ming Men, and travels downwards to the perineum, where it splits into the Conception Vessel and the Governor Vessel. GV 1 starts on the perineum, posterior to the anus, although both CV and GV channels are said to initially emerge at GV 1. The channel then travels posteriorly over the coccyx and midline of the sacrum, and up the midline through the spine, emerging at the skull at GV 16. From here the main pathway continues over the head to the apex at GV 20, but a branch also travels from GV 16 to meet at GV 20, but passes internally through the 'Sea of Marrow' – which is the brain. A further branch from GV 16 is said to descend to the Kidneys, passing through the inner Bladder point of BL 12. Much like the Conception Vessel having an aspect that travels up the posterior of the body, the Governor Vessel has a path that travels up the anterior. This shows how integrally linked these two channels are, and how Yin energy flows into Yang and vice versa. The main channel descends over the face in the midline, from GV 20, and passes over the philtrum of the upper lip, finishing inside the mouth under the top lip, at GV 28.
Area covered	Pelvis, rectal area, all spinal areas, all viscera through the SNS, skull, head, neck and brain.
Areas affected by treatment	Pelvic floor, gastroenterology in terms of lower bowel activity, *all* forms of back pain from coccydynia through to cervicogenic headaches, heat/inflammatory-based conditions – especially spinal, cognition and mental function, spirit and mental health, stress.
Key points	GV 2, GV 3, GV 4, GV 8, GV 10, GV 11, GV 14, GV 16, GV 20, GV 26.

Note: The GV points from GV 3 to GV 14 all follow the individual's spinal anatomy, and, as they are situated in the spaces between the spinous processes, they may be more obliquely superior in some places (notably around T5 and T6), and more upright in others (notably around the lumbar spine and T9 and T10).

GV 1   Changqiang   長強
Long and Strong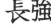

Luo-Connecting point of the Governor Vessel
Intersection of the Kidney, Gallbladder and Conception Vessel on the Governor Vessel

Myotome	None – superficial fascia
Dermatome	S4

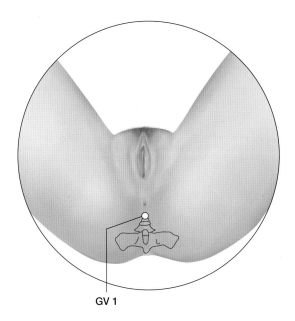

GV 1

Location
Midway between the tip of the coccyx and the anus.

Needling
0.5 to 1 cun perpendicular or upward oblique insertion.

Do not needle deeper or at a different angle.

Actions and indications
GV 1 is primarily used for *disorders of the anus and rectum*, including: haemorrhoids, diarrhoea, blood in the stools, constipation, rectal pain, and prolapse.

It also *regulates the spine and tonifies the Yang of the whole body* and can be used to treat: pain or swelling of the coccyx, lumbar pain, spermatorrhoea, and painful or turbid urination.

GV 1 has also been *traditionally used to calm and clear the mind* and treat spasm and epilepsy. It is an important *focus point for energy circulation* in Qigong practices.

> **Main Areas**—Anus. Coccyx. Spine.
> **Main Functions**—Benefits the anus and rectum. Regulates Qi and alleviates pain. Benefits the spine.

GV 2   Yaoshu   腰俞
Lumbar Shu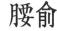

Myotome	None – superficial fascia
Dermatome	S3

Location
Located on the posterior midline, at the sacro-coccygeal hiatus.

To aid location, slide fingertip downward across the midline of the sacrum. The finger should naturally slip into the noticeable depression of the sacrococcygeal hiatus (inferior to the spinous process of the fourth sacral vertebra).

Needling
0.3 to 1 cun perpendicular or transverse-oblique superior insertion.

Actions and indications
GV 2 helps to *move Qi and Blood, dispel wind and dampness and alleviate pain from the channel pathway.*

It is of particular benefit to the *sacrum, lumbar region and legs*. It is also useful in the treatment of rectal pain, diarrhoea, dysuria and rectal prolapse, in common with GV 1.

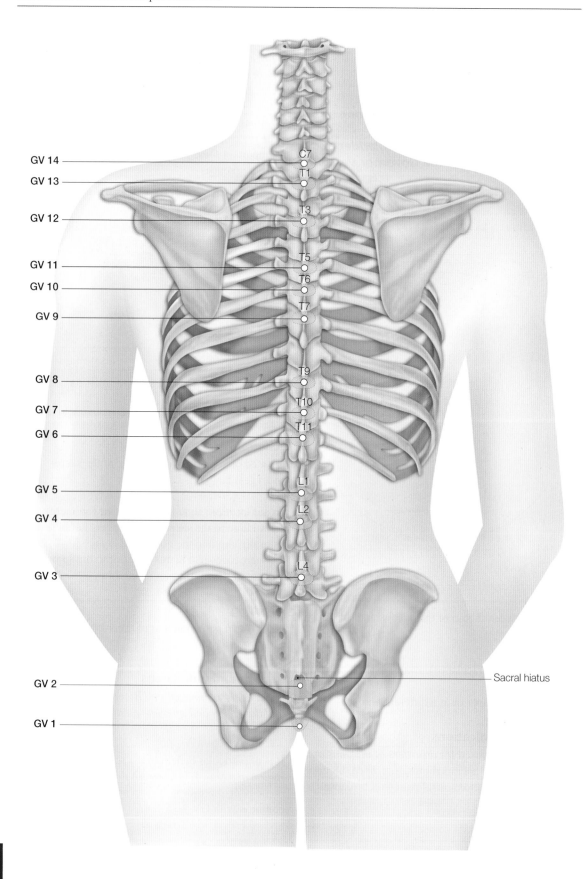

GV 14 — C7
GV 13 — T1
GV 12 — T3
GV 11 — T5
GV 10 — T6
GV 9 — T7
GV 8 — T9
GV 7 — T10
GV 6 — T11
GV 5 — L1
GV 4 — L2
GV 3 — L4
GV 2 — Sacral hiatus
GV 1

It is also mentioned as one of the *Seven Points for Draining Heat from the Extremities,* alongside LU 2, LI 15 and BL 40.

> **Main Areas**—Sacrum. Coccyx. Lumbar spine.
> **Main Functions**—Regulates Qi and Blood. Alleviates pain. Benefits the spine.

GV 3   Yaoyangguan 腰陽關
Yang Lumbar Gate

Myotome	None – superficial fascia
Dermatome	T12/L1

Location
On the posterior midline, below the spinous process of L4.

Note: To aid in understanding its location and function, GV 3 is level with the Large Intestine back-shu point (BL 25).

Needling
0.5 to 1 cun perpendicular insertion.

Actions and indications
GV 3 can be used to *dispel cold and regulate the lower jiao, benefit the lumbar region and legs,* and treat *disorders of the urogenital and gynaecological systems.*

Indications include: pain, weakness or paralysis of the lower limbs, lumbar pain, dysuria, urinary tract infections, diarrhoea, irregular menstruation, leucorrhoea, infertility, premature ejaculation, and impotence.

> **Main Areas**—Lumbar area. Spine. Lower limbs. Urogenital system. Uterus.
> **Main Functions**—Dispels dampness, heat and cold. Benefits the genitourinary system.

GV 4   Mingmen 命門
Life Gate

Myotome	None – superficial fascia
Dermatome	T9–T12

Location
On the posterior midline, below the spinous process of L2.

Note: To aid in understanding its location and function, GV 4 is level with the Kidney back-shu point (BL 23).

Needling
0.4 to 1 cun perpendicular insertion between the spinous processes of L2 and L3. The needle follows the angle defined by the shape of the spinous processes in a slightly superior direction.

Do NOT needle deeply. The needle should rest in or above the supraspinal ligament.

Actions and indications
GV 4 is one of the most *powerful points to tonify the Kidney Jing and Kidney Yang,* because of its location at the *Life Gate* (also known as the *Gate of Vitality*). For these purposes, moxibustion is the treatment of choice.

Indications include: chronic lumbar pain, stiffness of the spine, tinnitus, poor memory, chronic tiredness, debility, chronic conditions in general, premature ageing, irregular menstruation, amenorrhoea, leucorrhoea, abnormal uterine bleeding, infertility, impotence, premature ejaculation, spermatorrhoea, dysuria, incontinence, abdominal pain, haemorrhoids, diarrhoea, and prolapse of the rectum.

GV 4 is also important to *clear heat of interior, exterior, excess or deficient nature.* It treats such disorders such as steaming bone syndrome, (inflammatory bone disease), fevers, headaches, and epilepsy.

GV 4 is an *important focus point for energy circulation* in the Governor Vessel in Qigong practices.

> **Main Areas**—Lumbar area. Spine. Lower limbs. Urogenital system. Uterus. Entire body.
> **Main Functions**—Tonifies Kidney jing and Kidney Yang. Dispels cold and dampness. Alleviates pain. Clears heat. Benefits the lower jiao and genitourinary system. Increases fertility and vitality. Treats chronic diseases.

GV 5 Xuanshu

Suspended Pivot

Myotome	None – superficial fascia
Dermatome	T9–T12

Location
On the posterior midline, below the spinous process of L1.

Note: To aid in understanding its location and function, GV 5 is level with the Triple Energizer back-shu point (BL 22).

Needling
0.4 to 1 cun perpendicular insertion following the space between L1 and L2.

Actions and indications
GV 5 is used to *strengthen the Spleen and benefit the lumbar spine and the lower jiao.*

Symptoms include: abdominal distension, diarrhoea, undigested food in the stools, rectal prolapse, and pain or stiffness of the lumbar spine.

> **Main Areas**—Lumbar area. Spine.
> **Main Functions**—Strengthens the lumbar area. Alleviates pain. Boosts Spleen Qi and harmonises the Stomach.

GV 6 Jizhong

Spine Centre

Myotome	None – superficial fascia
Dermatome	T8–T11

Location
On the posterior midline, below the spinous process of T11.

Note: To aid in understanding its location and function, GV 6 is level with the Spleen back-shu point (BL 20).

Needling
0.4 to 1 cun perpendicular insertion following the space between T11 and T12.

Actions and indications
GV 6 can be used to *strengthen the Spleen, drain dampness and benefit the spine.*

Symptoms include: diarrhoea, jaundice, abdominal distension or pain, anorexia, epilepsy, and disorders of the spine, including pain and stiffness.

> **Main Areas**—Spine. Middle jiao.
> **Main Functions**—Strengthens the spine and alleviates pain. Boosts Spleen Qi.

GV 7 Zhongshu

Middle Spine Pivot

Myotome	None – superficial fascia
Dermatome	T8–T10

Location
On the posterior midline, below the spinous process of T10.

Note: To aid in understanding its location and function, GV 7 is level with the Gallbladder back-shu point (BL 19).

Needling

0.4 to 1 cun perpendicular insertion following the space between T10 and T11.

Actions and indications

Similar to GV 6 and BL 19.

> **Main Areas**—Spine. Stomach.
> **Main Functions**—Strengthens the spine. Alleviates pain.

GV 8   Jinsuo
Sinew Contraction

筋縮

Myotome	None – superficial fascia
Dermatome	T7–T9

Location

On the posterior midline, below the spinous process of T9.

Note: To aid in understanding its location and function, GV 8 is level with the Liver back-shu point (BL 18).

Needling

0.4 to 1 cun perpendicular insertion following the space between T9 and T10.

Actions and indications

The main actions of GV 8 are to *promote circulation of Liver Qi, calm the spirit, subdue wind and relieve spasm.*

Indications include: psychological disturbances, dizziness, epilepsy, fever, and spasm, stiffness or pain of the spine.

Combined with BL 18 bilaterally, this point gives a strong *anti-spasm effect for spinal musculature pain.*

> **Main Areas**—Spine. Liver.
> **Main Functions**—Relaxes the spine and alleviates pain. Regulates Liver Qi.

GV 9   Zhiyang
Reaching Yang

至陽

Myotome	None – superficial fascia
Dermatome	T6–T8

Location

On the posterior midline, below the spinous process of T7.

Note: To aid in understanding its location and function, GV 9 is level with the diaphragm back-shu point (BL 17).

Needling

0.5 to 1 cun perpendicular insertion between the spinous processes of T7 and T8. The needle follows the angle defined by the shape of the spinous processes in a slightly superior direction.

Actions and indications

GV 9 is an *important point to clear dampness and heat, particularly from the middle jiao*. It has been traditionally employed to treat *disorders of the Liver and Gallbladder*. Indications include: tightness, heaviness and pain of the chest, hypochondrium and abdomen, pain and swelling of the breasts, jaundice, nausea, dyspnoea, and cough.

GV 9 also *fortifies the Spleen* and treats generalised weakness and emaciation.

As a *local point*, GV 9 helps treat pain and stiffness of the spine.

> **Main Areas**—Spine. Diaphragm. Liver. Middle jiao.
> **Main Functions**—Clears dampness and heat. Regulates the Liver. Harmonises the middle jiao.

GV 10 Lingtai

Spirit Tower

Myotome	None – superficial fascia
Dermatome	T6

Location

On the posterior midline, below the spinous process of T6.

Note: To aid in understanding its location and function, GV 10 is level with the back-shu point for the Governor Vessel (BL 16).

Needling

0.4 to 1 cun perpendicular insertion following the space between T6 and T7.

Actions and indications

GV 10 can be of *benefit to the respiratory system and alleviate cough*. It has also been employed to *clear heat* and *detoxify poison* in the treatment of purulent boils (furuncles).

As a *local point*, it helps treat pain and stiffness of the spine. Combined with BL 16 bilaterally it is a strong combination for thoracic musculo-skeletal conditions.

Interestingly, T6 is the centre of the mobile joints of the spine, if you start at C1 and L5 and count in towards the middle. The region of T6 is also the area that *needs to be most mobile for the spinal cord*, as it is here that it is at its fattest within the spinal canal. *Lack of mobility here can lead to a lack of mobility in the rest of the spine, arms and also the emotions.* This is reflected in its name. This is due to the wide area of influence that the sympathetic chain has on the viscera through the sympathetic plexus that sits in front of the vertebrae in the thoracic column. There is a strong link between visceral feelings/ activities and emotional states with one feeding the other. A 'chicken and egg' situation.

Main Areas—Chest. Lungs. Spine. Spirit and Emotions.
Main Functions—Treats cough. Clears heat. Alleviates pain. Calms spirit. Frees emotions.

GV 11 Shendao

Shen Path

Myotome	None – superficial fascia
Dermatome	T5

Location

On the posterior midline, below the spinous process of T5.

Note: To aid in understanding its location and function, GV 11 is level with the Heart back-shu point (BL 15).

Needling

0.4 to 1 cun perpendicular insertion following the space between T5 and T6.

Actions and indications

The actions of GV 11 are primarily associated with *functions of the upper jiao organs and emotions*. As indicated in the name, the spiritual/ emotional way forwards can be influenced with the use of points in this region. It *strengthens the spirit*. Other indications include: dyspnoea, cough, asthma, depression, sadness, poor memory, fright palpitations, cardiac pain, epilepsy, and spasm.

As a *local point*, it helps treat pain and stiffness of the upper back and spine.

Main Areas—Chest. Heart. Spine.
Main Functions—Regulates upper jiao Qi. Calms the mind.

GV 12 Shenzhu
Body Pillar

身柱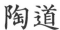

Myotome	None – superficial fascia
Dermatome	T2/T3

Location
On the posterior midline, below the spinous process of T3.

Note: To aid in understanding its location and function, GV 11 is level with the Lung back-shu point (BL 13).

Needling
0.4 to 1 cun perpendicular insertion following the space between T3 and T4.

Actions and indications
Similar to BL 13 and GV 11.

> **Main Areas**—Chest. Lungs. Spine.
> **Main Function**—Regulates upper jiao Qi.

GV 13 Taodao
Moulding Pathway

陶道

Intersection of the Bladder on the Governor Vessel

Myotome	None – superficial fascia
Dermatome	T1

Location
On the posterior midline, below the spinous process of T1.

Needling
0.4 to 1 cun perpendicular insertion following the space between T1 and T2.

Actions and indications
In common with adjacent Governor Vessel and Bladder channel points, GV 13 *releases the exterior, clears heat and alleviates cough*. It may be used as a *local point* to treat pain and stiffness of the upper back and neck.

> **Main Areas**—Chest. Lungs. Spine.
> **Main Function**—Regulates upper jiao Qi.

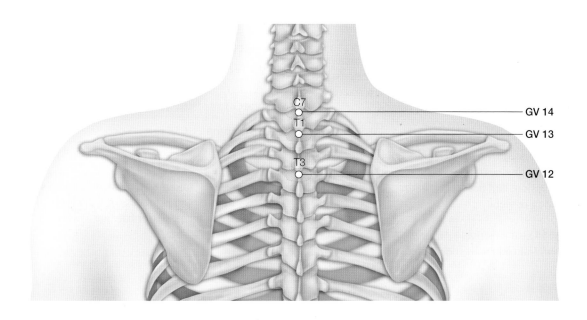

GV 14 Dazhui   大椎
Large Vertebra

*Intersection of all six Yang channels
on the Governor Vessel
Sea of Qi point*

Myotome	None – superficial fascia
Dermatome	C6–T1

Location
On the posterior midline, below the spinous process of C7.

Needling
0.5 to 1.2 cun perpendicular insertion between the spinous processes of C7 and T1. The needle follows the angle defined by the shape of the spinous processes, i.e. in a slightly superior direction.

Actions and indications
GV 14 is one of the *most important and commonly used points*. It is the intersection of all the Yang channels and is *important to regulate the movement of Yang Qi throughout the entire body*. It can *tonify or sedate the Yang Qi and regulates the ascending and descending of Yang Qi*.

It is *widely used to sedate excessive or rising Yang, subdue interior wind and clear heat*. Indications include: acute headache, migraine, high fever, convulsions, epilepsy, spasms, dizziness, hemiplegia, hypertension, tinnitus, pain and redness of the eyes, and redness of the face.

GV 14 can *help to lift the Yang Qi*, particularly when treated with moxibustion. Indications include: tiredness, poor concentration and memory, depression, dull headache, tinnitus, and diminished hearing or sight.

GV 14 also effectively *calms the Heart and the mind*. Indications include: palpitations, tachycardia, cardiac pain, tightness and pain of the chest, insomnia, mental restlessness, depression, and emotional disturbances.

GV 14 is *equally important to release the exterior* in cases of *wind heat and wind cold*. Symptoms include: chills and fever, runny nose, cough, and sore throat. It also *clears and tonifies the Lungs* and is useful to treat: asthma, wheeze, dyspnoea, shortness of breath, haemoptysis, and other symptoms of interior or chronic lung disease.

It is also a very important *local point* for *acute or chronic disorders of the cervical spine and upper back*. Symptoms include: pain and stiffness of the neck, upper back and shoulders, kyphosis, excessive protrusion of C7, stooped posture, and difficulty flexing the head and neck.

> **Main Areas**—Tai Yang area. Lungs. Chest. Heart. Mind. Cervical spine. Head.
> **Main Functions**—Regulates ascending and descending of Yang Qi. Clears heat. Subdues interior wind. Releases the exterior. Regulates Qi and Blood. Benefits the spine.

GV 15 Yamen
Gate of Muteness

*Intersection of the Yang Wei Mai
on the Governor Vessel
Sea of Qi point*

Myotome	None – superficial fascia
Dermatome	C3

Location
On the posterior midline, in the depression just superior to the spinous process of C2, approximately 0.5 cun within the posterior hairline.

To aid location, the spinous process of C2 is the first palpable spinous process below the external occipital protuberance.

Needling

0.3 to 0.5 cun obliquely in a caudal direction.

NEVER needle in a cephalad direction.

Actions and indications

GV 15 *dissipates wind of both exterior and interior origin* and is an important point to *open the sense organs* and *treat the back of the head, neck and brain*. It is particularly indicated for *disorders of the tongue*, including: paralysis, numbness, aphasia, and other speech disorders.

Other indications include: wind stroke, loss of consciousness, epilepsy, poor concentration and memory, heaviness of the head, deafness, headache, epistaxis, stiffness and pain of the neck, and degenerative disorders of the cervical spine.

> **Main Areas**—Tongue. Head. Spine.
> **Main Functions**—Subdues wind. Benefits the tongue. Opens the sense organs and benefits the brain.

GV 16 Fengfu
Wind Mansion

Intersection of the Yang Qiao Mai on the Governor Vessel
Sixth Ghost point
Sea of Marrow point
Window of the Sky point

Myotome	None – superficial fascia
Dermatome	C3

Location

Directly below the external occipital protuberance, in the depression between the attachments of the trapezius muscle, approximately 1 cun within the posterior hairline.

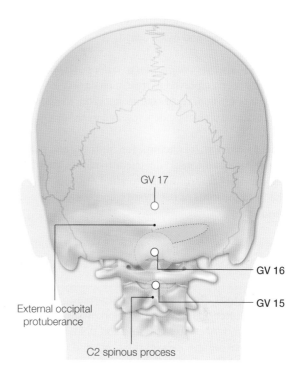

GV 17

GV 16

GV 15

External occipital protuberance

C2 spinous process

To aid location, palpate for the most tender spot which may be situated slightly further up or down the channel.

Needling

0.5 to 1 cun insertion, directed inferiorly. Do not apply strong manipulation.

Do NOT needle deeply or in a superior direction, because this poses considerable risk of injuring the spinal cord. Needling deeply in a superior direction may puncture the medulla oblongata, causing sudden death.

Actions and indications

GV 16 is a very important point for many *disorders of the head, brain and spine*. Its main functions are to *dispel exterior wind, descend excessive Yang, subdue interior wind and release spasm, clear the sense organs and nourish the Sea of Marrow (brain)*.

Indications include: sequelae of wind stroke, transient ischaemic attack, hemiplegia, numbness of the head and body, flaccidity or deviation of the tongue, aphasia, hypertension, dizziness, epilepsy, spasticity, vertigo, blurred or diminishing vision, headaches, epistaxis, tinnitus, sore throat, chills and fever, vomiting, and dyspnoea.

GV 16 is also very *important to calm the mind* and has been employed to treat such cases as: mental confusion, restlessness, agitation, insomnia, depression, suicidal tendencies, and even insanity.

As a *local point*, it is helpful for: stiffness and pain of the back of the neck, degenerative disorders of the cervical spine, difficulty rotating or bending the head forwards or backwards, and occipital headache.

It is an *important focus point for energy circulation* in the Governor Vessel in Qigong practices.

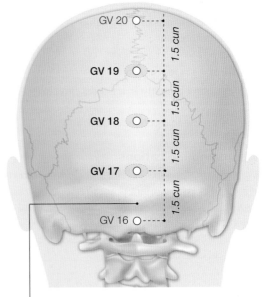

External occipital protuberance

Main Areas—Head. Brain. Sense organs. Spine.
Main Functions—Dissipates wind. Regulates Qi and Blood. Alleviates stiffness and pain. Clears the sense organs. Relaxes the body and calms the mind. Balances the nervous system.

GV 17   Naohu 腦戶

Cranium Door

---

*Intersection of the Bladder
on the Governor Vessel*

Myotome	None – superficial fascia
Dermatome	C2

Location
On the posterior midline, in the shallow depression directly superior to the external occipital protuberance, 1.5 cun superior to GV 16.

To aid location, GV 17 is one quarter of the distance from GV 16 to GV 20. Alternatively locate it further down towards the tip of the protuberance or slightly to the side.

Needling
0.1 to 0.3 cun perpendicular insertion.
0.3 to 1 cun transverse insertion upward or downward along the course of the channel.

A number of classical texts caution that needling GV 17 deeply will cause instant death. It is also known as the 'Kiss of the Dragon' point.

Actions and indications
Although GV 17 is not a very commonly used point, it can be useful to *dissipate wind, clear heat, clear the sense organs and benefit the eyes, regulate Qi and Blood, and alleviate pain.*

Indications include: headache, chills and fever, stiffness and pain of the neck, diminishing vision. redness and pain of the eyes, and excessive lacrimation.

GV 17 helps *clear and calm the mind* in cases of dizziness, epilepsy, depression, anxiety and insomnia.

Main Areas—Head. Sense organs.
Main Functions—Dispels wind. Clears heat. Calms the mind.

GV 18 Qiangjian
Unyielding Space

Myotome	None – superficial fascia
Dermatome	C2

Location
On the posterior midline, 1.5 cun directly superior to GV 17.

To aid location, GV 18 is halfway between GV 16 and GV 20.

Needling
0.3 to 0.8 cun subcutaneously in the direction of the channel.

Actions and indications
Similar to GV 17. GV 18 is not a commonly used point but it can be helpful in headaches and is generally indicated for disorders of the head and brain.

> **Main Areas**—Back of head. Brain.
> **Main Functions**—Sedates wind. Clears heat. Calms the mind.

GV 19 Houding
Behind the Vertex,
Behind the Crown

Myotome	None – superficial fascia
Dermatome	C2

Location
On the posterior midline, 1.5 cun directly inferior to GV 20.

Needling
0.3 to 0.8 cun subcutaneously in the direction of the channel.

Actions and indications
Headaches, high blood pressure. Helpful in *emotional stress states* giving rise to *headaches*.

> **Main Areas**—Head, Brain.
> **Main Functions**—Dispels wind. Clears heat.

GV 20 Baihui
One Hundred Convergences,
One Hundred Meetings

Intersection of the Bladder, Gallbladder, Triple Energizer and Liver channels on the Governor Vessel
Sea of Marrow point

Myotome	None – superficial fascia
Dermatome	C2

Location
At the vertex of the head, on the mid-sagittal line, 7 cun superior to the posterior hairline, 5 cun posterior to the ideal anterior hairline, at the midpoint of the line connecting the apex of the two ears (fold the ear forwards carefully to find the apex precisely).

According to classical sources, it is situated 'in a depression as large as the tip of the finger'.

Needling
0.3 to 1 cun transverse insertion posteriorly or anteriorly along the course of the channel.

Actions and indications
GV 20 is a *very important and dynamic point*. It is considered the *most Yang point of the body* (in this respect it is opposite to CV 1 and KI 1) and has the function of *descending excessive Yang and subduing interior wind*. It is very *important to clear the head and sense organs and also to calm the mind*.

Indications include: headache, pain at the vertex, heavy sensation in the head, dizziness, vertigo, wind stroke, loss of consciousness, numbness of the head and body, transient ischaemic attack, hemiplegia, spasticity, clenched jaw, hypertension, palpitations, feeling of heat, redness of the face, deafness, tinnitus, epistaxis, loss of sense of smell or taste, eye pain, blurred or diminishing vision,

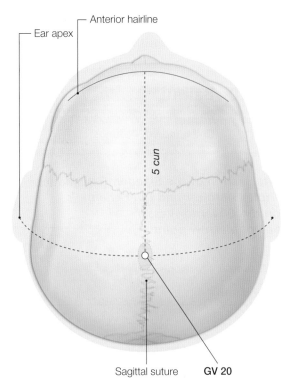

Ear apex
Anterior hairline
5 cun
Sagittal suture   GV 20

GV 21   Qianding

In Front of the Vertex

前頂

Myotome	None – superficial fascia
Dermatome	C2

Location
On top of the head, 1.5 cun anterior to GV 20.

Needling
0.3 to 0.8 cun subcutaneously in the direction of the channel.

Actions and indications
Similar to GV 20. Although GV 21 is not a very commonly used point, as GV 20 is used in preference, it can be helpful for headaches and is generally indicated for disorders of the head and brain. Traditionally it is also indicated for epilepsy and convulsions.

> **Main Areas**—Head. Brain.
> **Main Functions**—Sedates wind. Calms the mind. Alleviates pain.

blindness, epilepsy, sadness, fright, mental agitation, depression, and even insanity.

Additionally, GV 20 is *extensively employed to raise sinking Qi, increase Yang and benefit the Sea of Marrow.* Indications include: prolapse of the uterus, rectum or other organs, haemorrhoids, chronic diarrhoea, hypotension, *poor memory and concentration, and mental exhaustion.*

GV 20 is extensively employed in beauty treatment protocols to aid the raising of Qi and to help 'lift' flaccid areas. Also, moxibustion at GV 20 helps bring the colour back to a pale face.

GV 20 is also an important point of focus for vertically aligning the posture during Qigong practices and the Alexander technique uses this point as a focus.

> **Main Areas**—Head. Sense organs. Rectum. Uterus. Entire body.
> **Main Functions**—Descends excessive Yang and subdues wind. Lifts sinking Qi. Clears the head and sense organs. Calms the mind.

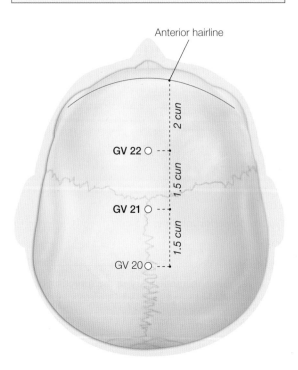

Anterior hairline
GV 22
GV 21
GV 20
2 cun
1.5 cun
1.5 cun

GV 22 Xinhui
Fontanelle Meeting

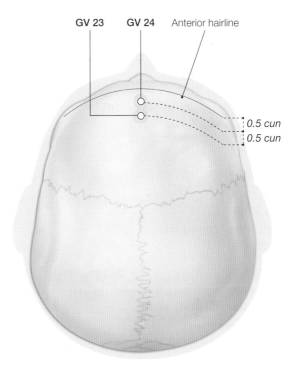

Myotome	None – superficial fascia
Dermatome	C2, trigeminal nerve

Location
On top of the head, 2 cun posterior to the anterior hairline.

Needling
0.3 to 0.8 cun subcutaneously in the direction of the channel.

Actions and indications
Similar to GV 21 and GV 23.

In common with GV 23, GV 22 has an effect on the nose, and is traditionally indicated for various associated symptoms including nasal discharge, blocked nose, poor sense of smell, and nosebleeds.

> **Main Areas**—Top of head. Nose. Brain.
> **Main Functions**—Benefits the nose. Alleviates pain. Sedates wind. Calms the mind.

GV 23 Shangxing
Upper Star

Tenth Ghost point

Myotome	None – superficial fascia
Dermatome	Trigeminal nerve

Location
On the mid-sagittal line, 1 cun posterior to the anterior hairline.

To aid location if the hairline has receded, this point is normally 4 cun superior to the eyebrows or the glabella. (3 cun from the eyebrows/ glabella gives the position of the ideal anterior hairline).

Needling
0.3 to 0.8 cun subcutaneously in the direction of the channel.

Actions and indications
GV 23 is an *important and widely used point for many disorders of the nose*. Its functions include *dissipating wind, reducing swelling, clearing heat, arresting bleeding*, and *clearing the head and face*.

Indications include: nasal obstruction or discharge, rhinitis, sinusitis, epistaxis, loss of sense of smell, headache, dizziness, diminishing vision, eye pain, and swelling or redness of the face.

GV 23 has also been employed to *calm the mind* and treat such cases as epilepsy, depression, and even insanity.

> **Main Areas**—Nose. Eyes. Face. Forehead.
> **Main Functions**—Dispels wind. Clears heat. Opens the nose. Clears the face and eyes. Calms the mind.

GV 24 Shenting

Shen Court

神庭

Intersection of the Bladder and Stomach on the Governor Vessel

Myotome	None – superficial fascia
Dermatome	Trigeminal nerve

Location

On the mid-sagittal line, 0.5 cun within the anterior hairline.

To aid location, the hairline is normally 3 cun superior to the eyebrows (or the glabella).

Needling

0.3 to 0.8 cun subcutaneously in the direction of the channel.

Actions and indications

GV 24 is an important point to *descend rising Yang, subdue interior wind, clear the head and calm the mind.*

Indications include: blocked or runny nose, epistaxis, eye pain, excessive lacrimation, chills and fever, headaches, vomiting, dizziness, wind stroke, hemiplegia, epilepsy, loss of consciousness, insomnia, depression, fright, and even insanity.

> **Main Areas**—Head. Mind. Nose. Eyes.
> **Main Functions**—Descends rising Yang and subdues wind. Calms the mind. Clears the face and eyes.

GV 25 Suliao

White Bone Hole

素髎

Myotome	None – superficial fascia
Dermatome	Trigeminal nerve

Location

At the tip of the nose, in the small depression between the two greater alar cartilages.

GV 25 is a sensitive location.

Needling

0.1 to 0.4 cun perpendicular insertion between the greater alar cartilages.
0.5 cun upward transverse insertion.
Prick to bleed.

Actions and indications

GV 25 is a *very dynamic and effective point to clear the sense organs, awaken the mind* and *restore consciousness.*

It *stimulates the lungs and breathing*, and effectively aids the body in the *detoxification process*. It is used extensively in smoking *cessation prescriptions* and is also indicated to *detoxify the blood, particularly following alcohol consumption.*

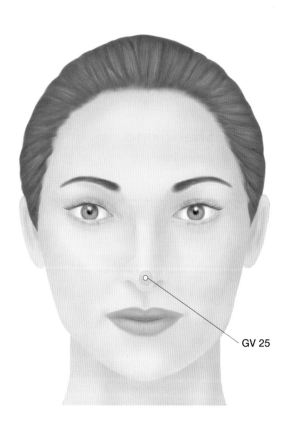

GV 25

GV 25 is very effective to *dissipate wind, clear heat and dispel stasis from the face*, and is particularly indicated to *open the nose and brighten the eyes*.

Indications include: acute or chronic disorders of the nose, epistaxis, nasal obstruction, polyps, loss of sense of smell, rhinitis, redness or swelling of the nose, dyspnoea, excessive lacrimation, and dryness, inflammation or swelling of the eyes.

GV 25 also effectively revives Yang, restores Qi and *powerfully stimulates the mind*.

Indications include: hypotension, palpitations, loss of consciousness, and other manifestations of shock. Although GV 26 and not GV 25 is categorised as the command point for the Consciousness, GV 25 may be equally, if not more, effective.

> **Main Areas**—Nose. Lungs. Eyes. Mind.
> **Main Functions**—Benefits the nose. Clears the face and eyes. Revives Yang, stimulates the mind and restores consciousness.

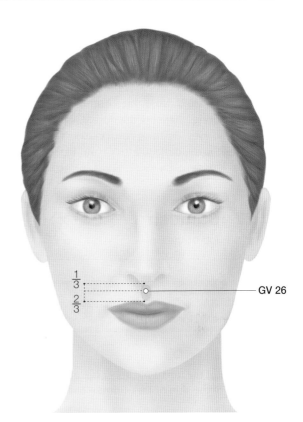

GV 26 Shuigou
Philtrum/Person Centre

水溝

Intersection of the Large Intestine and Stomach on the Governor Vessel
First Ghost point

Myotome	Facial nerve
Dermatome	Trigeminal nerve

Location
On the anterior midline, below the nose, approximately one third of the distance between the bottom of the nose and the top of the lip, a little above the midpoint of the philtrum. Situated in the orbicularis oris muscle.

Needling
0.2 to 0.3 perpendicular insertion.
0.2 to 0.4 upward oblique insertion.

Actions and indications
GV 26 is a *dynamic and important point to clear the face and nose, dissipate wind, clear heat, open the sense organs* and *restore consciousness*.

Indications include: loss of consciousness, (It is a point used to assess a patients *capacity to respond to painful stimuli*, if they are unconscious, by pinching or pressing this point with fingers), wind stroke, coma, spasticity, epilepsy, epistaxis, loss of sense of smell, runny nose, facial paralysis, deviation of the mouth, swelling of the face, thirst, halitosis, chills and fever, hypertension, depression, psychological disorders, hysteria, and even insanity.

Since GV 26 *strongly activates the Governor Vessel*, it is also effective for *disorders of the spine*, and is especially indicated for *acute lower backache and injury to the spine. Traditionally, for acute low back pain, it should be needled with the patient in standing and endeavouring to move around whilst the needle is in situ.*

As a *local point*, GV 26 is *effective to improve the appearance* and can help treat swelling or twitching of the upper lip, flaccidity or excessive tightness of the orbicularis oris muscle, and wrinkles of the upper lip.

> **Main Areas**—Mind. Nose. Face. Lumbar Spine.
> **Main Functions**—Benefits the nose. Clears the face and eyes. Restores consciousness and stimulates the mind. Regulates Qi and Blood. Alleviates lumbar pain.

GV 27 Duiduan
Top of the Lip

Myotome	Facial nerve
Dermatome	Trigeminal nerve

Location
At the centre of the top of the upper lip, at the intersection of the skin of the philtrum and the lip.

Needling
0.2 to 0.3 cun superior oblique insertion.
0.2 to 0.6 cun superior transverse insertion towards GV 26.

Actions and indications
Due to the delicate location of this point, it is seldom used in clinical practice for its traditional indications which emphasize heat in the mouth along with its associated symptoms.

It can be very useful in cases of neuralgia and facial pain, herpes and other skin conditions affecting this area. See also GV 26.

GV 27 is extremely sensitive and needle insertion can be very painful here.

> **Main Areas**—Upper Lip. Supralabial area. Mouth. Mind.
> **Main Functions**—Clears heat. Regulates Qi and alleviates pain. Calms the mind.

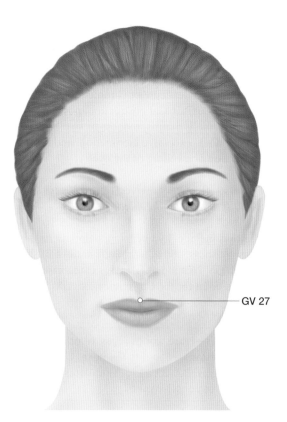

GV 27

GV 28 Yinjiao
Gum Intersection

Intersection of the Conception Vessel and Stomach on the Governor Vessel

Myotome	None
Dermatome	Trigeminal nerve

Location
Inside the mouth on the frenulum, at the junction of the upper lip and gum.

To aid location, the frenulum is the thin vertical band of tissue connecting the upper lip and gum at the midline.

Needling
0.1 to 0.3 cun superior oblique insertion.
Prick to bleed.

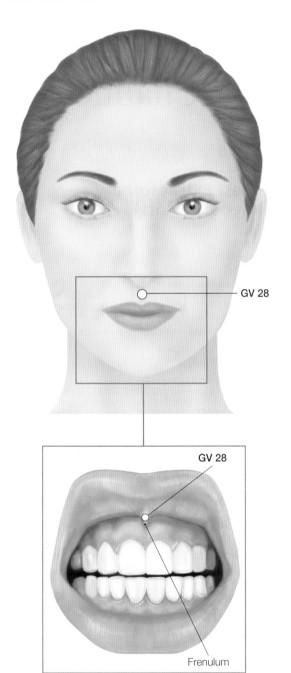

GV 28

GV 28

Frenulum

Actions and indications

GV 28 is primarily used to *clear heat* and treat *disorders of the gums and mouth*, although it also has a beneficial effect on the nose and eyes.

Indications include: acute inflammation of the gums, mouth ulcers, periodontitis, stomatitis, and disorders of the nose such as rhinitis and chronic nasal obstruction.

Main Areas—Gums. Mouth. Nose.
Main Functions—Benefits the gums. Clears heat.

22 Extra Non-Channel Points

(Alternative names: Extraordinary points, Miscellaneous points)

The Extra points (also known as 'Points outside the channels' or 'New Points') are points with special functions that do not belong to the main channel points, although some are situated on the path of one. For example, Yintang is on the Governor Vessel line but is not a specific GV point. Extra points have very specific actions, and many are extremely useful in clinical practice.

In terms of notation, when writing in clients' notes, it is preferable to use the *name* of the point instead of the numbering shorthand. The reason for this is that some texts may give a numerical status '1' for a particular Extra point, while others may give the same point the numerical status '3' – as has happened in the case of Yintang – a point between the eyebrows. In most texts, this point is referred to as 'Ex HN 3' (Extra Head Neck 3), but the author has come across at least two key texts that refer to it as 'Ex HN 1'.

To avoid any confusion, it is far better to use the name. There are also a lot of texts that do indeed use just the name and give no numerical status.

In general, the shorthand for notation in terms of indicating location is organised as shown below, as established by the World Health Organisation, and is the convention followed throughout this section:

HN – Head Neck
CA – Chest Abdomen
B – Back
UE – Upper Extremity
   (occasionally written as
AH – Arm Hand)
LE – Lower Extremity
   (occasionally written as
LF – Leg Foot)

Also, occasionally a text will use M as a prefix – meaning 'Miscellaneous'. For example, 'M HN 8' (Miscellaneous Head Neck 8) refers to Bitong, a point related to the nose; this could also be written as 'Ex HN 8' (Extra Head Neck 8). To reinforce the argument about discrepancies, this particular point can be found listed as 'M HN 14' in two texts, so you can imagine the potential confusion!

As well as giving the name, we will give the numerical listing found in the majority of texts and which is WHO accepted, and we will use 'Ex' as our prefix. Be aware, however, of the comment above about note-taking, and stick with the name – that never changes.

Extra Points of the Head and Neck (HN)

Ex HN 1 Sishencong 四神聰

Four Spirit Brightness,
Four Spiritual Alerts

Myotome	None – sited in galea aponeurotica of the cranium, so fascial
Dermatome	C2

Location
Four points either side of the vertex, 1 cun anterior, posterior and lateral to GV 20.

To aid location, GV 20 is 5 cun posterior to the ideal anterior hairline (and the ideal anterior hairline is 3 cun above the eyebrows/glabella).

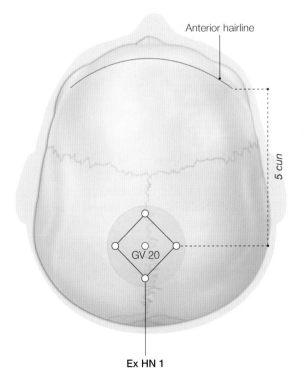

Anterior hairline

5 cun

GV 20

Ex HN 1

Needling
0.2 to 1 cun transverse insertion towards GV 20 (needle all four points). They will look like an inward tiara, pointing towards GV 20 at the centre.

Actions and indications
In common with GV 20, these four points are effective to *subdue interior wind, descend Yang, clear the ears, eyes and nose, and calm the mind.*

Indications include: headache, dizziness, vertigo, numbness, hemiplegia, wind stroke, aphasia, epilepsy, insomnia, depression, psychological disorders, poor memory, and disorders of the ears, eyes and nose such as epistaxis, tinnitus, and deafness.

They can be very useful for *learning difficulties, memory loss and lack of ability to concentrate.*

> **Main Areas**—Head. Mind.
> **Main Functions**—Clears the head and calms the mind. Subdues wind.

Ex HN 3 Yintang 印堂

Seal Hall

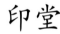

Myotome	Facial nerve
Dermatome	Trigeminal nerve

Location
At the glabella, midway between the eyebrows on the anterior midline. Situated in the procerus muscle.

Needling
0.3 to 0.7 cun oblique inferior insertion into the procerus muscle. You can pick up the muscle to insert the needle, although this is not mandatory. 0.4 to 1 cun oblique or transverse insertion medially towards BL 2 or BL 1.

Apply pressure to the point after removing the needle, because this can be a delayed bleeder.

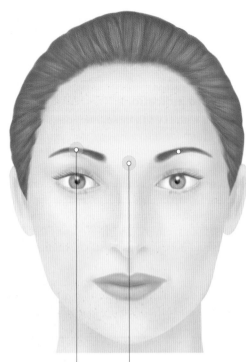

Ex HN 4   Ex HN 3

Actions and indications

Yintang is a *very important and extensively-used point to calm the mind* and *dispel wind, clear heat and alleviate pain from the face.* It effectively treats *disorders of the eyes, sinuses and nose.*

Indications include: anxiety, insomnia, depression, psycho-emotional disorders, hypertension, dizziness, epilepsy, frontal headache, tiredness and heaviness of the eyes, inflammation of the eyes, sinusitis, and disorders of the nose such as rhinitis and nasal congestion.

Yintang also helps *regulate the endocrine system* by stimulating the hypophysis and pineal gland, and can be used to treat hormonal imbalances.

Furthermore, it is a useful distal point for lumbar backache. Additionally, Yintang is an *important beauty point* for the area between the eyebrows.

Yintang can be used as a complementary point in many treatments, to draw the treatment together, or join the points.

Main Areas—Mind. Forehead. Eyes. Nose. Lumbar spine. Entire body.
Main Functions—Calms the mind and relaxes the body. Clears wind and heat from the face. Benefits the eyes and nose. Subdues wind. Complements the treatment.

Ex HN 4   Yuyao
Fish Waist

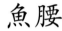

Myotome	Facial nerve
Dermatome	Trigeminal nerve

Location

In the depression at the centre of the eyebrow, directly above the pupil.

Needling

0.3 to 1 cun transverse insertion medially or laterally along the eyebrow. Pick up the skin to insert the needle into the muscle.

Apply pressure to the point after removing the needle.

Actions and indications

Yuyao is an excellent point to regulate *Qi, alleviate pain and benefit the eyes.*

Indications include: spasm of the eye muscles, flaccidity of the upper eyelid, paralysis of the orbicularis oculi muscle, inflammation and swelling of the eyes, frontal headache, migraine, facial pain, and trigeminal neuralgia.

Yuyao also has a calming effect on the mind, in common with Yintang (Ex HN 3).

Main Areas—Eyes. Forehead.
Main Functions—Regulates Qi and Blood. Alleviates pain and swelling. Benefits the eyes.

Ex HN 5　Taiyang
Sun (Supreme Yang)

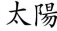

Myotome	Facial nerve
Dermatome	Trigeminal nerve

Location

In the depression of the temporal fossa, approximately 1 finger-breadth posterior to the midpoint between the outer canthus of the eye and the tip of the eyebrow.

It is sited in orbicularis oculi and may move up and down should the patient smile whilst it is in situ. At its posterior aspect, the edge of temporalis can be felt if the patient grits their teeth.

Needling

0.3 to 0.8 cun perpendicular insertion.
0.5 to 1.5 cun transverse posterior insertion.
0.5 to 1 cun oblique insertion.
Prick to bleed.

It is important to wait with palpation and ensure there is no pulse in this region.

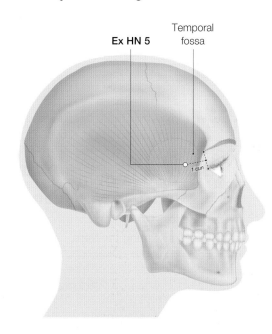

Ex HN 5　　Temporal fossa

1 cun

Do not puncture the branches of the zygomatico-orbital and superficial temporal artery. The pulse for these vessels should be felt more superficially towards the forehead.

Actions and indications

TaiYang is an *extremely useful and widely-used point* for temporal headache and disorders of the eyes. Its functions include: *regulating Qi and Blood, dissipating wind and clearing heat.*

Indications include: temporal headache, migraine, acute or chronic eye pain, redness, itching or swelling of the eyes, tired eyes, redness or swelling of the face, facial pain, trigeminal neuralgia, and facial paralysis.

> **Main Areas**—Temples. Eyes. Head.
> **Main Functions**—Regulates Qi and Blood. Alleviates pain and swelling. Benefits the eyes.

Ex HN 6　Erjian
Ear Apex

耳尖

Myotome	None – fascia of the ear
Dermatome	C2, trigeminal nerve

Location

At the apex of the ear. Fold the ear forwards to locate the apex precisely.

Needling

0.1 to 0.2 cun perpendicular insertion.
Prick to bleed (let two to five drops).

Actions and indications

Erjian is a *dynamic point to clear heat and descend rising Yang*. It also *soothes inflammation* and *dissipates swelling from the eyes and throat*. Furthermore, it has a *calming and pain-reducing effect*.

Indications include: high fever, hypertension, painful, inflamed eyes, sore, swollen throat, loss

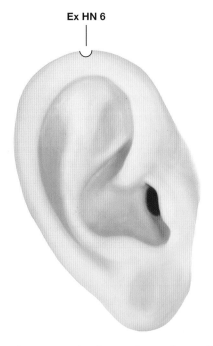

Ex HN 6

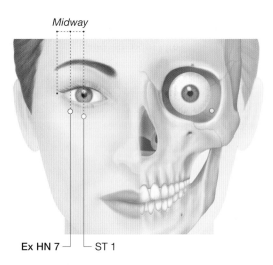

Midway

Ex HN 7 — └ ST 1

of consciousness, migraine, various pain conditions, and mental agitation.

> **Main Areas**—Eyes. Head. Liver. Entire body.
> **Main Functions**—Descends Yang and clears heat. Alleviates pain.

Ex HN 7 Qiuhou 球后
Behind the Eye Ball

Myotome	Facial nerve
Dermatome	Trigeminal nerve

Location
Between the eyeball and the infraorbital ridge, halfway between ST 1 and the lateral edge of the orbit.

Needling
0.5 to 1.2 cun perpendicular insertion, angled between the eyeball and the infraorbital ridge.

Support the eyeball with the tip of the finger and insert the needle slowly and carefully while the patient looks upward. Angle the needle slightly

downward and then perpendicularly along the inferior orbital wall under the eyeball. Do not manipulate the needle.

Qiuhou can bruise easily (see first aid for bruising for ST 1).

Qiuhou is one of the most sensitive and dangerous points to needle and therefore requires special skill and experience. Great care should be taken, as wrongly angled insertion can damage the eye. Use the thinnest needle possible.

Actions and indications
Benefits the eyes, in common with ST 1.

> **Main Area**—Eyes and area below.
> **Main Function**—Benefits the eyes and improves vision.

Ex HN 8 Bitong (also known as Shangyingxiang) 鼻通
Nose Passage
Penetrating the Nose

Myotome	Facial nerve
Dermatome	Trigeminal nerve

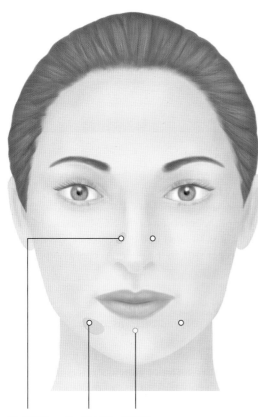

Ex HN 8   Ex HN 18   CV 24

Location

In the depression below the nasal bone, at the superior end of the nasolabial sulcus in the muscle nasalis.

Needling

0.3 to 0.5 cun transverse insertion towards the bridge of the nose.

Actions and indications

Bitong is an *important and widely-used point for disorders of the nose* and has similar functions to LI 20. It is especially indicated for: nasal congestion, rhinitis, sinusitis, nasal polyps, nasal discharge, and epistaxis.

Bitong also *soothes and clears the eyes*.

> **Main Area**—Nose.
> **Main Functions**—Clears wind and heat. Opens the nose.

Ex HN 14   Yiming
Clear Eyesight,
Dim Eyesight, Shielding Brightness

Myotome	C2/C3 and accessory nerve
Dermatome	C3

Location

Behind the ear lobe, 1 cun posterior to TE 17.

Needling

0.5 to 1 cun perpendicular insertion.

Actions and indications

Commonly used for *diseases of the eye*.

> **Main Areas**—Sub-occipital headaches. Eye conditions.
> **Main Function**—Clears and sharpens vision.

Ex HN 15   Bailao
Hundred Labours

Myotome	C5/C6
Dermatome	C3/C5

Location

With GV 14 as a marker, Bailao is 1 cun lateral and 2 cun superior of GV 14. It sits over C5/C6 facet joints, and is often sore due to the vast amount of neck musculature that attaches in this region.

Needling

0.5 to 1 cun obliquely inwards towards the spine.

Actions and indications

Useful for many cervico-thoracic neck problems, especially the more chronic kind where there may already be a poking chin and a forward hinge in the region of C6.

Main Areas—Mid to lower cervical spine, cervicogenic headaches.
Main Function—Reduces tension in lower cervical musculature.

Ex HN 18   Jiachengjiang 夾承漿
Adjacent to Saliva
Receptacle

Myotome	Facial nerve
Dermatome	Trigeminal nerve

Location
Approximately 1 cun lateral to CV 24, in the depression of the mental foramen.

To aid location, it is approximately below ST 4.

Needling
0.3 to 0.5 cun perpendicular insertion.
0.5 to 1.5 cun transverse insertion.

Actions and indications
Jiachengjiang is an *effective point to dissipate wind* and *regulates Qi and Blood* in the region.

Its main indications include: trigeminal neuralgia, facial pain, toothache, inflammation of the gums, deviation of the mouth, and facial paralysis.

Furthermore, it can be used to improve appearance in beauty treatments, in common with CV 24.

Main Areas—Mouth. Chin.
Main Functions—Regulates Qi and Blood. Dispels wind. Alleviates pain.

Ex HN 54   Anmian   安眠
Peaceful Sleep

Myotome	C1/C2, accessory nerve
Dermatome	C2/C3

Location
At the posterior border of the mastoid process, midway between GB 20 and TE 17, slightly posterior and superior to GB 12. Situated at the centre of the insertion of the SCM muscle. More deeply, it is situated in the splenius capitis muscle, and, deeper still, in the obliquus capitis superior muscle.

Needling
0.5 to 1 cun perpendicular insertion.

Do not puncture the branches of the great auricular nerve and the posterior auricular artery and vein. Needling deeply poses a risk of puncturing the

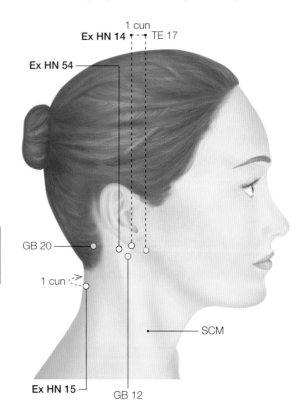

occipital artery and vein, and, posteromedially, in its deep position, the vertebral artery and vein.

Actions and indications

In common with adjacent points such as GB 12 and GB 20, Anmian *promotes relaxation by soothing Liver Qi and is extensively used to treat insomnia.* It also *clears heat and dispels wind from the head.* Indications include: mental restlessness, pain conditions, depression, dizziness, vertigo, migraine, hypertension, epilepsy, and tinnitus.

Furthermore, Anmian *clears the eyes and improves vision.*

> **Main Areas**—Mind. Head. Eyes.
> **Main Functions**—Promotes relaxation and sleep. Regulates Liver Qi. Benefits the eyes.

Extra Points of the Back (B)

Ex B 1A   Chuanxi
Gasping

Myotome	C7–T1
Dermatome	C5–T1

Ex B 1B   Dingchuan
Relieve Dyspnoea, Stop Wheezing

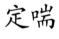

Myotome	C7–T1
Dermatome	C5–T1

Location

Chuanxi is 1 cun lateral to GV 14, and *Dingchuan* 0.5 cun lateral to GV 14.

To aid location, palpate superficially and then deeply to determine the most reactive site(s).

Needling

0.5 to 1 cun medial oblique insertion towards GV 14.

Actions and indications

Both Chuanxi and Dingchuan are widely employed to treat a variety of breathing complaints, including: acute wheezing, dyspnoea, coughing, and asthma.

> **Main Areas**—Chest. Lungs. Neck. Upper back.
> **Main Function**—Benefits the breathing and alleviates coughing.

Paravertebral Points and Other Extra Points of the Back

Ex B 2   Huatuojiaji
Hua Tuo's Paravertebral Points

華佗夾脊

Myotome	Segmentally, via dorsal rami, at level of each point
Dermatome	From C3–L5

Location

In the paraspinal groove, approximately 0.5 cun lateral to the posterior midline. They may be located either level with the lower borders, or the tips of the spinous processes of the cervical, thoracic and lumbar vertebrae. Some sources place these points slightly more medially, whilst others more laterally, up to 1 cun from the posterior midline. In clinical practice however, they should always be treated at the most responsive sites that elicit the desired sensation (see note further down).

The points shown on the left are approximately level with the facet joints; those on the right are approximately over the spinal nerve roots emerging from the intervertebral foramina. Therefore, in general, the former are more effective for disorders of the vertebrae, and the latter are more effective to regulate the nervous system and for interior disorders and neurological conditions.

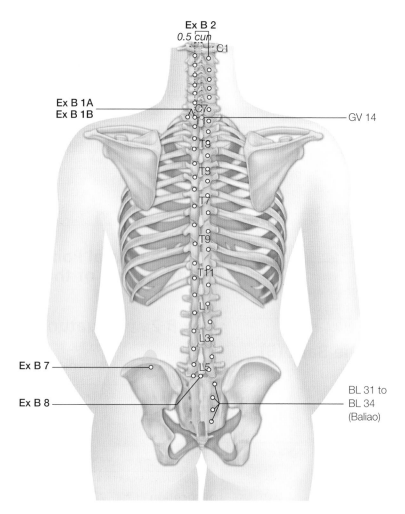

Ex B 2
0.5 cun
C1
Ex B 1A
Ex B 1B
C7
GV 14
T1
T2
T3
T4
T5
T6
T7
T8
T9
T10
T11
T12
L1
L2
L3
L4
Ex B 7
L5
BL 31 to
BL 34
(Baliao)
Ex B 8

Important note: Not only does the entire spine vary greatly from person to person, each vertebra is different and even the left and right spinal nerves emerging from each segment are not ever the same, even in the same person. Therefore, in order to correctly treat paraspinal points one must find the most reactive sites that elicit a specific reaction.

The term *Jiaji* or *Paravertebral points* was assigned to the seventeen pairs of points situated along the thoracic and lumbar spine by the renowned doctor *Hua Tuo* during the second century AD. This group of points has been expanded to include the points lateral to the seven cervical vertebrae, thus making twenty-four sets of points. Furthermore, the *Baliao* or *Eight Sacral Foramina points* (BL 31, BL 32, BL 33 and BL 34) can be considered part of the paravertebral point group.

Needling

0.5 to 1 cun oblique medial insertion towards the spine.
0.5 to 1 cun insertion at 10 degree angle toward midline in the cervical and thoracic regions.
Up to 2 cun perpendicular insertion in the lumbar and sacral spine.

Actions and indications

These dynamic points are *very important and extensively used in a wide range of disorders*. From a Chinese point of view, they are particularly *effective to dissipate Qi and Blood stasis, clear interior heat* and *regulate the internal organs*. They can be considered *alternative back-shu points*, whose functions they share.

374

They *effectively regulate the nervous system and are very useful in many disorders of the limbs and internal organs*. They are also *extensively employed to treat disorders of the spine* and *spinal nerves*, and are very useful in the *treatment of pain* (they are used in acupuncture anaesthesia). Furthermore, they calm the mind and induce physical relaxation. In terms of muscular access, the HTJ points will allow multifidus to be reached, which can be essential in effective treatment of chronic back pain in particular.

They are also the points of choice for conditions such as complex regional pain syndrome (previously RSI/complex upper limb working disorder/complex lower limb working disorder).

They have also been employed in a variety of severe stubborn diseases, including: aphasia, hemiplegia, paralysis, lupus erythematosus, ankylosing spondylitis, and multiple sclerosis.

Additionally, the paravertebral points are *useful diagnostically* both in terms of zangfu imbalance and in terms of spinal nerve or visceral referred pain.

> **Main Areas**—Entire body. Spine. Nervous system. Internal organs.
> **Main Functions**—Alleviates pain. Regulates the pertaining internal organs and the nervous system. Relaxes the body and mind.

Ex B 6 Yaoyi
Serving the Lumbar Region
腰宜

Myotome	Thoraco-lumbar fascia At depth QL T12/L1/L2
Dermatome	T12/L1

Location
3 cun lateral to the tip of the spinous process of L4. Often found in a dip where the thoraco-lumbar fascia is just attaching to the posterior iliac crest.

Needling
1 to 2 cun perpendicular. This point can be needled deeply because it has a multitude of layers of fascia to get through.

Actions and indications
This is an invaluable point for the treatment of *chronic back pain,* especially when the thoraco-lumbar fascia is tight and poorly nourished with lack of Blood and Qi flow. At depth, quadratus lumborum can be reached, which can be invaluable in the treatment of chronic lumbar back pain.

Ex B 7 Yaoyan
Lumbar Eyes
腰眼

Myotome	T8–L1, T12/L1
Dermatome	T10/T11

Location
At the centre of the wide depression inferior to the iliac crest, up to 4 cun lateral to the posterior midline, approximately level with GV 3 (below the spinous process of L4). Situated at the site of quadratus lumborum attachment onto the posterior iliac crest. This matches a known trigger point at this site that refers into the leg and buttock.

Some sources place this point below the iliac crest, which would site it in gluteus medius.

Needling
1 to 1.5 cun perpendicular insertion. To target the lower end of quadratus lumborum, the needle should be angled towards the sacrum.

Actions and indications
Yaoyan is an important point to strengthen the lumbar spine and reinforce the Kidneys. It also effectively *regulates Qi in the lower jiao and alleviates pain.*

Indications include: chronic or acute lower back pain, sciatica, irregular menstruation, and frequent urination.

> **Main Areas**—Lower back. Uterus. Urinary system.
> **Main Functions**—Alleviates pain. Regulates Qi in the lower jiao.

Ex B 8 Shiqizhui 十七椎

Seventeenth Vertebra

'Sneeze Point' (so named as to say it quickly sounds like a sneeze)

Myotome	None – superficial fascia
Dermatome	T12/L1

Location

On the posterior midline, in the lumbosacral joint, between the spinous process of L5 and S1.

Important note: In some cases L5 and S1 are fused, making it seem that there are six sacral vertebrae. In these cases use GV 3, between L4 and L5 instead.

Also, in about 7% of people there is a sixth lumbar vertebra, and in others, S1 is not fused with S2, making it appear there are six lumbar vertebrae. In these cases, palpate the points between the spinous processes of L5–L6 and L6–S1 or L5–S1 and S1–S2 to determine which are more reactive during pressure palpation.

Needling

0.5 to 1.5 cun perpendicular insertion into the space between L5 and S1. Only a very slight change of angle will miss the exact point that produces deqi extending outwards across the entire lower back reaching the abdomen.

Actions and indications

Shiqizhui is an invaluable point in the treatment of *acute or chronic lower back pain and weakness of the lumbosacral joint*, particularly when there is stenosis or disc compression between L5 and S1.

It is also widely-used to treat acute dysmenorrhoea and pelvic pain, and is also effective for pain relief during labour.

It has also been traditionally employed to *fortify the Kidneys* and *benefit the genitourinary system*.

> **Main Areas**—Lower back. Uterus. Urinary system.
> **Main Functions**—Alleviates pain. Regulates Qi in the lower jiao.

Extra Points of the Chest and Abdomen (CA)

Ex CA 1 Zigong (also known as Zhigong or Zigongxue) 子宫

Child's Palace

Myotome	T7–T12
Dermatome	T11/T12

Location

3 cun (one hand-width) lateral to CV 3, 4 cun below the umbilicus.

Needling

0.5 to 1.5 cun perpendicular insertion.

Actions and indications

Zigong is an *important point for disorders of the ovaries and uterus*, including: infertility, irregular menstruation, abnormal uterine bleeding, leucorrhoea, endometriosis, uterine prolapse, and abdominal pain.

> **Main Areas**—Uterus. Ovaries. Abdomen.
> **Main Functions**—Increases fertility. Regulates menstruation. Benefits the uterus.

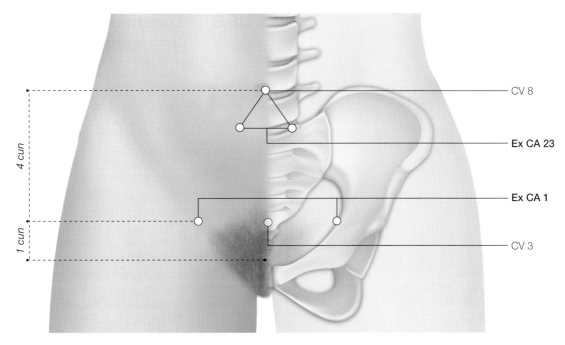

Ex CA 23   Sanjiaojiu   三角灸

Moxibustion

Triangle

Furthermore, it is recommended to treat the point on the left side for disorders of the right, and vice versa.

> **Main Areas**—Abdomen. Intestines.
> **Main Functions**—Regulates Qi. Alleviates pain. Stops diarrhoea.

Myotome	T7–T12
Dermatome	T10–T12

Location

Three points on each corner of an equilateral triangle, with the apex point at the navel (CV 8). The sides of the triangle are traditionally measured as equal to the width of the patient's smile.

Needling

No needling.
Moxibustion only as a regimen.

Actions and indications

These points *effectively regulate Qi in the abdomen, alleviate abdominal pain and stop diarrhoea.* They are also indicated to treat hernias and *symptoms of upsurging Qi* such as nausea and thoracic oppression. Functions somewhat similar to CV 8.

Extra Points of the Upper Extremity (UE)

Ex UE 7 Yaotongdian   腰痛點

Lumbar Pain Point

Myotome	C8/T1
Dermatome	C7/C8

Location

Three points on the dorsum of the hand, in the depressions between the second, third, fourth and fifth metacarpal bones. Approximately 1 cun distal to the transverse wrist crease, in the depressions just distal to the bases of the metacarpals.

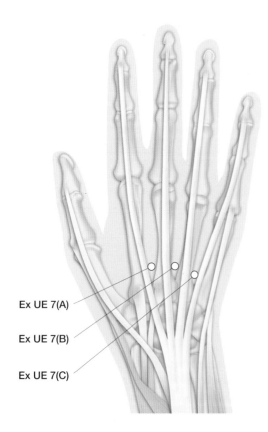

Ex UE 7(A)

Ex UE 7(B)

Ex UE 7(C)

To aid location, there are often one or more small palpable nodules in the region between the metacarpals. The best treatment site is usually at the most painful nodule.

Points (A) and (C) are more effective for stiffness or injury to the paraspinal muscles in the lower back and pain next to the spine, whereas the middle point (B) is more effective for pain on the spine itself.

Needling
0.5 to 1 cun perpendicular insertion.

Actions and indications
These points are very *effective to treat acute lower backache.*

Main Area—Lower back.
Main Functions—Regulates Qi and Blood. Alleviates stiffness and pain.

Ex UE 8   Luozhen
Stiff Neck (Outer PC 8)    落枕

Myotome	C8/T1
Dermatome	C7

Location
On the dorsum of the hand, between the second and third metacarpal bones, about 0.5 cun proximal to the MCP joints.

To aid location, it is at the site of most tenderness (often, there is a small palpable 'nodule' at the epicentre that can be very painful on pressure).

Also, if the patient makes a loose fist, the skin is stretched and a visible depression appears. Luozhen is usually at the epicentre of this depression.

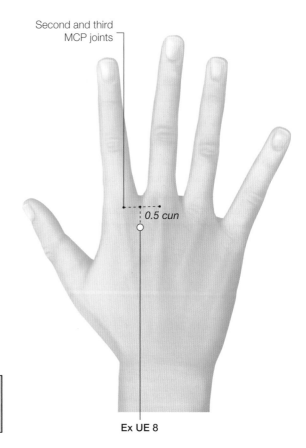

Second and third MCP joints

0.5 cun

Ex UE 8

Needling

0.3 to 1 cun perpendicular or oblique proximal insertion.

Actions and indications

Luozhen is a very dynamic and effective point to *release pain and stiffness of the neck and arm.*

> **Main Areas**—Neck. Upper limbs.
> **Main Functions**—Regulates Qi and Blood. Alleviates pain and stiffness.

Ex UE 9   Baxie   八邪
Eight Evils

Myotome	C8/T1
Dermatome	C7/C8

Location

Eight points on the webs between each of the fingers, distal to the MCP joints and approximately

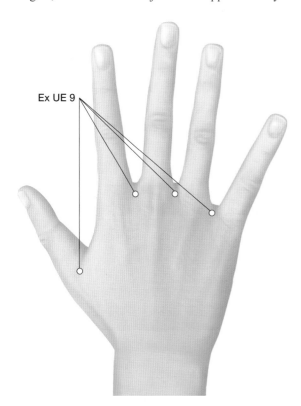

Ex UE 9

0.5 cun proximal to the margin of the webs. They are usually located and treated with the hand in a loose fist.

Needling

0.5 to 1 cun perpendicular insertion between the shafts of the metacarpal bones. Needle with the fingers relaxed in a loose fist.
Prick to bleed.

Actions and indications

These are important points for *disorders of the fingers and MCP joints*, including arthritis and injury, swelling, stiffness and contraction of the fingers.

They are also used to *clear heat* and treat headache, earache, toothache, sore throat, pain of the eyes and fever.

> **Main Areas**—Head. Redness of throat. Hand and Finger conditions.
> **Main Function**—Alleviates pain and stiffness of the hands and fingers.

Ex UE 10   Sifeng   四縫
Four Seams

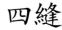

Myotome	None – superficial fascia
Dermatome	C7/C8

Location

Four points at the midpoint of the transverse creases of the proximal IP joints of the second to fifth fingers, on the palmar aspect of the hands.

Usually there are two main creases; these points are located at the deeper of the two creases, which is usually the proximal one.

To aid location, define the creases by flexing the fingers.

Needling

Most texts recommend pricking these points to draw a little blood or thin yellow fluid. However, acupressure and moxibustion can also be employed.

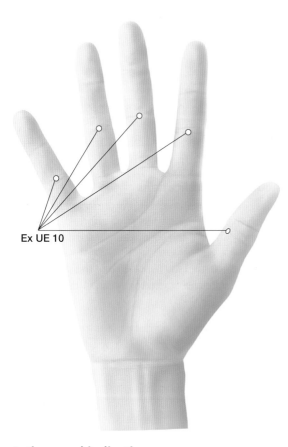

Ex UE 10

Ex UE 11   Shixuan

Ten Diffusions

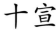

Myotome	None – superficial fascia
Dermatome	C7/C8

Location
Ten points at the tip of each finger, 0.1 cun from the centre of the free margin of the nail.

Needling
Most texts recommend pricking these points with a three-edged needle to draw a little blood, and then applying moxibustion.

However, shallow perpendicular needling, sustained pressure or strong tapping of the fingertips can also be effectively employed. Moxa pole therapy and rice-grain moxibustion can be useful.

Ex UE 11

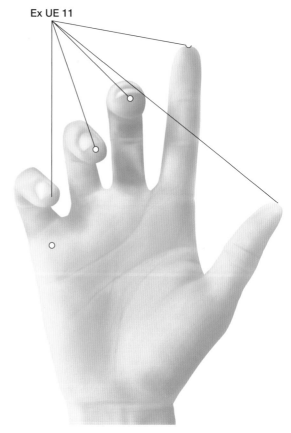

Actions and indications
These points are extensively used to treat a *wide range of paediatric disorders*, particularly in relation to *nutrition and the digestive system*. They *boost the middle jiao and Spleen*, helping *improve the transformation and transportation of food essences and body fluids, thus helping nourish the body* and *relieve accumulation and abdominal swelling*.

Indications include: eating disorders in children, malnutrition, emaciation, swelling and pain of the abdomen, diarrhoea, vomiting, food stagnation, lack of appetite, infantile colic and indigestion, and respiratory disorders such as coughing and asthma.

They effectively treat *pain and stiffness of the fingers*.

> **Main Areas**—Abdomen. Chest. Fingers.
> **Main Functions**—Boosts the middle jiao and tonifies the Spleen. Relieves accumulation.

Actions and indications

These points are *very dynamic* and have similar functions to the jing-well points, including: *clearing the sense organs, face, head and throat, restoring consciousness, dispelling exterior wind, clearing heat and subduing interior wind*. They are also *employed to treat children*.

Indications include: loss of consciousness, fainting, wind stroke, hypertension, heat stroke, high fever, seizures, infantile convulsions, acute pain or swelling of the throat, vomiting, and diarrhoea.

Additionally, these points can be useful to treat *numbness and pain of the fingers*.

Main Areas—Brain. Senses. Abdomen.
Main Functions—Restores consciousness. Subdues wind and stops seizures. Clears the brain and sense organs. Clears heat and dispels exterior wind.

Ex UE 48   Jianqian (also known as Jianneiling)   肩前

Front of the Shoulder

Myotome	C5/C6
Dermatome	C3/C4

Location

In the depression between the coracoid process and the head of the humerus, midway between the end of the anterior axillary fold and LI 15.

Usually, it is located with the arm hanging down freely at the sides. However, it is sometimes easier to find the tender point if the arm is abducted.

Needling

0.5 to 1 cun perpendicular insertion.
1 to 1.5 cun oblique inferior insertion.

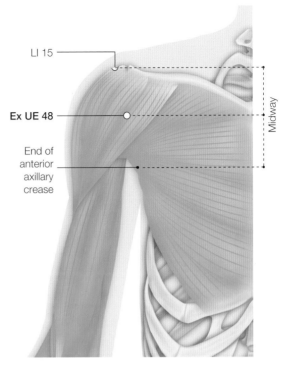

LI 15

Ex UE 48

End of anterior axillary crease

Midway

Do not puncture the supraclavicular nerve and, more deeply, the anterior humeral circumflex artery and vein.

Actions and indications

JianQian is a very useful point for chronic or acute stiffness and pain of the shoulder joint.

Main Areas—Shoulder. Upper arm.
Main Functions—Regulates Qi and Blood. Alleviates stiffness and pain.

Extra and New Points of the Lower Extremity (LE)

Ex LE 2   Heding   鶴頂

Crane's Summit

Myotome	None – in fascia of rectus femoris
Dermatome	L3

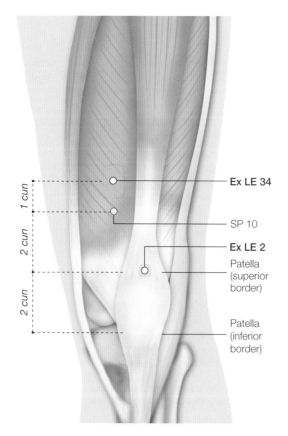

Ex LE 34

SP 10

Ex LE 2

Patella
(superior
border)

Patella
(inferior
border)

1 cun

2 cun

2 cun

Ex LE 5   Xiyan
Eyes of the Knee

膝眼

Myotome	None – sited over fat pads of knee
Dermatome	L3–L5 junction at knee

Location

A pair of points just below the patella, one in the medial and one in the lateral depression formed by the patellar ligament when the knee is flexed.

To aid location, these points are approximately one finger-width from the border of the patellar ligament.

The medial point is known as *Nei Xiyan, Ex LE 4 (Inner Eye of the Knee)*, and the lateral point, *Wai Xiyan (Outer Eye of the Knee)*, which is also called *Dubi (Calf's Nose)* or *ST 35.*

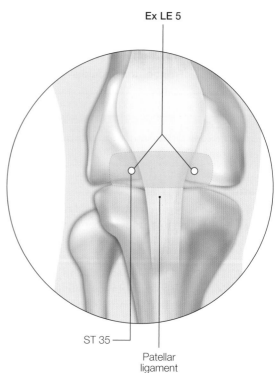

Ex LE 5

ST 35

Patellar
ligament

Location

In the small depression just above the midpoint of the superior border of the patella.

Needling

0.5 to 1 cun perpendicular or transverse insertion under the patella.

Actions and indications

Heding is an effective point for disorders of the knee and patella, including swelling, stiffness and pain.

Main Areas—Knees. Patella.
Main Function—Alleviates stiffness and pain.

Needling

1 to 2 cun perpendicular insertion, angled slightly medially, towards the centre of the knee joint, or BL 40.

1 to 2 cun oblique superior medial insertion under the patella.

Actions and indications

These points are *extremely helpful in many disorders of the knees,* including chronic or acute pain, stiffness and swelling. Stimulation of these points, particularly in their deep position (use needles or Qigong therapy), is *beneficial to the synovial cartilages and menisci* inside the knee joint and helps in cases of degenerative conditions and inflammation.

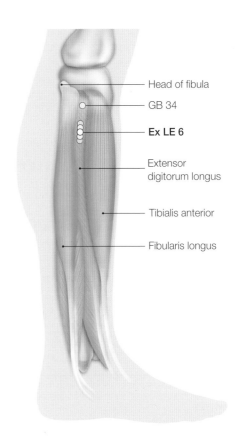

Head of fibula

GB 34

Ex LE 6

Extensor digitorum longus

Tibialis anterior

Fibularis longus

> **Main Areas**—Knees. Lower limbs.
> **Main Functions**—Regulates Qi and Blood. Alleviates stiffness, swelling and pain.

Ex LE 6 Dannangxue 膽囊穴
Gallbladder Point

Myotome	L4–S1
Dermatome	L5

Location

On the right leg, 1 to 2 cun distal to GB 34, at the most tender site on pressure palpation.

Needling

0.5 to 1.5 cun perpendicular insertion.

Actions and indications

Dannangxue is a *very important and extensively used point for many disorders of the gallbladder and bile duct* and is especially indicated for both acute and chronic cholelithiasis and cholecystitis.

It also treats such symptoms as nausea, poor digestion of fats, obesity, and pain of the hypochondrial area.

Dannangxue is *useful diagnostically,* because it often becomes tender in cases of gallbladder disharmony.

As a *local point,* it can be treated bilaterally in cases of pain, weakness or paralysis of the lower limbs.

> **Main Areas**—Gallbladder. Digestive system.
> **Main Functions**—Regulates Qi, dispels stasis and alleviates pain. Benefits the gallbladder.

Ex LE 7 Lanweixue 闌尾
Appendix Point

Myotome	L4–S1
Dermatome	L5

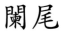

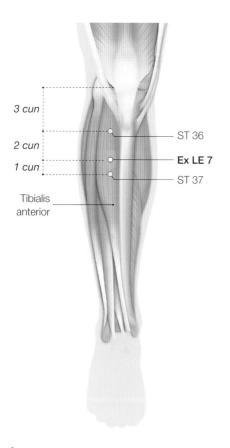

3 cun

2 cun

1 cun

ST 36

Ex LE 7

ST 37

Tibialis anterior

As a *local point*, it can be treated bilaterally, for cases of pain, weakness or paralysis of the lower limbs.

> **Main Areas**—Appendix. Large Intestine. Shin.
> **Main Functions**—Clears heat, dampness and fire poisons from the Large Intestine. Alleviates pain.

Ex LE 10   Bafeng
Eight Winds

Myotome	None – superficial fascia
Dermatome	L5/S1

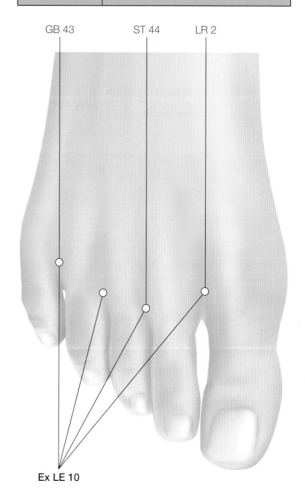

GB 43   ST 44   LR 2

Ex LE 10

Location
Approximately 2 cun below the right ST 36 at the most tender site during pressure palpation. However, this location can be treated bilaterally for channel disorders and pain.

Needling
0.5 to 1.5 cun perpendicular insertion.

Actions and indications
Lanweixue is a *very important and extensively used point for the treatment of acute and chronic appendicitis*. It may be used to treat other digestive symptoms such as bloating and indigestion.

It is also *useful diagnostically*, because it becomes tender if there is inflammation of the intestine.

The Bafeng point group includes LR 2, ST 44, and GB 43.

Location

Eight points on the dorsal surface of the foot, located in the webs between each of the toes, distal to the MTP joints. Approximately 0.5 cun proximal to the margin of the webs.

Needling

0.3 to 1 cun oblique insertion, directed between the metatarsal bones.
0.3 to 0.5 cun perpendicular insertion.

Actions and indications

These are all *very dynamic points* and are *extensively employed to clear interior heat and descend excessive Yang*. They have been used in a *large variety of disorders,* including: headache, tinnitus, inflammation of the eyes, toothache, hypertension, fever, hepatitis, gastritis, constipation, seizures, and menstrual disorders (see also: LR 2, ST 44, and GB 43).

However, they are of *primary importance as local points for pain, swelling and stiffness of the MTP joints and toes*. They also *improve Qi and Blood circulation in the entire lower limbs* and may be useful in the treatment of atrophy and paralysis.

> **Main Area**—MTP joints.
> **Main Functions**—Alleviates stiffness and pain. Regulates Qi and Blood. Clears heat.

Resources

AACP: 2019. *Let Qi Flow: An AACP Masterclass Guide to the 12 Meridians*. AACP/Dorset Press, UK.

Appleyard, I.: 2020. Acupuncture and the Opioid Crisis. *Acupuncture in Physiotherapy*, 32(1), pp. 43–5.

Aung, S. & Chen, W.: 2007. *Clinical Introduction to Medical Acupuncture*. Thieme, Stuttgart.

Benias, P. et al.: 2018. Structure and Distribution of an Unrecognized Interstitium in Human Tissues. *Sci Rep*, 8, 4947. www.nature.com/scientificreports, accessed Dec. 2020.

Bertschinger, R.: 1991. *The Golden Needle and Other Odes of Traditional Acupuncture*. Churchill Livingstone, Edinburgh.

Bradnam, L.: 2003. A Proposed Clinical Reasoning Model for Western Acupuncture. *New Zealand Journal of Physiotherapy*, 31(1), pp. 40–5.

British Medical Association: 2000. *Acupuncture: Efficacy, Safety and Practice*. Harwood, Amsterdam.

Buck, C., Deadman, P., Hicks, A. & Weeks, P.: 2019. Acupuncture in the West: Diversity and Orthodoxy. *Journal of Chinese Medicine*, 121, pp. 57–64.

Chen, E.: 1998. *Cross-Sectional Anatomy of Acupoints*. Churchill Livingstone, Edinburgh.

Cheng-Tsai, Liu, Zheng-Cai, Liu & Ka Hua: 1999. *A Study of Daoist Acupuncture & Moxibustion*. Blue Poppy Press, Boulder, Colorado.

Cheng, X.: 1999. *Chinese Acupuncture and Moxibustion*. Foreign Languages Press, Beijing.

Clavey, S.: 1995. *Fluid Physiology and Pathology in Traditional Chinese Medicine*. Churchill Livingstone, Edinburgh.

Deadman, P.: 2016. *Live Well Live Long: Teachings from the Chinese Nourishment of Life Tradition*. JOCM, Hove.

Deadman, P., Baker, K. & Al-Khafaji, M.: 2007. *A Manual of Acupuncture, Second edition*. JOCM, Hove.

Ding, L., Professor: 1991. *Acupuncture, Meridian Theory and Acupuncture Points*. English translation by Y. Benlin and W. Zhaorong, Nanjing College of Traditional Chinese Medicine and Nanjing International Acupuncture Training Centre. Foreign Languages Press, Beijing.

Focks, C: 2008. *Atlas of Acupuncture*. Churchill Livingstone, Edinburgh.

Ellis, A., Wiseman, N. & Boss, K.: 1989. *Grasping the Wind*. Paradigm Publications, Brookline, Massachusetts.

Ellis, A., Wiseman, N. & Boss, K.: 1991. *Fundamentals of Chinese Acupuncture, revised edition*. Paradigm Publications, Brookline, Massachusetts.

Ernst, E. & White, A.: 1993. *Acupuncture: A Scientific Appraisal*. Butterworth-Heinemann, Oxford.

Fang, J. et al.: 2009. The Salient Characteristics of the Central Effects of Acupuncture Needling: Limbic-Paralimbic-Neocortical Network Modulation. *Hum Brain Mapp*, 30(4), pp. 1196–206. Doi: 10.1002/hbm.20583.

Filshie, J. & White, A.: 1998. *Medical Acupuncture: A Western Scientific Approach*. Churchill Livingstone, Edinburgh.

Han, J.S. & Sun, S.L.: 1990. Differential Release of Enkephalin and Dynorphin by Low and High Frequency Electroacupuncture in the Central Nervous System. *Acupunct Sci Int J*, 1, pp. 19–23.

Harris, R., Zubieta, J.-K., Scott, D.J., Napadow, V., Gracely, R. & Clauw, D.J.: 2018. Traditional Chinese Acupuncture and Placebo (Sham) Acupuncture are Differentiated by Their Effects on the μ–Opioid Receptors. *Acupuncture in Physiotherapy*, 30(1), pp. 11–23.

Hecker, H.-U., Steveling, A., Peuker, E., Kastner, J. & Liebchen, K.: 2001. *Color Atlas of Acupuncture: Body Points, Ear Points, Trigger Points*. Thieme, Stuttgart.

Helms, J.M.: 1995. *Acupuncture Energetics: A Clinical Approach for Physicians*. Thieme, Stuttgart.

Hempen, C.-H. & Chow, V.W.: 2006. *Pocket Atlas of Acupuncture*. 2006 Thieme, Stuttgart.

Hoppenfeld, S.: 1976. *Physical Examination of the Spine and Extremities*. Appleton-Century-Crofts, East Norwalk, Connecticut.

Hopwood, V.: 2004. *Acupuncture in Physiotherapy*. Butterworth-Heinemann, London.

Huan, Z.Y. & Rose, K.: 2001. *A Brief History of Qi*. Paradigm Publications, Brookline, Massachusetts.

Huang, M. et al.: 2012. Characterizing Acupuncture Stimuli Using Brain Imaging with fMRI: A Systematic Review and Meta-analysis of the Literature. *PLoS One*, 7(4), e32960 (plosone.org).

Huang, M. et al. 2018. Critical Roles of TRPV2 Channels, Histamine H1 and Adenosine A1 Receptors in the Initiation of Acupoint Signals for Acupuncture Analgesia. *Sci Rep*, 8, 6523. Doi: 10.1038/s41598-018-24654-y.

Hui, K.K., Marina, O., Liu, J., Rosen, B.R. & Kwong, K.K.: 2010. Acupuncture, the Limbic System, and the Anticorrelated Networks of the Brain. *Autonomic Neuroscience: Basic & Clinical*, 157(1–2), pp. 81–90.

Hui, K.K.S. et al.: 2007. Characterization of the 'Deqi' Response in Acupuncture. *BMC Complementary and Alternative Medicine*, 7(33).

Johns, R.: 1996. *The Art of Acupuncture Techniques*. North Atlantic Books, Berkeley, California.

Johnson, P.: 2018. 'But Where Exactly Is It?' – The Pitfalls of Teaching and Learning Point Location. *Journal of Chinese Medicine*, 117, pp. 32–7.

Juhan, D.: 1987. *Job's Body: A Handbook for Bodywork*. Station Hill Press, Barrytown, New York.

Katz, J. & Rosenbloom, B.: 2015. The Golden Anniversary of Melzack and Wall's Gate Control Theory of Pain: Celebrating 50 Years of Pain Research and Management. *Pain Res Manag*, 20(6), pp. 285–6. Doi: 10.1155/2015/865487.

Kellgren, J.H.: 1938. Observations on Referred Pain Arising from Muscle. *Clin Sci*, 3, pp. 175–90.

Kellgren, J.H.: 1938. Referred Pains from Muscle. *Br Med J*, 1(4023), pp. 325–7.

Kendall, F.P., McCreary, E.K. & Provance, P.G.: 1993. *Muscles: Testing and Function, Fourth edition*. Lippincott, Williams & Wilkins, Baltimore.

Keown, D.: 2014. *The Spark in the Machine: How the Science of Acupuncture Explains the Mysteries of Western Medicine*. Singing Dragon, London.

Keown, D.: 2019. *The Uncharted Body: A New Textbook of Medicine*. Original Medicine Publications, Tunbridge Wells.

Kong, J., Gollub, R., Huang, T., Polich, G., Napadow, V., Hui, K., Vangel, V., Rosen, B. & Kaptchuk, T.J.: 2007. Acupuncture de qi, from qualitative history to quantitative measurement. *Journal of Alternative and Complementary Medicine*, 13(10), pp. 1059–70.

Korostyshevskiy, V.: 2015. Locating Active Acupuncture Points: The Solution to a Paradox in Acupuncture Research. *Journal of Chinese Medicine*, 108, pp. 32–6.

Lade, A.: 1989. *Acupuncture Points: Images and Functions*. Eastland Press, Seattle, Washington.

Langevin, H. & Yandow, J.: 2002. Relationship of Acupuncture Points and Meridians to Connective Tissue Planes. *Anat Rec (New Anat)*, 269, pp. 257–65.

Langevin, H., Bouffard, N., Churchill, D. & Badger, G.: 2007. Connective Tissue Fibroblast Response to Acupuncture: Dose-Dependent Effect of Bidirectional Needle Rotation. J. Altern Complement Med., 13(3), pp. 355–60.

Larre, C. & Rochat de la Vallée, E.: 2003. *The Extraordinary Fu*. Monkey Press, London.

Larre, C. & Rochat de la Vallée, E.: 2005. *The Seven Emotions: Psychology and Health in Ancient China*. Monkey Press, London.

Lian, Y.-L., Chen, C.-Y., Hammes, M. & Kolster, B.C.: 2006. *The Pictorial Atlas of Acupuncture: An Illustrated Manual of Acupuncture Points*. Edited by H. P. Ogal and W. Stor. Translation from German by C. Grant. Konemann, Cologne.

Lifang, Q. & Garvey, M.: 2015. Early Chinese Perspectives of the Mind: An Evolutionary Account of the Shen in Chinese Medical Psychology. *Journal of Chinese Medicine*, 109, pp. 37–52.

Lin, Z.-H.: 2008. *Pocket Atlas of Pulse Diagnosis*. Thieme, Stuttgart.

Longmore, M., Wilkinson, I. & Torok, E.: 2001. *Oxford Handbook of Clinical Medicine, Fifth edition*. Oxford University Press.

Maciocia, G.: 1995. *Tongue Diagnosis in Chinese Medicine*. Eastland Press, Seattle, Washington.

Maciocia, G.: 1989. *The Foundations of Chinese Medicine: A Comprehensive Text for Acupuncturists and Herbalists, First edition*. Churchill Livingstone, Edinburgh.

Maciocia, G., foreword by Professor Zhou Zhong Ying: 1994. *The Practice of Chinese Medicine: The Treatment of Diseases with Acupuncture and Chinese Herbs, First edition*. Churchill Livingstone, Edinburgh.

MacPherson, H., Hammerschlag, R., Lewith, G. & Schnyer, R.: 2007. *Acupuncture Research: Strategies for Establishing and Evidence Base*. Elsevier, Philadelphia, Pennsylvania.

MacPherson, H., Altman, D.G., Hammerschlag, R., Li, Y., Wu, T., White, A. & Moher, D.: 2010. Revised Standards for Reporting Interventions in Clinical Trials of Acupuncture (STRICTA): Extending the CONSORT Statement. *Acupunct Med*, 28(2), pp. 83–93. Doi: 10.1136/aim.2009.001370.

MacPherson, H. et al.: 2017. Unanticipated Insights into Biomedicine from the Study of Acupuncture. *Acupuncture in Physiotherapy*, 28(2), pp. 11–20.

Mason, C.: 2019. Acupuncture Dosage: Adapting Treatment Prescriptions for Safety and Optimal Therapeutic Effect. *Acupuncture in Physiotherapy*, 31(1), pp. 25–36.

Mayor, D.: 2008. *Electroacupuncture*. Butterworth-Heinemann, Oxford.

McCracken, T.: 2005. *Black's Concise Atlas of Human Anatomy*. A & C Black, London.

McDonald, J.: 2015. Evidence-Based Methods of Point Selection: Using Historical Literature and Modern Research to Inform Point Selection. *Journal of Chinese Medicine*, 109, pp. 5–22.

McDonald, J.: 2019. Why Randomised Placebo-Controlled Trials are Inappropriate for Acupuncture Research. *Journal of Chinese Medicine*, 119, pp. 47–54.

Melzack, R. & Wall, P.D.: 1965. Pain Mechanisms: A New Theory. *Science*, 150, pp. 971–9.

Mendell, L.: 2014. Constructing and Deconstructing the Gate Theory of Pain. *Pain*, 155(2), pp. 210–6. Doi: 10.1016/j.pain.2013.12.010.

Mi, Huang-fu: 1994. *The Systematic Classic of Acupuncture and Moxibustion* (A Translation of the Jia Yi Jing by Yang Shou-zhong and Charles Chace), Blue Poppy Press, Boulder, Colorado.

Moore, K.L., Dalley, A.F.: 1999. *Clinically Oriented Anatomy, Fourth edition*. Lippincott Williams & Wilkins, Philadelphia.

Palmer, M.: 2001. *Yin and Yang: Understanding Chinese Philosophy of Opposites and How to Apply It to Your Everyday Life*. Piatkus, London.

Park, H., Park, J., Lee, H. & Lee, H.: 2002. Does Deqi (Needle Sensation) Exist? *Am J Chin Med*, 30, pp. 45–50.

Pattenden, L.: 2018. Extra Points: Clearing up the Confusion. *Acupuncture in Physiotherapy*, 30(1), pp. 57–65.

Phillips, J.: 2018. Modern Acupuncture Technique: Propagation of Needling Sensation, Tonification and Sedation. *Journal of Chinese Medicine*, 117.

Platzer, W.: 2003. *Color Atlas and Textbook of Human Anatomy, Vol. 1*: Locomotor System. Thieme Medical Publishers, Stuttgart.

Putz, R., Pabst, R. & Weiglein, A. H.: 2001. *Sobotta Atlas of Human Anatomy, 13th edition*. Lippincott, Williams & Wilkins, Baltimore.

Reichstein, G.: 1998. *Wood becomes Water: Chinese Medicine in Everyday Life*. Kodansha, New York.

Reid, T.: 2015. The Limitations and Misuses of Evidence Based Medicine: A Critical Evaluation. *Journal of Chinese Medicine*, 108, pp. 15–31.

Rochat de la Vallée, E.: 2006. *A Study of Qi in Classical Texts*. Monkey Press, London.

Rohen, J.W., Yokochi, C. & Lutjen-Drecoll, E.: 2002. *Color Atlas of Anatomy: A Photographic Study of the Human Body, 5th edition*. Lippincott, Williams & Wilkins, Baltimore.

Ross, J.: 1998. *Acupuncture Point Combinations: The Key to Clinical Success*. Churchill Livingstone, Edinburgh.

Schleip, R., Findley, T., Chaitow, L. & Huijing, P.: 2012. *Fascia: The Tensional Network of the Human Body*. Churchill Livingstone, Edinburgh.

Schnorrenberger, C. & Schnorrenberger, B.: 2011. *Pocket Atlas of Tongue Diagnosis*. Thieme, Germany.

Schuenke, M., Schulte, E. & Shumacher, U.: 2005. General Anatomy and Musculo-skeletal System. Thieme, Stuttgart.

Shah, J., Thaker, N., Heimur, J., Aredo, J.V., Sikdar, S. & Gerber, L.: 2015. Myofascial Trigger Points Then and Now: A Historical and Scientific Perspective. *PM&R*, 7(7), pp. 746–61. Doi: 10.1016/j.pmrj.2015.01.024.

Shanghai College of Traditional Medicine: 1981. *Acupuncture: A Comprehensive Text*. Translated and edited by J. O'Connor and D. Bensky. Eastland Press, Seattle, Washington.

Travell, J.G. & Simons, D.G.: 1983. *Myofascial Pain and Dysfunction: The Trigger Point Manual, First edition*. Williams & Wilkins, Baltimore, Maryland.

Unschuld, P.U.: 1986. *Nan-Ching: The Classic of Difficult Issues (Comparative Studies of Health Systems and Medical Xare)*. University of California Press, London.

Unschuld, P.U.: 2003. *Huang Di Nei Jing Su Wen: Nature, Knowledge, Imagery in an Ancient Chinese Medical Text*. University of California Press, London (with Appendix: 'The Doctrine of the Five Periods and Six Qi in the Huang Di nei jing su wen').

Vianna, E., Weinstock, J., Elliott, D., Summers, R. & Tranel, D.: 2006. Increased Feelings with Increased Body Signals. *Soc Cogn Affect Neurosci*, 1(1), pp. 37–48. Doi: 10.1093/scan/nsl005.

Vincent, C.A., Richardson, P.H., Black, J.J. & Pither, C.E.: 1989. The Significance of Needle Placement Site in Acupuncture. *J Psychosom Res*, 33, pp. 489–96.

Wang, S.J., Yang, H.Y., Wang, F. & Li, S.T.: 2015. Acupoint Specificity on Colorectal Hypersensitivity Alleviated by Acupuncture and the Correlation with the Brain-Gut Axis. *Neurochemical Research*, 40(6), pp. 1–9.

Watson, T.: 2008. *Electrotherapy: Evidence-Based Practice*. Churchill Livingstone, Edinburgh.

White, A. & Ernst, E.: 2004. A Brief History of Acupuncture. *Rheumatology*, 43(5), pp. 662–3. Doi: 10.1093/rheumatology/keg005.

White, P. et al.: 2008. Southampton Needle Sensation Questionnaire: Development and Validation of a Measure to Gauge Acupuncture Needle Sensation. *J Altern Complement Med*, 14(4), pp. 373–9. Doi: 10.1089/acm.2007.0714.

Williams, P.L., Bannister, L.H., Berry, M.M., Collins, P., Dyson, M., Dussek, J.E., & Ferguson, M.W.J., eds.: 1995. *Gray's Anatomy, 38th (international) edition*. Churchill Livingstone, Edinburgh.

Wiseman, N. (translator and compiler): 1990. *Glossary of Chinese Medical Terms and Acupuncture Points*. Paradigm Publications, Brookline, Massachusetts.

Wiseman, N. & Ye, Feng: 1998. *A Practical Dictionary of Chinese Medicine*. Paradigm Publications. Brookline, Massachusetts.

Wong, E.: 2011. *Taoism: An Essential Guide*. Shambhala, Boston, Massachusetts.

Wood, J.: 2019. Acupuncture Pain and the Emotional Mind. *Acupuncture in Physiotherapy*, 31(1), pp. 37–42.

Wu, N.L. & Wu, A.Q.: 1997. *The Yellow Emperor's Canon of Internal Medicine* (*Huang Di Nei Ching*). China Science Technology Press, Beijing.

Xinghua, B.: 2001. *Acupuncture: Visible Holism*. Butterworth-Heinemann, Oxford.

Xinnong, C.: 1990. *Chinese Acupuncture and Moxibustion*. Foreign Language Press, Beijing.

Zhen, L.S.: 1985. *Pulse Diagnosis*. Paradigm Publications, Brookline, Massachusetts.

Zhong, Y.X. & Chu, J.: 1995. *Fundamentals of Chinese Medicine, revised edition*. Translated and amended by N. Wiseman and A. Ellis. Paradigm Publications, Brookline, Massachusetts.

About the Authors

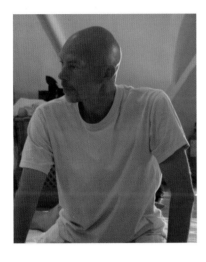

Chris Jarmey (1954–2008) first became interested in Oriental philosophies at the age of 9, being particularly drawn to Buddhist and Daoist practices. This led him at the age of 14 into the exploration and practice of both Indian yoga and a Chinese martial art known as Kenpo.

Throughout the next 30 plus years, Chris spent his time researching and practicing bodywork-based healing methods alongside the extensive practice of Buddhist and Daoist Qigong, yoga, and meditation methods.

In 1975, Chris began his study of Western approaches to healing and rehabilitation, as a means to contrast and supplement his experience of Eastern methods. He qualified as a state registered physiotherapist in 1978, with a special interest in therapeutic exercise systems. Shortly afterwards he embarked upon extensive study and research into osteopathic methodology, following this with training with Carlo De Paoli in Western herbal medicine based on traditional Chinese medicine principles.

Concurrent with his above studies, from 1978 to 1981, Chris evaluated the healing effects of yoga, shiatsu and qigong within NHS hospitals and medical rehabilitation centres, with good results.

Between 1981 and 1985, Chris lived and studied in a number of yoga centres and ashrams in India, the UK and the USA, to broaden and deepen his experience of Indian hatha yoga and related arts. In the late 1985 he founded The European Shiatsu School to offer a comprehensive practitioner training course in this effective form of bodywork.

Chris continued to practice and teach shiatsu and qigong until his sudden tragic and premature death in 2008 from an inherited cardiac myopathy.

During his career, Chris wrote a number of authoritative texts on anatomy and bodywork including shiatsu, acupuncture, qigong and meditation, notably *The Concise Book of Muscles* (Lotus Publishing) and *Shiatsu: The Complete Guide* (Harper Collins).

Ilaira Bouratinos, Dip.AcDS, received her diploma in acupuncture from the London School of Acupuncture and Traditional Chinese Medicine and subsequently founded the Oriental Medicine and Shiatsu Training Centre in Athens in 1994.

She teaches acupuncture, shiatsu, and a variety of other bodywork methods, both in Greece and internationally.

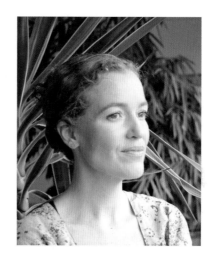

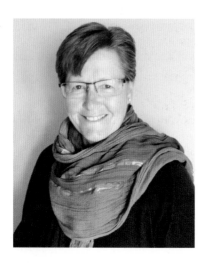

Lynn Pearce, BA, MCSP, LicAc, Cert Med Ed, is an accredited lecturer within the Acupuncture Association of Chartered Physiotherapists (AACP), a clinician of 39 years, and an acupuncture practitioner of 31 years.

Qualifying as a physiotherapist from Addenbrooke's Hospital in Cambridge in 1982, Lynn developed an early interest in acupuncture and its role in musculo-skeletal medicine. Initial study at the Centre for Complementary Therapies in Southampton led to her following a more Chinese medical model training at the British College of Acupuncture, gaining her Licentiate in 1993.

She was lead tutor for the Traditional Chinese Medical Model component on the MSc in Acupuncture at Coventry University and was presented with the AACP Tutor of the Year at the AACP Excellence Awards, 2016. She has been a regular and popular presenter at AACP conferences and runs CPD events on a number of acupuncture-related subjects.

She has contributed to *Complementary Therapies for Physical Therapists: A Theoretical and Clinical Exploration* (ed. Charman, B., 2000), the Complementary Therapies and Healthcare Practice module for MacMillan Open Learning (1997) and produced papers on technique and dose, for use in the AACP Foundation Course in Acupuncture.

Lynn is also a qualified Clinical Canine Massage Therapist and member of the K9 Massage Guild, and endeavours to apply the theories and skills contained in this book in her bodywork on her canine clients.